HANDICAPPED CHILDREN
AND YOUTH

HANDICAPPED CHILDREN AND YOUTH

A Comprehensive Community and Clinical Approach

Edited by

Helen M. Wallace, M.D., MPH
Robert F. Biehl, M.D., MPH
Allan C. Oglesby, M.D., MPH
Graduate School of Public Health
San Diego State University
San Diego, California

Lawrence T. Taft, M.D.
University of Medicine and Dentistry of New Jersey
Rutgers Medical School
New Brunswick, New Jersey

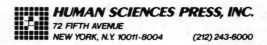
HUMAN SCIENCES PRESS, INC.
72 FIFTH AVENUE
NEW YORK, N.Y. 10011-8004   (212) 243-6000

Printed in the United States of America
987654321

Library of Congress Cataloging-in-Publication Data

Handicapped children and youth.

  Includes index.
  1. Handicapped children—Care and treatment—United
States. 2. Handicapped children—Services for—United
States. I. Wallace, Helen M. [DNLM: 1. Community
Health Services—United States. 2. Handicapped.
3. Rehabilitation—in infancy & childhood. WS 368 H236]
RJ138.H34 1987   362.4'0973   86-20922
ISBN 0-89885-333-8

CONTENTS

CONTRIBUTORS

Baer, Marion Taylor, Ph.D., R.D., Nutritionist, University Affiliated Program for Developmental Disabilities, Children's Hospital, Los Angeles,

Bailey, E. J., Ph.D., Assistant Professor of Special Education, Center on Human Development, University of Oregon, Eugene

Barnard, Kathryn E., R.N., Ph.D., Professor of Nursing, University of Washington, Department of Parent-Child Nursing; Child Development and Mental Retardation Center, Seattle, Washington

Bender, Leonard F., M.D., M.S., President and Chief Executive Officer, Rehabilitation Institute, Inc.; Professor and Chairman, Department of Physical Medicine and Rehabilitation, Wayne State University School of Medicine, Detroit, Michigan

Biehl, Robert F., M.D., MPH, Associate Director, Division of Services for Crippled Children, University of Illinois, Chicago, Illinois; Adjunct Professor of Public Health, Graduate School of Public Health, San Diego State University, California

Bricker, Diane, Ph.D., Professor of Special Education, Director of Early Intervention Program, Center on Human Development, University of Oregon, Eugene

Byers-Brown, Betty, M. Ed., FCST, Assistant Professor of Pediatrics, Rutgers University Medical School, New Brunswick, New Jersey

Capute, Arnold J., M.D., MPH, Vice President for Medical Affairs, The Kennedy Institute for Handicapped Children; Associate Professor of Pediatrics, Johns Hopkins School of Medicine, Baltimore, Maryland

Cohen, Herbert J., M.D., Director, Rose F. Kennedy Center, University Affiliated Facility; Director, Children's Evaluation and Rehabilitation Center; Professor of Pediatrics and Rehabilitation Medicine, Albert Einstein College of Medicine, Bronx, New York

Conway-Callahan, Melinda K., T.R.S., M.P.A., Director, Therapeutic Recreation Services, Rehabilitation Institute, Inc.; Instructor, Department of Recreation and Park Services, Wayne State University, Detroit, Michigan

Crocker, Allen C., M.D., Director, Developmental Evaluation Clinic, Childrens Hospital, Boston; Associate Professor of Pediatrics, Harvard Medical School

Davis, Martin J., D.D.S., Director, Division of Pediatric Dentistry; Chief, Comprehensive Care Section, Columbia University School of Dental and Oral Surgery, New York City

Dumars, Kenneth W., M.D., Professor of Pediatrics, University of California Medical School, Irvine; Chief, Division of Developmental Disabilities and Clinical Genetics

Duran-Flores, Deborah, M.S. Ed., O.T.R., Senior Occupational Therapist, Division of Developmental Disabilities and Clinical Genetics

Foster, Carol, Ph.D., Assistant Adjunct Professor, Division of Developmental Disabilities, Clinical Genetics, Department of Pediatrics, University of California, Irvine

Freeman, John M., M.D., Professor, Neurology and Pediatrics, The Johns Hopkins University School of Medicine; Director, Epilepsy Center, Johns Hopkins Medical Institution, Baltimore, Maryland

Gafford, Ludmilla Suntzeff, MSPA, ACSW, Associate Professor, Chief of Social Work, The University of Tennessee Center for the Health Sciences, Child Development Center, Memphis, Tennessee

Hills, Heidi L., D.M.D., Director, Postdoctoral Program in Pediatric Dentistry, Columbia University School of Dental and Oral Surgery, New York City

Ireys, Henry T., Ph.D., Assistant Professor of Pediatrics and Psychiatry, Albert Einstein College of Medicine, Bronx, New York

Krajicek, Marilyn J., Ed.D., R.N., University of Colorado Health Sciences Center, Denver

Laney, Mary D., Ph.D., CCC, Assistant Professor of Pediatrics, Rutgers University Medical School, New Brunswick, New Jersey

Levine, Melvin, D., M.D., Professor of Pediatrics, University of North Carolina School of Medicine, Chapel Hill

Loberg, David E., Ph.D., President, The Woods Schools, Langhorne, Pennsylvania

Lynch, Eleanor Whiteside, Ph.D., Professor, Department of Special Education, San Diego State University, California

Magrab, Phyllis R., Ph.D., Child Development Center, Georgetown University, Washington, DC

Magyary, Diane L., CRN, PNP, Ph.D., Assistant Professor, University of Washington Department of Parent-Child Nursing, School of Nursing; Child Development and Mental Retardation Center, Seattle, Washington

Milstein, Barbara, J.D., Senior Attorney for the Center on Law and Social Policy, Washington, DC

Moore, Marie L., M.S., O.T.R., F.A.O.T.A., Assistant Professor and Program Director of Nursing and Allied Health, Division of Allied Health, Occupational Therapy Department, Tuskegee University, Alabama

Morris, Hughlett, Ph.D., Professor of Speech Pathology, The University of Iowa, Iowa City

Murphy, Ann, M.S.W., Director of Social Work, Developmental Evaluation Clinic, Children's Hospital, Boston; Clinical Assistant Professor of Social Work, Boston University

Oglesby, Allan C., M.D., MPH, Professor and Head, Division of Maternal and Child Health, Graduate School of Public Health, San Diego State University, California

Palmer, Frederick B., M.D., Developmental Pediatrician, The Kennedy Institute for Handicapped Children; Associate Professor of Pediatrics, Johns Hopkins University School of Medicine, Baltimore, Maryland

Peppe, Kathryn K., R.N., M.S., Administrative Staff Nursing Consultant, Division of Maternal and Child Health, Ohio Department of Health, Columbus

Rosenbaum, Sarah, J.D., Attorney and Director of the Health Division, Children's Defense Fund, Washington, DC, and Senior Attorney, Center on Law and Social Policy

Sells, Clifford, J., M.D., MPH, Professor of Pediatrics, Director of the Clinical Training Unit, Child Development and Mental Retardation Center, Seattle, Washington

Shapiro, Bruce K., M.D., Developmental Pediatrician, Kennedy Institute for Handicapped Children; Associate Professor of Pediatrics, Johns Hopkins University School of Medicine, Baltimore, Maryland

Shimizu, Hiroshi, M.D., Associate Professor and Director, Division of Audiology and Speech-Language Pathology, Department of Otolaryngology—Head and Neck Surgery, The Johns Hopkins University School of Medicine, Baltimore, Maryland

Spiro, Alfred J., M.D., Professor of Neurology and Pediatrics; Director, Pediatric Neurology; Director, MDA Muscle Disease Clinic, Albert Einstein College of Medicine, Bronx, New York

Sternfeld, Leon, M.D., MPH, Medical Director, United Cerebral Palsy Research and Educational Foundation, Inc., New York City

Stills, Stanley, M.S., MFCC, Staff, Division of Developmental Disabilities and Genetics, University of Californnia Medical School, Irvine

Taft, Lawrence T., M.D., Professor and Chairman, Department of Pediatrics, University of Medicine and Dentistry of New Jersey, Rutgers Medical School, New Brunswick

Vining, Eileen P. G., M.D., Assistant Professor, Neurology and Pediatrics, The Johns Hopkins University School of Medicine, Baltimore, Maryland

Wachtel, Renee C., M.D., Developmental Pediatrician, Kennedy Institute For Handicapped Children; Associate Professor of Pediatrics, Johns Hopkins University School of Medicine, Baltimore, Maryland

Wallace, Helen M., M.D., MPH, Professor of Maternal and Child Health, Graduate School of Public Health, San Diego State University, California

Weinrich, Ernest, MSW, UCPA Western District Office, Burlingame, California

Wolraich, Mark L., M.D., Professor of Pediatrics, University of Iowa Medical School, Iowa City

PREFACE

The 1960s, 1970s, and 1980s witnessed the rapid development of community services for handicapped children, youth, and their families. As a result, various separate "systems" of public services for handicapped children and youth exist; these include the official crippled children's services, services available to those with developmental disabilities, special education services, services for young handicapped children provided through the Head Start program, and services for disabled teenagers and adults through the state vocational rehabilitation agencies. In addition, a number of voluntary agencies provide services for categorical handicapped children and their families. Because these various services exist separately in communities, it is essential for professional health stafff working in communities to become very familiar with them, so that handicapped children and youth and their families may be referred promptly for diagnosis, treatment, habilitation care. It is the intent of this book to reach physicians, dentists, nurses, social workers, nutritionists, and therapists (physical, occupational, speech) in an effort to assist them to work and function more effectively in working with community services for handicapped children and youth.

Helen M. Wallace, M.D., MPH
Robert F. Biehl, M.D., MPH
Lawrence T. Taft, M.D.
Allan C. Oglesby, M.D., MPH

Part I

THE PROBLEM

Chapter 1

DEFINITIONS

Robert F. Biehl

This book deals with society's recognition and management of handicapping conditions in its children and youth. These problems have been with us throughout the ages; however, not until recently has any serious attempt been made to address them in a unified or coordinated manner. One factor that has at times facilitated and at others inhibited this process is the way in which the problems have been conceptualized and defined. To the extent that definitions include or exclude groups of children, they influence the size and character of treatment populations, the cost and shape of programs, the support of legislators and advocacy groups, and the eligibility of individuals for services. This chapter will address various definitions of developmental disability, the relationship of disability to defect and handicap, and the advantages and disadvantages of categorical and functional definitions as they pertain to programs for the developmentally disabled.

DEVELOPMENTAL DISABILITY

The concept of developmental disability as a specific entity is relatively new. It was not until 1970, with amendment of Public Law 88-164, that the term was defined in American legislation. And it was not until 1973, with passage of the landmark Developmental Disabilities Assistance and Bill of Rights Act, that it became firmly established as a national priority. The concept grew from a desire to target resources to a specific group of chronic conditions that were perceived to have common characteristics and needs. Originally, the conditions targeted had important constituencies, which were at first hesitant to risk changes that might dilute the resources available to their specific disabilities. The initial definitions of developmental disability, therefore, preserved a categorical approach, helping to ensure the support of the advocates for the conditions identified. An example of this categorical approach is found in the definition used in Public Law 94-103:

> The term "developmental disability" means a disability which—
>
> (A) (i) is attributable to mental retardation, cerebral palsy, epilepsy, or autism;
>   (ii) is attributable to any other condition of a person found to be closely related to mental retardation because such condition results in similar impairment of general intellectual functioning or adaptive behavior to that of mentally retarded persons or requires treatment and services similar to those required for such persons; or
>   (iii) is attributable to dyslexia resulting from a disability described in clause (i) or (ii) of this subparagraph; and
> (B) originates before such person attains age eighteen;
> (C) has continued or can be expected to continue indefinitely; and
> (D) constitues a substantial handicap to such person's ability to function normally in society.

Although this definition contained features that cross categories—i.e., onset in the developmental period, prolonged duration, and substantial handicap—the specific designation of mental retardation, cerebral palsy, epilepsy, and autism served to exclude many other important handicapping conditions. Birth defects, sensory disorders, chronic medical illness, disabling injury, and mental health disorders other than autism were all at risk of exclusion unless they could be redescribed under one of the specified categories.

Subsequent definitions sought to remedy this difficulty by basing inclusion on an individual's functional limitations rather than the category of the disabling condition. An example of this functional approach is found in the definition used in Public Law 95-602:

> The term "developmental disability" means a severe, chronic disability of a person which—
> (A) is attributable to a mental or physical impairment or combination of mental and physical impairments;
> (B) is manifested before the person attains the age twenty-two;
> (C) is likely to continue indefinitely;

(D) results in substantial functional limitations in three or more of the following areas of major life activity:
(i) self-care, (ii) receptive and expressive language, (iii) learning, (iv) mobility, (v) self-direction, (vi) capacity for independent living, and (vii) economic sufficiency; and

(E) reflects the person's need for a combination and sequence of special interdisciplinary, or generic care, treatment, or other services which are of life-long or extended duration and are individually planned and coordinated.

This newer definition retained the features of early onset, chronic duration, and substantial severity but replaced the categorical labels with seven areas of functional limitation. It then went further to note the probable need for targeted individuals to receive individually planned services from coordinated interdisciplinary sources.

DISABILITY, DEFECT AND HANDICAP

Central to the newer functional definition of developmental disability is an understanding of the relationship between the terms *defect* or impairment, *handicap* or functional limitation, and *disability*. Although these terms are often used loosely, and on occasion interchangeably, they have meanings that are useful to distinguish. Webster (1971) defines *defect* as a "lack," "fault," or "flaw," disability as a "physical or mental illness, injury or condition which incapacitates," and *handicap* as "a disadvantage that makes achievement unusually difficult, especially a physical disability that limits the capacity to work." In health care we have traditionally thought of defects in terms of intrinsic impairments of the body or intellect; for example, a birth defect or mental deficiency. In the broader community context of this work, however, it should be remembered that extrinsic social and economic impairments exist that also have profound influence on the capacity of an individual to develop and function successfully.

When a defect interferes with a required human activicty, it becomes a disability. Thus, the paraplegia of an infant with spina bifida becomes a disability as soon as it limits age-appropriate mobility at about 6 months; the inability of the same infant to achieve fecal continence does not become a disability until the second year of life, when control is expected; and associated reading difficulty might not be recognized as a disability until school age. Using an extension of this reasoning, a child with a defect such as cleft lip and palate may be relieved of feeding disability following successful surgical repair.

Handicap embodies the concept of a disability for which the individual is unable to develop adequate compensatory strategies.

Whether or not adequate compensation occurs, i.e., whether disability results in handicap, depends on a number of factors, including the following (WHO, 1980):

1. The existence of acceptable alternative behaviors, habilitating treatment, and/or effective adaptive equipment.
2. The disabled person's physical, intellectual, and psychological ability to accept and/or use available help.
3. The capacity and willingness of society to make help available.
4. The attitudes of society and its tolerance of individuals recognized as different.

Table 1-1 provides an excellent list of the diversity of uncompensated intrinsic disabilities, *intrinsic handicaps*, that have been recognized to interfere with important human activities (adapted from Agerholm 1975).

The terms *defect*, *disability*, and *handicap* also have value in the understanding of prevention. It should be recognized that primary, secondary, and tertiary prevention can be conceptualized as efforts to prevent, respectively, the development of defects, disabilities, and handicaps. In this context, primary prevention activities, such as accident avoidance, immunizations, and prenatal care, seek to prevent the development of defects resulting from accidents, infections, and problems of pregnancy; secondary prevention activities, such as phenylketonuria screening and early identification of cerebral palsy, seek to find defects and treat them before they produce disability; and tertiary prevention or habilitation activities, such as special education and use of adaptive equipment, seek to reduce or prevent the handicap caused by an existing disability.

THE ROLE OF DEFINITION IN PROGRAM DEVELOPMENT

A health care program typically develops to meet a perceived need in the population. In most cases, the advocacy of strong supporters is necessary before even the most needed program can be implemented. Definition plays an important role both in the assessment of need and in the gaining of support for implementation.

ASSESSMENT OF NEED

Need in health care has traditionally been described in terms of the number of new cases (*incidence*) or existing cases (*prevalence*) of a specific health problem. This approach assumes that the needs of all individuals within a given diagnostic category are sufficiently similar that they can be

Table 1-1. Intrinsic Handicaps and Features

Type	Possible Features
Locomotor handicap	A. Impaired mobility in environment B. Impaired postural mobility C. Impaired manual dexterity D. Reduced exercise tolerance
Visual handicap	A. Total loss of sight B. Impaired (uncorrectable) visual acuity C. Impaired visual field D. Perceptual defect
Communication handicap	A. Impaired hearing B. Impaired talking C. Impaired reading D. Impaired writing
Intellectual handicap	A. Mental retardation B. Loss of learned skills C. Impaired learning ability D. Impaired memory
Invisible handicap	A. Metabolic disorders requiring permanent therapy (e.g. diabetes, cystic fibrosis) B. Epilepsy, and other unpredictable losses of consciousness C. Special susceptibility to trauma (e.g. haemorrhagic disorders, bone fragility, susceptibility to pressure sores) D. Intermittent prostrating disorders (e.g. migraine, asthma, vertigo)
Aversive handicap	A. Unsightly distortion or defect of part of the body B. Unsightly skin disorders and scars C. Abnormal movements of body (athetosis, tics, grimacing, etc.) D. Abnormalities causing socially unacceptable smell, sight or sound

summed to produce an accurate assessment of the needs of the whole population. In acute illness this assumption works reasonably well. Diagnostic labels such as appendicitis, streptococcal pharyngitis, and fractured femur describe conditions that have basic management needs that vary very little from one individual to the next. Indeed, the needs for services in many categories are so uniform that health insurers now group them into *diagnostically related groups* and reimburse providers not for the individual services actually provided but rather for treatment of a typical episode of illness. Categorical definitions therefore can simplify the process of needs assessment by allowing use of an existing data base that counts diagnoses. When variation within a diagnostic category is minimal, credible cumulative estimates are achieved that provide reasonable basis for program planning.

When dealing with chronic disabilities such as cerebral palsy, epilepsy, and mental retardation, there is an inclination to follow the same approach. The information that exists about the extent of developmental disability in the population is also largely documented in terms of diagnostic categories, and it is tempting to define total population need as the product of prevalence and the needs of a typical case. The problem this presents becomes apparent when one compares the characteristics of acute and chronic illness (Table 1-2).

As indicated in Table 1-2, the uniformity found in acute conditions disappears when one considers chronic disabilities. Within each diagnostic category, chronic conditions contain wide variation in severity and markedly different individual needs that reflect individual spectra of disability, developmental level, and societal expectations. Typical cases characteristic of a whole category do not exist. In addition, the problems and needs of a single individual commonly overlap categories. It is not unusual for a child identified as having cerebral palsy in one data base to be counted as mentally retarded in another and as epileptic in yet a third. This lack of uniformity within diagnostic categories of chronic disabilities and propensity for multiple enumeration in existing data bases confound the ability to use unmodified categorical information in needs assessment and program planning for this group of conditions.

SUPPORT FOR IMPLEMENTATION

Advocacy groups typically form to serve a specific categorical condition. The categorical label provides a source of identity for the organization and serves as a rallying point for membership acquisition, fund raising, and political action. Definition of the focus of a new program in terms of the categorical interests of existing advocacy groups provides potential access to the support of those groups. To the extent that the group perceives the program to be an extension of its own efforts, it may champion the cause and may even provide resources. Strict functional definition of a program, even when the focus clearly includes the population supported by the advocacy group, can be seen as a source of competition for resources and de-emphasis of the importance of the specific condition. This will certainly reduce the support from the group and may result in attempts to impede the program. The importance of this difference in effect was not ignored when Congress framed the early definitions of developmental disabilities.

Table 1-2.   Characteristics of Acute and Chronic Illness

Characteristics	Acute Illness	Chronic Illness
Duration	Brief	Prolonged; often life-long crossing many developmental periods
Scope	Often limited to single organ or system; little effect upon self-image or independence	Typically involves multiple functions/systems; strong impact upon self-esteem, independence
Presentation & Course	Limited variation; course highly predictable; often tendency for improvement without medical help	Much variation within diagnostic categories; tendency to lose further function without help
Impact	Limited	Coping skills and resources of individual and family stressed over prolonged periods
Management	Commonly managed by single discipline (medicine)	Often involves many disciplines—each with own terminology
Cost of Mismanagement	Often not recognized; unnecessary studies and overmanagement costs occur over limited duration	Unnecessary costs accumulate over time. Drain on limited resources may preclude needed measures

DEFINITION AND ELIGIBILITY

The definitions used to describe a targeted population for a service delivery program also define the characteristics that make an individual eligible for those services. When the definitions are written in categorical terms, the individual must acquire the categorical label before program services will be provided. This can present certain individual and organizational problems: (a) the individual must accept a label that may not accurately or fully describe his condition or reflect his individual needs; (b) by its nature, a label tends to assume uniformity and detract from the development of appropriate individualized planning; (c) the label categorizes the individual as someone apart from the mainstream and tends to limit opportunities for normalization; (d) intrinsic organically based labels tend to minimize the significance of societal and environmental factors in both the etiology of handicap and its management; and (e) inappropriately labeled individuals may find the label difficult if not impossible to remove or modify, thus incurring the potential risk of a self-fulfilling prophecy.

Organizationally, categorical definitions carry additional risks when, as in the case of the developmental disabilities, multiple disciplines are involved in provision of services and each discipline develops its own criteria for diagnosis. Multihandicapped individuals may find that they are eligible to receive services for only a portion of their disability or from only one provider discipline. Patients with severe impairments that do not fall neatly into the criteria for the targeted categories may find themselves excluded, whereas less impaired individuals with more typical presentations receive full services.

Functional definitions avoid most of these barriers by assigning eligibility on the basis of functional limitation rather than diagnosis. Unfortunately, current functional definitions contain significant ambiguity and permit considerable room for interpretation of what comprises *severe* disability, *substantial* limitation, economic *sufficiency*, and so on. This ambiguity results in concern that programs based on functional definitions may be too difficult to implement with uniformity and fairness, that overly permissive eligibility determinations may overwhelm available resources, or conversely, that overly rigid determinations may result in exclusion of numbers of disabled individuals who met previous categorical definitions. The political implications of these latter concerns are obvious and relate directly to a program's fiscal viability and base of support.

SUMMARY AND CHALLENGE

Developmental disability refers to a diverse group of conditions, with the features of early onset and long duration, that have the potential to impair human function significantly. Such conditions may be intrinsic or extrinsic to the individual and may produce varying degrees of handicap depending on factors that also may be intrinsic or extrinsic. Early definitions of developmental disability used categorical terms that helped assure the support of advocacy groups and appeared to simplify the process of needs assessment but restricted eligibility for services, ignored extrinsic factors, and limited the opportunity for individual planning and normalization. More recent attempts to use functional definitions have removed some of the risks caused by labeling and provided a mechanism for targeting of resources to those with greatest need. The functional approach is less familiar to health care workers, however, and is perceived to be more difficult to implement and control, open to broader individual interpretation, and politically less attractive. Despite these perceptions, the characteristics of chronic disabilities clearly require the development of programs that permit a degree of individual fit not possible with categorical definitions. The challenge of future program designers will be to create functional definitions that do not alienate support groups and that are sufficiently precise and unambiguous to assure uniform application at a level supportable by available resources.

REFERENCES

Agerholm, M. (1975). Handicaps and the handicapped. *Journal of the Royal Society of Health, 1, 3*.

Webster's third new international dictionary of the English language, unabridged. (1971). Springfield, MA: G. and C. Merriam Co.

World Health Organization. (1980). *Early detection of handicap in children: Report on a WHO working group, 15-18 May 1979*, Copenhagen: World Health Organization, Regional Office for Europe.

Chapter 2

IMPACT OF HANDICAPPING CONDITIONS ON THE CHILD AND FAMILY

Ann Murphy
Allen C. Crocker

TRANSITIONS IN SOCIAL CONCEPTS OF HANDICAPS AND THEIR TREATMENT

The impact of a chronic illness or handicapping condition on a child and his family is the result of multiple factors that have changed over time. In the not too distant past there was little professional concern with the meaning of an illness to an individual, its implications for his personal development, or the stresses imposed on the family. There was limited scientific information about handicaps and their causes. All to often they were associated in the public mind with moral issues, such as sin and retribution, or with poor family stock. Treatments were relatively ineffective, and rehabilitation was an undeveloped concept. Often the behavior of affected individuals was stereotyped. They might be perceived as ridiculous or frightening. On the other hand, persons with physical handicaps were sometimes idealized as patient and philosophical about their plight, offering an example to others. In contrast, illnesses with a less visible impact on appearance or function often posed fewer social barriers than they would today. The range of extant conditions has shifted over time. Improvements in treatment have resulted in the elimination of some chronic illnesses once common and have sustained life for individuals who formerly died at an early age. Poliomyelitis and retrolental fibroplasia are no longer prevalent; children with Down syndrome or cystic fibrosis have a much improved life expectancy. Knowledge about the origins of illness and increasingly sophisticated methods of treatment have resulted in a sense of control and less resignation about disabilities being due to fate or God's will. Individuals and families are more aware that it does not have to be that way. The public's expectations of treatment have often exceeded its potential. Faith in professionals has been superseded by an awareness that their competence must be assessed. Second opinions and informed consent are increasingly important aspects of communication between patient and professional. The patient and family must share in the decision about the relative risks and benefits in a plan of care.

Society has increasingly assumed responsibility for providing a minimum standard of living for its citizens. It is controversial to what extent an individual is expected to provide for his own needs through insurance or savings and what is a public function. Medical treatment of an illness or disability, particularly in a child, is becoming a presumption rather than a privilege. Access to public subsidies is often determined by a complex and often confusing set of eligibility criteria.

A Developmental Approach to Treatment

The initial focus of concern in professional work with families and children was apt to be on the degree of compliance they demonstrated with the recommendations of health professionals. It is only in recent years that concepts from mental health and child welfare were applied to medical care of the child (Freud, 1952). There has been an increased concern with the psychological state of the individual. Knowledge about the impact of a chronic illness or deformity on a child's developing self-concept and the psychological implications of therapeutic procedures increasingly influence the mode and timing of medical treatment of children. The enhanced recognition of the importance of family participation and support resulted in adaptations of medical programs and institutional approaches to include the family's preferences and values. In earlier times the primary contact person was typically the mother. The father, brothers and sisters, and grandparents have now emerged as significant family members whose attitudes, concerns, and contributions must be considered (Drotar, 1981).

The Normalization Movement

The role of a handicapped person in the family and the community has been greatly influenced by progress in scientific knowledge and treatment of disease. Another important influence has been the changing social structure, from large extended families with a stable base in a rural community to the highly mobile nuclear family or single-parent family all of whom are employed outside the home. Historically, although expectations of improvement and change were modest, a handicapped person might have a contributing role and social acceptance from neighbors who had known him since early childhood. Caretaking might be shared among many family members. Families might be valued for providing a protected environment. The future was within the extended family unit. If this was not possible, there was a network of publicly supported facilities that would provide education and care. Such institutions were organized to meet the needs of individuals with a single disability. Sometimes the program was of high quality, but the ultimate outcome, except for the unusual individual, was a sheltered living situation. Some institutions, particularly those for mentally retarded or mentally ill persons, were used for people who did not fit into the community. Often the care was poor, but it was a socially accepted alternative for a stressed family to use. They were encouraged by professionals to use institutionalization as a resource to protect the integrity of the family. Handicapped persons were often assumed to be the cause of family problems, and placement was routinely recommended as the treatment of choice (Aldrich, 1947).

At the initiative of families, affected individuals, and professionals who challenged the status quo there has now been a major shift in the role of the handicapped person in society. It has become an entitlement for a disabled person to participate in all age-appropriate activities, education, and social institutions. Consequently, it is a public responsibility to eliminate all social and physical barriers to normal functioning. Programs should be individualized and integrated whenever possible. The family and the community are now thought of as the appropriate milieu for the handicapped and chronically ill person, particularly a child. The service system should be designed to maintain the person in a natural situation (Wolfensberger, 1972, 1983). Institutions are being eliminated as options. There has been a growth of new professions, such as early-intervention workers, parent trainers, advocates, and the like, to assist individuals and their families in actualizing their full potential. However, the service systems and funding mechanisms are much less developed than the philosophy. Services are often age-specific or are not well adapted to working or less motivated parents. There are many uncertainties in the new climate of optimism (Gliedman & Roth, 1980).

IMPACT OF HANDICAPPING CONDITIONS ON THE CHILD

The disorders under discussion in this text are the bases for exceptionality in the children involved. This specialness can have profound and intrusive effects on all aspects of their lives. Being different can have a high personal cost. In later chapters much specific information is presented on individual disabilities; some general comments will be provided here.

First-Order Effects

Function and activity.   It is implicit in the concept of "developmental disabilities" that restrictions exist among several important functions. PL 95-

602 (the Rehabilitation, Comprehensive Services, and Developmental Disabilities Amendments of 1978) includes in the basic definition early-onset, long-lasting "mental or physical impairment" or combinations, often involving limitations in language, learning, and/or mobility. The panoply of untoward outcomes resulting from pernicious influences on genetic, prenatal, perinatal, and childhood development includes numerous bodily and central nervous system disabilities. Not surprisingly, the same force (e.g., a genetic disorder, a setting for congenital malformation, or prematurity) can affect many functions. In a population of young people with mental retardation, for example, about one-third also will have physical disability and motor function problems, 10 percent may have seizures, and a similar number will have sensory handicaps. A group of children with cerebral palsy will have a prevalence of mental retardation at 50 percent or more, and those with epilepsy will show retardation at an increased rate (perhaps 25 percent). For general discussion of multiple disabilities, see Nelson and Crocker (1983) and Crocker (1987a). Impairment in communication skills is widespread, documenting the sensitivity of language function to alterations in nervous system or physical integrity. It is this tendency for common origins of handicaps, and their frequent multiplicity, that has led to the design of joint efforts in service systems, education, public planning, and prevention programs.

Health problems.   There is a vulnerability in issues of health that is also intrinsic to many of the syndromes with disabilities. This has stimulated a philosophy of "alike/unalike" consideration in the need for medical care. For most such children the usual (alike) components of health management pertain, such as immunization, prompt attention to acute infection, and surveillance for general disorders. There is also, however, a requirement for particular vigilance regarding unusual (unalike) incidence or types of impediments. Several examples can be given. The child with Down syndrome has special involvement with congenital heart disease, chronic serous otitis media, atlantoaxial instability, ocular refractive errors, hypothyroidism, gastrointestinal anomalies, hip dysplasia, and leukemia. Patients with the mucopolysaccharidoses may have difficulty with hernias, hearing problems, arachnoid cysts, seizures, airway obstruction, and cardiac failure. Those with myelodysplasia are often troubled with hydrocephalus, paraplegia, scoliosis, complications of neurogenic bladder and bowel disability, skin trauma, seizures, and so on. In cerebral palsy there may be concern with weakness, spasticity, contractures, dislocations, strabismus, seizures, hearing impairment, and/or nutritional difficulty.

Provision of appropriate supportive medical care can be a challenge. Most primary care pediatricians have rather small numbers of these special-needs children in their practices and have limited familiarity with optimal health maintenance principles (Crocker, 1987b; Shonkoff, Dworkin, Leviton, & Levine, 1979). The most significant requirements for specialty medical referrals are in the areas of neurology, orthopedics, cardiology, nutrition, ophthalmology, audiology, otolaryngology, and reconstructive surgery.

Behavioral aberrations. Young persons with developmental disabilities are in a compromised situation regarding adaptation to the world around them; it is thus not unexpected that their behavioral responses may be individual and atypical. It is often commented that about one-half of persons with significant mental retardation, for example, have important emotional disorders, with behavioral implications. This extends from the common "inappropriate behavior" of the youth with Down syndrome, to the frequent symptoms of depression in the retarded young adult (Szymanski & Biederman, 1984), and on to the occasional "dual diagnosis" of the seriously retarded adult who has manifestations of troubling mental illness (Szymanski & Grossman, 1984). All of this greatly compromises progress in the implementation of programs of developmental training and therapy and tends to alienate public and professional support; it also leads to unhappiness for the involved client. Further, there is incomplete understanding of behavioral factors that may be indigenous to certain developmental disability syndromes, not merely adaptational components. These would include impulsive or hyperkinetic characteristics in some situations of cerebral pathology, autistic-like behavior in untreated phenylketonuria or severe congenital rubella, and the exquisite social and communicative isolation of the child with infantile autism.

Reproductive constraints. A background concern exists regarding reproductive possibilities for the young person with developmental disorders, however well supported their course may be. In some instances this issue may derive from basic factors inherent in their condition. For example, no males with Down syndrome or fragile-X syndrome have ever been known to have fathered children, and young women with Down syndrome have enormously reduced fertility. Females with classical phenylketonuria will have up to 90 percent incidence of abnormal offspring (mental retardation, microcephaly, congential heart disease), the picture of so-called maternal PKU, if their elevated serum phenylalanine levels are not controlled by dietary therapy begun before conception of the infants. It is probable, but not fully known, that fertility levels are generally reduced in many syndromes with multiple congenital anomalies and other conditions of serious central nervous system disease. Certainly, in current cultural circumstances the opportunities for parenthood are diminished when major mental retardation exists, for complex reasons and justifications. Some of the issues are related to genetic factors, as in certain infrequent dominantly inherited conditions, but usually the altered dynamic is social and personal. It must be noted that we as a society have not resolved our conflicts about reproductive opportunities for disabled persons; present guidelines for sex education, social behavior, birth control, and sterilization are confused.

Survival issues. Going beyond concerns about function, health, and behavior, there are some pervasive elements in the developmental disabilities that impact directly on mortality. This population is beleaguered by threats to their existence, both basic and by complication. A fatal outcome at an early age is unavoidable in many of the large-molecule inborn errors of metabolism (the lipidoses and mucopolysaccaridoses) and in the muscular dystrophy syndromes. Tumorous extensions of the phakomatoses, (neurofibromatosis, tuberous sclerosis) may take the lives of children and adults. Renal failure is the most common cause of early death in myelodysplasia. Compromised long-term survival in some persons with Down syndrome is a topic of very active current discussion, as the meaning of Alzheimer-like cerebral changes is studied. A late-emerging panencephalitis is sometimes expressed in young people with congenital rubella. Of particular concern, however, are the cumulative effects of medically important elements in the developmental disorders. There are depleting consequences from recurrent pulmonary infections, with or without aspiration in gastroesophageal reflux, from urinary tract and other infections, and from chronic undernutrition. The altered life circumstances of persons with severe profound mental retardation and serious physical or motor function handicaps render them vulnerable (and sometimes injured). There is a special obligation for supporting medical services to attend to erosive elements in the course of persons with disabilities.

Second-Order Effects and Consequences

The presence of a disabling condition or chronic illness has a cascade of repercussions on the life-style and options of the involved child. The improved circumstances that have evolved in the past 20 years have done much to buffer the stress of exceptionality, but troubling realities persist. An altered self-image and the experience of segregation and rejection are the central elements. Such young people are indeed a particular and incompletely understood minority group, as had been documented by Gliedman and Roth (1980) and the Vanderbilt study (Hobbs, Perrin, & Ireys, 1985).

It is in the world of education that a child's difference is most tellingly displayed. Separation from the majority of his peers has been reduced by the "least restrictive environment" mandate of PL 94-142. Current review shows, however, that most youngsters with Down syndrome are still in segregated classes (Fredericks, 1987). The opportunities for social interaction, extracurricular activities, and athletics are constrained by transportation arrangements and other practical matters. Further, interruption in the educational schedule may be forced by hospital admissions, periods of home care, and the need for special therapies.

Beyond the school, these children face an array of barriers, some physical and some attitudinal. The concept that "anatomy is destiny" often intrudes in the choice of friends, recreation, vocational possibilities, the right to drive a car, and religious activities. Even in the environment of his home the special child may experience a congenial synchrony or the opposite, dependent on what has been referred to as "the match" ["the critical encounter between a child's unique stylistic and cognitive repertoire and the personal needs, expectations, and values of the parent" (Crocker & Levine, 1983)] or "the goodness of fit" ["the degree of consonance or dissonance between the child and parent" (Ulrey, 1981)]. As a tragic outcome of disordered match or fit, there can even be a situation of neglect or abuse, as documented to be at an increased incidence of child abuse in children with developmental disabilities.

IMPACT OF HANDICAPPING CONDITIONS ON THE FAMILY

Loss and the Grieving Process

A disability is experienced as a loss of actual of potential functions and social roles. Grieving is a normal response to significant loss (Solnit & Stark, 1961). The process of grieving can be conceptualized as a sequence through which individuals adapt to internal and external changes resulting from the loss. The initial reaction is one of shock and disbelief that such a catastrophe even has occurred. The more unanticipated and the more significant the loss, the more intense and prolonged the period of shock is likely to be. When the denial cannot be maintained, the person may experience intense anger and/or guilt as a means of fixing responsibility for the loss either to others or to himself. This may be followed by feelings of sadness as the reality and permanence of the change are assimilated with acceptance of the consequent need for adaptation. The grieving process may be reactivated by events or life stages that require new adaptations to the loss. These may be anniversaries, developmental milestones, and social events that are altered by the original loss. Although it is possible to speculate on characteristic reactions to loss and disability, it is important to stress that the specific responses of individuals are determined by their interpretation of the loss. The extent and pattern of grieving will be colored by the type of loss, how critical it is to their psychological and social functioning, previous experiences with loss, personal coping strategies and resources, and the social supports available to them (Caplan, 1976; Rapoport, 1965). Featherstone (1980) has pointed out the universality of certain parental reactions: guilt, fear, loneliness, and anger.

Congenital and Acquired Disabilities

The time of life in which a handicap occurs is of critical importance for the development of the individual. A birth defect that markedly alters the child's appearance or is known to compromise intellectual development can impair his initial acceptance as a family member. Parents have an idealized image of the child during the pregnancy that is reassessed at the time of birth when they claim him as their own. Major defects can be disruptive to the process of "bonding" unless discussion of the diagnosis and its implications are sensitively handled (Kennell, 1974; Rappaport, 1965). If the child has major medical problems that require separation or technical management, it is important that the parents' role and participation in caretaking be maintained as much as possible to facilitate the family ties. Congenital disabilities that are diagnosed at a somewhat later stage often have been preceded by a growing awareness of the parents that something is wrong. They may postpone seeking professional consultation to defer having their fears confirmed. On the other hand, many parents describe professionals who did not take seriously the concerns they had about their child's development. Belated clarification of these symptoms may have contributed unnecessary stress to an already tense parent–child relationship. Parents may be more threatened if developmental problems are brought to their attention by an outside organization such as the school. This challenges their perception of the child as being normal, and they may try to avoid confronting the disability by attributing the cause to the inadequacies of the educational system. A congenital disability requires a parent to deal with the loss of the fantasied child they had planned to have.

Children with congenital problems may not perceive themselves as disabled until they are four or five years of age. They may be anxious about the special care or treatment they require and may be well aware that other persons view them as sick. Their first awareness that they lack something or are different may come from being unable to do things that their peers do, but this awareness may be confined to specific activities and functions. The more pervasive implications of their disability as a permanent impairment of classes of function, or one that carries with it alterations of roles and social status, evolve over time. It is often easier to integrate into the self-concept a disability that is concrete or specific to one organ, such as a deformed limb or a heart condition. Problems that involve cognitive abilities or communication or those that significantly impair facial appearance are more central to issues of self-esteem. A cognitive impairment may complicate a child's ability to develop compensatory mechanisms (Cobb, 1970). The family must share this discovery and adaptation with the child, as each grows and learns.

A child who has lost abilities or functions in a sudden fashion, secondary to major illness or accident, poses different and perhaps more challenging issues of adaptation for himself and his family. The older a person is, the more established is his sense of self and his network of relationships and social roles. In addition to losses in body function and abilities, the child may have to change schools, relinquish roles in his family, and perhaps experience the loss of significant relationships with others who cannot adapt to the individual's diminished level of functioning. The disability may require revision of life goals. The individual and his family are probably more vulnerable to being fixated in the grieving process. Overwhelmed with anger, depression, or denial, they may have considerable difficulty in engaging in a rehabilitation program. This would require the individual to shift his self-concept to incorporate the change in his body and to acknowledge the need to revise goals and develop compensatory skills. He might be unable to accept the need for adaptive equipment or participation in programs designed for handicapped persons. Adolescents and young adults who especially prize their independence have serious problems adapting to a disability that may require them to assume passive and dependent roles. Families also have particular problems with such major transitions. They may feel a responsibility to protect the affected person from the reality of the change. They may blame themselves for the illness or accident, or harbor bitter feelings toward others who may have been at fault, with or without pursuit of legal recourse. They also may have major problems in revising their relationship with the child to accommodate the new limitations.

The situation of progressive disorders has its own special concerns. Most such conditions are hereditary in nature and carry troubling considerations for the parents regarding their own involvement and the meaning for family building. There is often a shock from the unexpected encounter with a rare and unfamiliar disease and a sudden entry into the territory of genetic counseling, possible planning for prenatal diagnosis in upcoming pregnancies, and a bewildering array of clinical circumstances (Crocker & Cullinane, 1972). The illness itself may have a desultory course, wherein the child gradually loses function, has demanding care requirements, and ultimately dies. For the family there is depression, alarm, and sense of futility. The service system responds with varying degrees of resourcefulness, particularly regarding assistance in home health care (Mackta, 1984). Parent support groups have a very strategic role in contributing to the reintegration of such households. Continuity in developmental and educational services must be well defended (Crocker, 1983a; Weyhing, 1983).

The Lives of the Parents

Much has been written about the stress generated by having a handicapped child as a family member—its potential for disrupting family relationships, goals, and integrity, (Crnic, Friedrich, & Greenberg, 1983). A handicapped child does require revision of expectations and roles within a family. Many disabilities have major care needs, multiple hospitalizations, extensive home treatments, and financial costs that deplete a family's resources. Mobility may be restricted by the fact that health insurance is often job-related, and specialized care and educational programs may be restricted to certain geographical areas. Community resources often are less available for older children when their families need more help. The child's physical growth can complicate home care. A parent may be required to serve as a companion to an adolescent whose social relationships would be best served by a peer group. Parents may have to assume developmentally inappropriate roles, such as assisting with personal hygiene, that may perpetuate dependency and make a normal parent-child relationship difficult. With advancing age the parents may have increasing apprehension about their own vulnerability to illness and be uncertain about who will assume the role of caretaker if they cannot. They may never be able to look forward to privacy in their own relationship. If the disability is congenital, the parents may decide to limit their family for fear of recurrence. Alternatively, they may increase the family and have another child to compensate for the family member with a disability. Certain disabilities may subject the family to curious stares or inappropriate questions. The social image and acceptability of the family may be affected.

Although the presence of a handicapped child may alter family roles, the integrity of the family can be preserved if there is good communication and adequate community supports (Murphy, 1983; Murphy, Pueschel, & Schneider, 1972). In families where there have been preexisting stresses a handicapped child can accentuate them or even become a focus for family problems. Conversely, some families describe personal growth or strengthening of family bonds that occurred as a result of dealing with the needs of a handicapped child. They state that the experience altered their value system and increased their sensitivity to others (McCubbin et al., 1980; Wikler, Wasow, & Hatfield, 1983). On balance there has not been an increased rate of divorce documented in studies of families where there are children with disabilities (Lansky, Cairns, Hassanein, Wehr, & Lowman 1978; Sabbeth & Leventhal, 1984; Silbert, Newberger, & Fyler, 1982), although it is admitted that this may not be an adequate indicator of marital adjustment in general.

Implications for Brothers and Sisters

As is obvious, but only recently given notable designated attention, there is a vigorous sharing of the effects of the special child's presence by the brothers and sisters in the family (Powell & Ogle, 1985). There are many areas to be considered in their responses, including the following:

1. Alteration in the normalcy of family rhythm, conformity, and image (an adapted home, loss of some flexibility, need to attend to other than their own gratification).

2. Competition for parental resources and attention (priorities for parents' energies and time, demands for family funds).

3. Misconceptions that the normal child may carry (puzzlement about causation, possible genetic issues, what will happen to the involved child).

4. Need for the young person to act as a surrogate parent

(share in care, baby-sitting, conflict in social activities, possible lifelong responsibility).

5. Obligation to meet enhanced parental expectations (need to "make up" for frustrations, prove parental normalcy).

6. Bewilderment in response to parents' conflicts, griefs, and the like (alteration of role model, insecurity about family stability).

These dynamics are further compounded by mixed messages that are often given to the normal children, such as double standards about compliance and behavior, rights and competencies of the affected child, and the complex effects of mutual stress (Crocker, 1981).

It is of interest that the majority of studies regarding the personal adaptation of brothers and sisters shows a favorable outcome (Crocker, 1983b). Further, Featherstone (1980) has documented a number of positive effects of such family life, including increased acceptance of the spectrum of human differences, new perceptions about the meaning of accomplishment, and a less casual acceptance of good health. Inclusion of brothers and sisters in discussions of child study and service planning has useful results, as do individual counseling and group sessions with similarly involved peers (Murphy, Pueschel, Duffy, & Brady, 1976). Significant communication about these programs is now available in a special newsletter.[1]

IMPACT OF THE SYSTEM OF SERVICES

The initial diagnosis of a handicap is a critical period for parents in forming constructive attitudes toward their child's development. It is also an opportune time to develop good working relationships with professional people who will be involved in their child's care through the years.

When a handicap is identified at birth, usually the parents and professional staff have had no opportunity for preparation. The staff in maternity hospitals often have little current knowledge about habilitation of handicapped children. If there is no medical intervention readily available, they may be preoccupied with their own sense of failure at delivering a child they cannot help. The specialist who informs the parents may have had no previous relationship with them. The family may be devastated and look to the professional staff to help them assess the implications of the diagnosis for the development of their child. Crisis theory stresses that interventions given at this juncture can be far more influential than help offered after the crisis has been resolved (Rapoport, 1965).

---

[1] Sibling Information Network Newsletter, 249 Glenbrook Road, Box U-64, Department of Educational Psychology, The University of Connecticut, Storrs, CT, 06268.

Professionals need to develop the ability to listen as well as inform. Families will give important clues to their concerns and reactions by the types of questions they raise. It is important to explore their misconceptions because if they are not elicited and clarified, these ideas may continue as a more significant influence on their behavior than the information provided by the expert. Families need to hear about the child's strengths as well as his defects so that they can obtain a sense of the whole child. If the child has an unusual appearance or has a diagnosis that has a negative social image, the parents may need support in bonding with the child because their anxieties can interfere with contact. They may need positive role models and assistance in interacting with the child. Although most parents will want to assume responsibility for the child's care if given assistance, professionals must individualize their expectations of parents. Some parents need more time before they can make a commitment; others are unable to relate to a child with significant disability. If after exploration of their concerns, the parents are unable to care for the child, a referral to a child welfare agency for planning is indicated. Many families find this a difficult transition because they associate such agencies with inadequate and neglectful parents. However, it is well established that handicapped children, like all children, thrive best in a family situation.

It is important to plan for communication between the acute hospital or diagnostic center and the local community. If possible, community resources that can support the parents in the care of the child should be identified and contacted. It is desirable to arrange a meeting, if possible, so parents can begin to form relationships with key professionals and be assured they will have available the supports they need. Many parents complain that pediatricians do not offer assistance with developmental questions and tend to focus on acute illness. Sometimes doctors seem to need to stress the handicap and its limitations rather than the potential, more positive aspects of the child's development. Professionals are often overly concerned that parents will not realize the full extent of a cognitive disability. Diagnoses are usually made in medical settings. Often there is no knowlege of or trust in community-based educational systems, such as early intervention programs, that can offer important supports to parents in child rearing. The opportunity to meet with other parents of children with similar disabilities can provide parents with an additional network of supports.

In this regard, parent self-help groups and consumer organizations can offer priceless assistance in the achievement of reassurance and confidence (see the current directory of special interest groups published by the National Center for Education in Maternal and Child Health, 1985).[2] Often parents with handicapped children are very isolated and lack the orientation

---

[2] "A National List of Voluntary Organizations in Maternal and Child Health," published by the National Center for Education in Maternal and Child Health, Washington, DC, 20057.

and feedback about child rearing that is available to parents of normal children. Some parents will be resistant to such contact as they are not ready to identify with resources and programs designed for handicapped persons. They may need more time to assimilate their child as an individual with a disability. Ideally, families should have a visible network of accessible and developmentally appropriate resources to supplement their care of the disabled child and to help them establish appropriate short-term and long-term goals. These would include a source of local medical care, respite care, financial counseling, transportation, and education and recreation opportunities. The recent years have seen a dramatic enhancement in the understanding and availability of assisted home care for children with handicaps, rendering many situations manageable that were previously believed to be the purview of hospital environments only (Halamandaris, 1985; Kohrman, 1984). Some families are able to seek out appropriate services and advocate for themselves. However, next steps are usually not apparent to parents, and their energies may be absorbed in handling current responsibilities and crises. Transitions from early intervention programs that are family-centered to public school, which focuses on the child, are difficult. Further, there is little anticipatory guidance about issues of adolescence and young adulthood to assist the family in preparing for the future.

In family adaptation to the presence of a child with significant disability there is clearly a mixture of stress and personal growth. As a part of what some would consider an evolution but which Turnbull and Summers (1987) call a revolution, families have come on line in a posture of affirmation and accomplishment. This has occurred with help from professionals, to be sure, but the major credit must go to their own spirit of love, self-help, and mutual assistance. Parents have unexpectedly learned, for example, the techniques of sign language, pulmonary physical therapy, advocacy for educational programs, quality assessment of medical care, and design of legislation to secure rights. Most particularly, they have learned to value the troubled children where professionals have traditionally doubted. They have ended up teaching the teachers.

REFERENCES

Aldrich, C. (1947). Preventive medicine and mongolism. *American Journal of Mental Deficiency*. 52, 127–129.

Caplan, G. (1976). The family as a support system. In G. Caplan & M. Killilea (Eds.), *Support systems and mutual help* (pp. 19–36). New York: Grune & Stratton.

Cobb, H. (1970). The attitude of the retarded person towards himself. In M. G. Schreiber (Ed.), *Social work and mental retardation* (pp. 125–136). New York: John Day.

Crnic, K. A., Friedrich, W. N., & Greenberg, M. T. (1983). Adaptation of families with mentally retarded children: A model of stress, coping, and family ecology. *American Journal of Mental Deficiency*, *88*, 125–138.

Crocker, A. C. (1981). The involvement of siblings of children with handicaps. In A. Milunsky (Ed.), *Coping with crisis and handicap* (pp. 219–223). New York: Plenum.

Crocker, A. C. (1983a). Inborn errors of metabolism. In J. Umbreit (Ed.), *Physical disabilities and health impairments* (pp. 233–239). Columbus, OH: Charles E. Merrill.

Crocker, A. C. (1983b). Sisters and brothers. In J. A. Mulick & S. M. Pueschel (Eds.), *Parent-professional partnerships in developmental disabilities services* (pp. 139–148). Cambridge, MA: Ware Press.

Crocker, A. C. (1987a). The spectrum of medical care in the developmental disabilities. In I. L. Rubin & A. C. Crocker (Eds.), *Developmental disabilities: Medical care of children and adults*. Philadelphia: Lea & Febiger.

Crocker, A. C. (1987b). Systems of health care delivery: Private practice. In I. L. Rubin & A. C. Crocker (Eds.), *Developmental disabilities: Medical care of children and adults*. Philadelphia: Lea & Febiger.

Crocker, A. C., & Cullinane, M. M. (1972). Families under stress: The diagnosis of Hurler's syndrome. *Postgraduate Medicine*, *51*, 223–229.

Crocker, A. C., & Levine, M. D. (1983). The right to be different. In M. D. Levine, W. B. Carey, A. C. Crocker, & R. T. Gross (Eds.), *Developmental-behavioral pediatrics* (pp. 1220–1223). Philadelphia: W. B. Saunders.

Drotar, D. (1981). Psychological perspectives in chronic illness. *Journal of Pediatric Psychology*, *6*, 211–228.

Featherstone, H. (1980). *A difference in the family: Life with a disabled child*. New York: Basic Books.

Fredericks, H. D. (1987). Elementary school. In S. M. Pueschel, C. Tingey, J. E. Rynders, A. C. Crocker, & D. M. Crutcher (Eds.), *New perspectives on Down syndrome*. Baltimore: Paul H. Brookes.

Freud, A. (1952). The role of bodily illness in the mental life of the child. *Psychoanalytic Study of the Child*, *7*, 69–81.

Gliedman, J., & Roth, W. (1980). *The unexpected minority: Handicapped children in America*. New York: Harcourt Brace Jovanovich.

Halamandaris, V. J. (Ed.). (May, 1985). Pediatric home care (special issue). *Caring*, *4* (5).

Hobbs, N., Perrin, J. M., & Ireys, H. T. (1985). *Chronically ill children and their families*. San Francisco: Jossey-Bass.

Kennell, J. (1974). Evidence for a sensitive period in the human mother. In M.H. Klaus, T. Leger, & M. A. Trause (Eds.), *Maternal attachment and mothering disorders: A round table* (pp. 39–43). Sausalito, CA: Johnson & Johnson.

Kohrman, A. (1984). Pediatric home care: A ten-point agenda for the future. In *Home care for children with serious handicapping conditions* (pp. 98–105). Washington, DC: Association for the Care of Children's Health.

Lansky, S. B., Cairns, N. U., Hassanein, R., Wehr, J., & Lowman, J. T. (1978). Childhood cancer: Parental discord and divorce. *Pediatrics, 62*, 184–188.

Mackta, J. (Ed.). (1984). *One day at a time.* Cedarhurst, NY: National Tay-Sachs & Allied Diseases Association.

McCubbin, H., Joy, C., Cauble, A. E., Comeau, J., Patterson, J., & Noodle, R. (1980). Family stress and coping: A decade review. *Journal of Marriage and the Family, 42*, 855–871.

Murphy, A. (1983). Community services and resources within the family. In J. A. Mulick & S. M. Pueschel (Eds.), *Parent-professional partnerships in developmental disabilities services* (pp. 149–172). Cambridge, MA: Ware Press.

Murphy, A., Pueschel, S. M., Duffy, T., & Brady, E. (1976). Meeting with brothers and sisters of children with Down's syndrome. *Children Today, 5*, 20–23.

Murphy, A., Pueschel, S. M., & Schneider, J. (1972). Group work with parents of children with Down's syndrome. *Social Casework, 54*, 114–119.

Nelson, R. P., & Crocker, A. C. (1983). The child with multiple handicaps. In M. D. Levine, W. B. Carey, A. C. Crocker, & R. T. Gross (Eds.), *Developmental-behavioral pediatrics* (pp. 828–839). Philadelphia: W. B. Saunders.

Powell, T. H., & Ogle, P.A. (1985). *Brothers and sisters: A special part of exceptional families.* Baltimore: Paul H. Brookes.

Rapoport, L. (1965). The state of crisis: Some theoretical considerations. In H. J. Parad (Ed.), *Crisis intervention: Selected readings* (pp. 22–31). New York: Family Service Association of America.

Sabbeth, B. F., & Leventhal, J. M. (1984). Marital adjustment to chronic childhood illness: A critique of the literature. *Pediatrics, 73*, 762–768.

Shonkoff, J. P., Dworkin, P. H., Leviton, A., & Levine, M. D. (1979). Primary care approaches to developmental disabilities. *Pediatrics, 64*, 506–514.

Silbert, A. R., Newberger, J. W., & Fyler, D. C. (1982). Marital stability and congenital heart disease. *Pediatrics, 69*, 747–750.

Solnit, A. J., & Stark, M. H. (1961). Mourning and the birth of a defective child. *Psychoanalytic Study of the Child, 16*, 523–537.

Szymanski, L. S., & Biederman, J. (1984). Depression and anorexia nervosa of persons with Down syndrome. *American Journal of Mental Deficiency, 89*, 246–251.

Szymanski, L. S., & Grossman, H. (1984). Dual implications of "dual diagnosis." *Mental Retardation, 22*, 155–156.

Turnbull, A. P., & Summers, J. A. (1987). From parent involvement to parent support: Evolution to revolution. In S. M. Pueschel, C. Tingey, J. E.

Rynders, A. C. Crocker, & D. M. Crutcher (Eds.), *New perspectives on Down syndrome*. Baltimore: Paul H. Brookes.

Ulrey, G. (1981). Emotional development of the young handicapped child. *New Directions for Exceptional Children*, *5*, 33–51.

Weyhing, M. C. (1983). Parental reactions to handicapped children and familial adjustments to routines of care. In J. A. Mulick, & S. M. Pueschel (Eds.), *Parent-professional partnerships in developmental disabilities services* (pp. 125–138). Cambridge, MA: Ware Press.

Wikler, L., Wasow, M., & Hatfield, H. (1983). Seeking strengths in families of developmentally disabled children. *Social Work*, *28*, 313–315.

Wolfensberger, W. (1972). *The principle of normalization in human services*. Toronto, Canada: National Institute on Mental Retardation.

Wolfensberger, W. (1983). Social role valorization: A proposed new term for the principle of normalization. *Mental Retardation*, *21*, 234–239.

This work was supported in part by D.M.C.H. Project 928, and A.D.D. Grant #03DD0135, D.H.H.S.

Part II

SOCIETAL RESPONSES AND RESOURCES

Chapter 3

BRIEF HISTORY OF PROGRAMS AND SERVICES FOR HANDICAPPED CHILDREN AND YOUTH IN THE UNITED STATES

Helen M. Wallace

Organized public concern and responsibility for handicapped children in the United States have been expressed to a great extent only in the last 50 years, since the enactment of the Social Security Act in 1935. Prior to that time, services for handicapped children had largely consisted of residential care, both public (provided in the form of large residential state hospitals financed by the states) and private (paid for by families).

SOCIAL SECURITY ACT—TITLE V

Title V of the Social Security Act, enacted in 1935, authorized federal funds for the states to extend and improve maternal and child health services and also authorized federal funds for the states to extend and improve "services for locating, and for medical, surgical, corrective and other services and care for and facilities for diagnosis, hospitalization, and after care for children who are crippled or who are suffering from conditions leading to crippling" (Social Security Act, 1978 ed.).

RISE AND CONTRIBUTION OF VOLUNTARY AGENCIES

During the 1930s and 1940s, the fact that President F. D. Roosevelt had serious residua from poliomyelitis led to the formation of the National

Foundation For Poliomyelitis, a voluntary agency dedicated to the purpose of prevention of the disease and to the development of diagnostic, treatment, rehabilitation, and continuing care services for individuals suffering from the effects of poliomyelitis.

The 1940s and 1950s witnessed the rise of other voluntary agencies; examples are numerous and include the American Heart Association, which was concerned with the diagnosis and treatment of children with rheumatic fever and rheumatic heart disease, and prophylaxis against future attacks of rheumatic fever. Other examples are the United Cerebral Palsy Association, concerned with advocacy, legislation, training, prevention, and provision of services for children and adults with cerebral palsy; and the National Association for Retarded Citizens, with its broad concerns for individuals with mental retardation.

IMPACT OF PRESIDENT KENNEDY ON THE FIELDS OF MENTAL RETARDATION AND OF HANDICAPPED CHILDREN

The election of President J. F. Kennedy in 1960 led to the immediate formation of the President's Panel on Mental Retardation (1962), which produced the report/blueprint for the future. This report had far-reaching effects on the development of action and services for the prevention of mental retardation (MR), the care of the mentally retarded, and handicapped children and youth in general, including

> development of state planning for MR (which became Title XVII of the Social Security Act);
>
> inclusion of some mentally retarded children and youth for care under state crippled children's (CC) programs;
>
> inclusion of more mentally retarded youth and adults in state vocational rehabilitation programs;
>
> development of 25 university-affiliated facilities for MR, for the care of patients, and for training of personnel;
>
> development of three university research centers for research into causes and prevention of MR;
>
> expansion of a small number of existing community centers to a large number, for the evaluation, diagnosis counseling, treatment, and habilitation of children with MR;
>
> early support for the field of genetics, including diagnosis, counseling, and research;
>
> support for Maternity and Infant Care projects for high-risk women and their infants, as one effort to reduce MR;

support for Children and Youth projects for the comprehensive care of high-risk children and youth of poor
families.

Much of this legislation was supported by the voluntary agencies concerned
with the handicapped, particularly the National Association for Retarded
Citizens, the United Cerebral Palsy Association, and the Epilepsy Foundation of America.

COLLABORATIVE PERINATAL STUDY

The Collaborative Perinatal Study, supported by the National Institute
of Neurological Diseases and Stroke, was conducted by 14 collaborating
medical schools in the United States (Niswander & Gordon, 1972). This was
a study of 55,908 pregnant women and their children, begun January 1, 1959,
and ended in December 1965, on the causes and possible prevention of cerebral palsy and other central nervous system manifestations as the subsequent effects of maternity and newborn care.

DEVELOPMENTAL DISABILITIES LEGISLATION (PL 91-517)

The Developmental Disabilities Services and Facilities Construction Act
was originally passed in 1970 and subsequently amended in 1975 and 1978.
It covers developmental disabilities, including MR, cerebral palsy, epilepsy,
and autism. It provides federal funds to the states for basic state grants for
services, for protection and advocacy, for some university-affiliated facilities
for the handicapped, and for special projects.

EDUCATION FOR ALL HANDICAPPED CHILDREN ACT (PL 94-142)

PL 94-142, originally enacted in 1973, was a landmark legislation, providing federal funds to the states and requiring the states to make available
free appropriate public education and related services for handicapped children and youth from the age of three years to twenty-one years. In addition,
children under three years of age may be served if an individual state elects
to do so.

REHABILITATION ACT OF 1973

The Rehabilitation Act of 1973 replaced the earlier Vocational Rehabilitation Act. It provides federal funds to the states for basic state grants for

training of personnel, for service projects, and for independent living for the moderately to severely disabled. Disabled youth are covered by this program.

INCLUSION OF HANDICAPPED CHILDREN IN HEAD START

Head Start is a federally financed program, begun in 1965 as part of the Economic Opportunity Act anti-poverty programs. It provides a combination of socialization, education, social services, health services and care, and parent education to four-year-old children of poor disadvantaged families. Since 1976 10 percent of the children in Head Start are required to be handicapped.

SUPPLEMENTAL SECURITY INCOME DISABLED CHILDREN'S PROGRAM

In 1976 Congress established a separate categorical program to assist disabled children receiving Supplemental Security Income (SSI) benefits. Under this program, the Social Security Administration refers blind and disabled children under age sixteen receiving SSI benefits to state CC agencies for services.

SUMMARY

In summary, during the 50 years since 1935, considerable progress has been made in the development and expansion of services for handicapped children and youth and their families in the United States. This has occurred through major federal legislation providing federal funds to the states and requiring certain basic services in the fields of health, education, vocational training assistance, and independent living. At the same time, there have been efforts made to improve the quality of life for the handicapped and to incorporate them into the mainstream of society. During this period, a major trend has been in the de-institutionalization of handicapped children and youth, without sufficient alternative services developed in the community to assist those de-institutionalized and their families. Progress in care has been achieved by the combined efforts of public and voluntary agencies. Some attention has been paid to prevention, largely through efforts in genetics, family planning, and improvement in maternal and perinatal care. Nevertheless, it is clear that there are many handicapped children and youth in the United States without access to the basic care and services provided for others.

REFERENCES

Niswander, K. R., & Gordon, M. (1972). *The women and their pregnancies*. Philadelphia: W. B. Saunders.

President's Panel on Mental Retardation. (1962). *A proposed program for national action to combat mental retardation*. Washington, DC: U.S. Government Printing Office.

Social Security Act. (1978 ed.). Title V. Section 501. Washington, DC: U.S. Government Printing Office.

Chapter 4

ORGANIZATION AND PROVISIONS OF MAJOR PUBLIC PROGRAMS FOR HANDICAPPED CHILDREN AND YOUTH AND THEIR FAMILIES

Helen M. Wallace

At present there is not yet a comprehensive approach to the care, management, and assistance provided for handicapped children and youth and their families. Rather, there appears to be a number of separate parallel systems of care. These include the following:

1. Official state Crippled Children's programs.
2. State education efforts at implementation of PL 94-142, the Education for All Handicapped Children Act.
3. State developmental disabilities services and programs, serving children, youth, and adults with developmental disabilities.
4. State programs to provide vocational rehabilitation services for disabled youth and adults.
5. Head Start, serving handicapped three to five-year-olds who are in the Head Start program.

All of these state and local programs and services for handicapped children and youth are tied to and supported by federal legislation and appropriations.

It would be hoped that it would be possible to pull together, coordinate, and integrate these separately legislated/funded approaches to make it possible to provide a unified approach for the benefit of handicapped children and youth and their families.

OFFICIAL CRIPPLED CHILDREN'S PROGRAM

The official Crippled Children's (CC) Program is a partnership program between the federal and the state governments. It is designed to promote early identification of handicapped children and to provide evaluation, diagnosis, treatment, rehabilitation, continuing care, and case management services for handicapped children and youth and their families.

Legislative Base

Title V, Part 2, of the Social Security Act enacted in 1935, established the federal authorization for the state CC programs, as follows: To enable the states to extend and improve "services for locating crippled children and for medical, surgical, corrective, and other services and care for the facilities for diagnosis, hospitalization, and aftercare for children who are crippled or who are suffering from conditions leading to crippling."

Title V of the Social Security Act served as the federal legislative authority for the state CC programs until 1981. In 1981, the Omnibus Budget Reconciliation Act established the Maternal and Child Health (MCH) Block Grant.[1] The MCH Block Grant continued the federal legislative authority, as reproduced above, and also added responsiblity for disabled children under the Supplemental Security Income (SSI) program, as follows: "Provide rehabilitative services for blind and disabled individuals under the age of 16 receiving benefits under Title XVI of this Act." The MCH Block Grant became effective October 1, 1981. It gave the states greater discretion, within certain legislated limitations, to determine programmatic needs, set priorities, allocate funds, and establish oversight mechanisms. At the same time, it curtailed the opportunity of the federal funding agency to provide consultation and technical assistance to the states. It also reduced the requirement of accountability from the state CC programs.

Administration

The federal responsibility for the state CC Programs is located in the Division of Maternal and Child Health, U.S. Department of Health and Human Services, Rockville, Maryland, and in its ten regional offices.

Each state and territory has an official CC program, which is administered by the state CC agency (SCCA). In 47 states the CC agency is located in the state health department. In the remaining ten, the CC agency is lo-

---

[1] Title V of the Social Security Act Amendments.

cated in other state agencies, such as the state university (three); the state welfare department (six); the state education department (one).

Funding and Expenditures

The state CC programs are funded primarily by a combination of federal and state funds. In 1981 the sources of funds expended by the state CC programs were as follows:

Source	Amount	%
State	$224 million	63
Federal[2]	103	29
Fees & Reimbursement	13	3.7
Local	6	1.6
Other	11	3.1
TOTAL	$356 million	

Federal funds for the support of state CC Programs are allocated to each state by a formula. Each state receives Fund A, which consists of a grant of $70,000, plus an additional amount determined by the number of children under twenty-one years of age; Fund A is matched by the state. Fund B, which is unmatched by the state, is determined by the financial needs of the state.

Under the MCH Block Grant, the state CC programs have received a proportionately larger percentage of the available federal funds. The state CC programs continue to have high priority. There has been a trend toward consolidating the Supplemental Security Income (SSI) program for disabled children into the state CC program (GAO, 1984).

Functions

Functions of the official CC programs include the following:
1. Advocacy.
2. Promoting the development, improvement, expansion, and extension of health and medical care services for handicapped children and youth of all kinds and their families throughout all sections of the state.
3. Receiving and administering the federal funds for CC programs from the MCH Block Grant.
4. Stimulating and improving earlier case finding of handicapped children and youth.

[2] From both the MCH Block Grant and Supplemental Security Income.

5. Promoting the development of and participation in the delivery of expert evaluation, diagnostic, treatment, and rehabilitative services for handicapped children and youth, using the interdisciplinary approach.

6. Promoting and providing demonstration services to demonstrate new patterns of delivery of comprehensive health care of handicapped children and youth.

7. Promoting and providing follow-up and continuity of health care of handicapped children and youth, providing case management.

8. Stimulating efforts to prevent the occurrence of handicapping conditions in children and youth (primary prevention) and to prevent the damaging effects of handicapping conditions (secondary prevention).

9. Evaluating health services provided to handicapped children and youth and their families.

10. Uncovering unmet needs and services for handicapped children and youth.

11. Conducting studies of needs and services for handicapped children and youth, collecting, analyzing, and disseminating data.

12. Participating in education of parents and the public.

13. Participating in education of members of the health professions.

14. Setting and raising standards of health care for handicapped children and youth and conducting quality assurance.

15. Drafting suggested legislation in regard to the health care of handicapped children and youth.

16. Working closely with other official, voluntary, and private agencies and universities to coordinate care for handicapped children and youth, e.g., education, vocational rehabilitation, voluntary agencies, various medical specialty groups, Title 19, and developmental disabilities: (a) participating in evaluation of handicapped children and youth for special educational placement; (b) referral and participating in evaluation of handicapped youth for vocational rehabilitation services; (c) assisting the Department of Social Services in planning for the care of handicapped children under the Title 19 program.

17. Promoting the coordination of services for handicapped children and youth in the state.

18. Promoting regional planning for services for handicapped children and youth.

19. Promoting the development of genetic diagnostic and counseling services.

20. Planning and participating in third-party payment from Title 19, Vocational Rehabilitation, Blue Cross, Blue Shield, etc.

21. Improving residential care of the handicapped.

22. Administering the SSI program for disabled children.

Quality of Care

State CC programs represent one of the first attempts to enter the field of medical care. They have provided experience in the development and testing of effective new methods of planning, organizing, and implementing community programs designed to bring health services of high quality to vulnerable children and youth. There has been particular emphasis on quality of care.

Staff

SCCAs usually have a multidisciplinary staff, consisting of a director, usually a physician (pediatrician); nurses; social workers; physical therapists; occupational therapists; psychologists; experts in the field of communicative disorders; nutritionists; and dentists. These staff members carry out the functions of the state CC program listed above. A small core staff primarily carries administrative functions (planning, implementing, evaluating, coordinating); the majority primarily carries clinical functions in providing patient care (assessment, treatment, management of patients and families).

Children Cared for in State CC Programs

Each state determines the conditions for which the state CC program will provide services. Each state establishes its own diagnostic and financial eligibility criteria. Thus, there is considerable variation in the number and types of children cared for.

In general, the state CC case loads include children requiring care throughout childhood and adolescence, and those with handicaps so incapacitating that the cost of care is beyond the resources of the family.

There have been changes in the types of children cared for in state CC programs over the years; less children seen with conditions resulting from infections (osteomyelitis, tuberculosis, poliomyelitis) and orthopedic conditions; more children with congenital defects, neurological conditions, multiple handicaps, and such conditions as cystic fibrosis, hemophilia, leukemia, and the mentally retarded who are also "crippled."

In 1982, 44 SCCAs provided services to approximately 540,000 children with handicapping conditions (ASTHO Foundation, 1984), a rate of 8 children per 1,000 under twenty-one years of age. Thirty-six SCCAs reported a total of 1.6 million encounters for the children under their care, an average of 4.2 encounters[3] per child.

Demographic Characteristics

Of the total number of children seen in 1982, 37 percent were new patients, and 63 percent were return or carry-over patients. Forty-one percent of all children served had been under SCCAs care for more than 3 years.

The age distribution of children served by SCCA in 1982 was as follows:

Age Group	Percent of Total
Less than 1 year	7.4
1–4 years	28.3
5–11 years	33.6
12–19 years	26.4
20–21 years	4.3

The largest age group served during 1982 was that of children aged five to eleven years. One reason may be that the children may have been diagnosed on entry into the school system (i.e., hearing, vision, and learning disorders). Another reason may be that treatment requires a certain level of development (i.e., cardiac, orthopedic, and orofacial conditions).

The distribution of children served by SCCAs in 1982 by family income status is as follows:

Family Income Status	Percent of Total
At or below poverty level	57.5
Poverty to 150% of poverty level	20.2
150–200% of poverty level	13.0
Over 200% of poverty level	9.2

More than three-fourths of the children served were from families at or below 150 percent of the poverty level. This is in accord with the intent of the SCCAs to make services available to low-income families or to those with limited access to health services.

Payment sources for the services provided for children cared for by SCCAs in 1982 were as follows:

[3] An encounter is defined as a face-to-face contact between a patient and a provider of health care services who exercises independent judgment in the care and provision of health services to the patient.

Payment Source	Median Percent
SCCA	69
Private insurance	22
Medicaid	5
Self-pay	+
+ less than 1%	

Diagnostic Conditions

Children served by the SCCAs in 1982 had the following diagnostic conditions.

Diagnostic Category	Percent of Children Served
Hearing	25.0
Orthopedic	24.5
Cardiac	11.3
Chronic medical	6.4
Vision	6.4
Orofacial and dental	6.1
Speech/language	4.5
Mental retardation	3.4
Learning disorders	2.8
Emotional disturbances	1.2
Other medical/surgical	15.3
Other neuropediatric–developmental	13.4
Unknown	5.4

The most frequently reported categories were hearing, orthopedic, chronic medical, and vision. Among infants under one year of age, orthopedic and cardiac were the most frequently reported; in the one to four-year age group, orthopedic, hearing, and cardiac were the most frequently reported; in the five to eleven-year age group, hearing, orthopedic and vision were most frequently reported, as they were in the twelve to nineteen and over-nineteen age groups.

Services Provided

All state CC programs must provide diagnostic services without charge.

The chronic nature of most handicapping conditions requires a multifaceted, multidisciplinary program of ongoing care. In addition to high-quality evaluation, diagnostic, and treatment services, many handicapped children require long-term case management and careful coordination of a broad range of health, social, educational, vocational, and rehabilitative services. These management programs include planning, individualized care, counseling, monitoring patient status, periodic reassessment, and coordinating services.

Funds of CC programs are used to provide direct services in the following ways: (a) through state-operated and -staffed clinics; (b) under contractual or fee-for-service arrangements with private practicing medical specialists; (c) a combination of full-time state staff and part-time private medical specialists working together in state-operated clinics. Regardless of the method used, all state CC programs are designed to provide evaluation, diagnosis, treatment, and rehabilitative services to children with handicapping or chronic conditions. All use a multidisciplinary approach in care. The CC programs assume responsibility for case management; they prepare an individualized service plan, arrange for the delivery of needed medical, health, and support services, and modify the plan as needed to reflect changes in the child's condition.

In addition to these patient care services, state CC programs also provide other broad services, which are listed below.

Other Services and Activities of SCCAs

Direct patient services. In addition to providing treatment and care to children in ambulatory and inpatient settings, SCCAs provide a number of other direct patient services. These include laboratory tests, social work, speech therapy, physical therapy, hearing therapy, dental care, public health nursing, occupational therapy, outreach, transportation, nutrition, vision therapy, and home health care.

Indirect services. SCCAs provide a wide variety of other types of services designed to expand, strengthen, and improve the delivery of care to handicapped children and youth and their families on a statewide basis. These include coordination; education/counseling, technical assistance; planning; administration and management; collecting, recording, analyzing, and disseminating data; setting standards; evaluation of care and services; leadership; resource development and allocation; assessment of scope and nature of needs and problems; quality assurance; and research.

In 1982 SCCAs provided professional health care in an *ambulatory* setting to 76 percent of the children served. Ten percent of the children served by SCCAs were hospitalized in 1982 for diagnosis and/or treatment. Other services most frequently provided were *clinical management*[4] (72 percent of children served) and case management[5] (57 percent).

Family counseling and training were provided to 31 percent of the children served. Special types of adaptive care (braces, prosthetics, and hearing

---

[4] *Clinical management* includes planning, arranging, and coordinating services related to the medical care and health of the child.
[5] *Case management* usually involves interdisciplinary coordination of all needed services, including medical, social, and educational; liaison and coordination of efforts among state and local agencies and professionals involved in the child's total care.

aids) were provided to 10 percent, and family support services (home visits, homemaker services, and transportation) to 7 percent of the children.

Eligibility

Eligibility criteria for care under state CC programs represent a serious obstacle to reaching and providing care for all handicapped children and youth who need it. Each state sets its own eligibility criteria—in both diagnostic conditions and financial eligibility. This not only prevents some children and youth from receiving the prompt necessary care, it also creates confusion in the understanding and utilization of state CC services because of serious inconsistencies from one state to another.

Unmet Needs

1. There is great need to broaden eligibility (both diagnostic and financial) so that state CC programs may provide the needed services for all handicapped children and youth who require them.

2. As a corollary, the financing of state CC programs requires major expansion.

3. There is need for extension of state CC services to all sections of each state so that all handicapped children and youth will have equal access to quality services. There is need for more emphasis on statewide planning.

4. There is need for futher development and use of a plan of regionalized care and services.

5. There is need for better planning, working together, and coordinating of services with the developmental disabilities program, the field of education and special education in the implementation of PL 94-142, the vocational rehabilitation program, the Medicaid–EPSDT program, the state MCH program, the mental health programs, and private agencies serving handicapped children and youth.

6. There is need for a systematic planned evaluation of the component parts of state CC programs.

SSI DISABLED CHILDRENS PROGRAM

In 1976 Congress established a separate categorical program to assist disabled children receiving SSI benefits. Under this program the Social Security Administration refers blind and disabled children under sixteen years of age receiving SSI benefits to SCCAs for counseling and other services. The SCCAs establish individual service plans for these children and provide referrals for services. In addition, they provide medical, social, developmental, and rehabilitative services mainly to children under seven years of age.

EDUCATION OF HANDICAPPED CHILDREN—PL 94-142

PL 94-142, the Education for All Handicapped Children Act, was enacted by Congress in 1975, in an effort to make it possible for all handicapped children of school and preschool age to receive a free appropriate public education. The original act of 1975 was landmark legislation, comparable in significance in the field of handicapped children and youth to Title V of the Social Security Act of 1935.

PL 94-142, as enacted in 1975, reported that there were more than 8 million handicapped children in the United States and that their special educational needs were not being fully met, as more than half did not receive appropriate educational services. One million were excluded entirely from the public school system; many handicapped children were participating in regular school programs where handicaps were undetected; and because of lack of adequate services within the public school system, families were often forced to find services outside the public school system, often at great distance from their residence and at their own expense. It is the purpose of PL 94-142 to assure that all handicapped children have available to them a free appropriate public education that emphasizes special education and related services to meet their unique needs based on an individualized program plan, to assure that the rights of handicapped children and their parents or guardians are protected, to assist states and localities to provide for the education of all handicapped children, and to assess and assure the effectiveness of efforts to educate handicapped children. The term *related services* means transportation and such developmental, corrective, and other supportive services (including speech pathology and audiology, psychological services, physical and occupational therapy, recreation, and medical and counseling services) as may be required to assist a handicapped child to benefit from special education; and it includes the early identification and assessment of handicapping conditions in children. PL 94-142 requires that handicapped children and youth receive their education in the least restrictive environment. It requires that an "individualized education program" be developed for each child, with annual goals. It provides federal funds to assist the states to implement the requirements of the act. It provides procedural safeguards to protect the rights of the child and to assure the provision of appropriate education for each child, with right of appeal by the family.

Number and Type of Handicapped Children Served

In the school year 1982–83, slightly more than 4 million children were served, an increase over 1981–82. There were increases in the categories of learning disabled, emotionally disturbed, and visually handicapped, and decreases in the other categories.

Age

States in 1982–1983 continue to report increases in the number of preschool handicapped children served, especially those aged three through five. Thirty-eight states mandated services to at least some portion of the birth-through-age-five population; and where mandated, a larger population of this age group was served in 1982–1983.

Secondary and Postsecondary Age

An expansion of services to secondary- and postsecondary-age handicapped students has occurred, partly because of increased recognition of the importance of a successful transition from school to work and community life, and the need to preserve educational gains from earlier education. There was a 9 percent increase in services for students aged eighteen through twenty-one in 1982–1983 over the previous year. All states have mandates to provide services to handicapped students through age seventeen, and 24 states have mandates to serve handicapped youths through the age of twenty-one if they have not graduated from high school. There is a growing trend toward expansion of vocational services and use of community resources to provide vocational training to this age group.

Least Restrictive Environment

Less than 7 percent of all handicapped children are educated in either separate schools or separate environments. Of the more than 93 percent who are educated in regular schools, about two-thirds receive their education in the regular classroom with nonhandicapped peers.

Funding

States use a mixture of federal, state, and local funds to finance services for handicapped children and youth. For fiscal year 1985, the following federal funds were appropriated by Congress for the education of the handicapped:

State grants	$1,135,000,000
Early childhood	22,500,000
Secondary & transitional services	6,300,000
Postsecondary	5,300,000
Personnel development	61,000,000

COLLABORATIVE DEMONSTRATION PROJECTS BETWEEN OFFICIAL STATE CC PROGRAMS AND STATE DEPARTMENTS OF EDUCATION

In 1978 funding was provided for a three-year period through state official CC programs in Connecticut, Hawaii, Iowa, Louisiana, Oregon, and Utah. It was intended to improve communication and coordination in state and local service delivery systems for handicapped children (Nelkin, 1983). The six state projects demonstrated how to formalize agency cooperation to improve services for children with handicaps. The major focus of the projects was the preschool population, and efforts were directed primarily at the local community level. The six state projects involved a variety of services and model programs. In-service training was emphasized. Formal interagency agreements were developed; both private and public service providers were involved in development of interagency collaborative efforts; creative, effective use of existing resources through interagency collaboration eliminated duplication of efforts, diminished confusion for parents, and saved funds.

Description of Projects

The six state projects have served both preschool and school-age populations, but the major focus of the collaborative efforts was on the preschool population. These collaborative efforts were directed primarily at the local community level. The six projects involved a wide variety of services and model programs.

Major programs or models developed by the states include the following:

Connecticut
  Medical/Developmental Child Find
  Community resource team
  Curriculum task force

Hawaii
  Kona Infant and Child Development Program
  Health Support Service Demonstration Project

Iowa
  Integrated evaluation and planning clinics
  Common interagency communication system
  Regional community child centers

Louisiana
  Training of medical personnel in evaluation and IEP process
  Criteria for determining infants at risk
  Model for comprehensive medical assessment

Oregon
   Computer-assisted reference file of services for handi-
   capped Interdisciplinary evaluation clinics
   In-service training program

Utah
   Handicapped Child Data Project
   Newborn Questionnaire Project

Unmet Needs

Among unmet needs are the following:

1. There is great need for education, MCH, CC programs, and vocational rehabilitation and services to work more closely together to provide comprehensive care for handicapped children and youth.

2. The term *related services* in the implementation of PL 94-142 needs to include all essential relevant services for each child, including medical and health participation.

3. The individualized education plan for each child needs to be comprehensive and easily understood and interpreted by staff concerned and by parents.

4. Services and programs for the secondary and postsecondary age groups need strengthening so that the earlier gains made by the youth will not be lost. All states should mandate programs through age twenty one.

DEVELOPMENTAL DISABILITIES

History

In 1963 Congress enacted PL 88-164, the first federal categorical construction program for the mentally retarded. PL 88-164 provided federal funds to (a) build research centers for preventing and combating mental retardation; (b) construct public or nonprofit clinical facilities [i.e., university-affiliated facilities (UAFs)] that would provide inpatient/outpatient services, demonstrate how specialized services could be provided, and provide clinical training for physicians and others working with the retarded; and (c) encourage states to build community facilities for the retarded.

In 1970 Congress amended PL 88-164, which expired in 1970, by enactment of PL 91-517. The emphasis shifted from construction to planning and services and to developing a network of services for the disabled. This law broadened the target population to include cerebral palsy, epilepsy, and other neurological conditions closely related to mental retardation. A new term, *developmental disability*, was adopted to describe the new target group.

In 1973 PL 94-103, the Developmentally Disabled Assistance and Bill of Rights Act, was enacted. This act continued support of state grants and UAFs. Two new programs were added: a state protection and advocacy program and a special projects program. *The state formula grants* were for planning, administration, delivering services, and constructing facilities for the developmentally disabled (DD). *The state protection and advocacy program* was designed to establish and guard the rights of the DD and assure that they have quality services for maximum physical, psychological, and social development. *The UAF program* was to support the operation of demonstration facilities and provide interdisciplinary training to strengthen staff resources to serve the DD. The *special projects program* was to support the demonstration of new or improved techniques for delivering services and assist with meeting the special needs of the disadvantaged DD.

Administration of Developmental Disabilities

Administration of the developmental disabilities program is a shared responsibility among national and state officials.

At the *national* level, there is a developmental disabilities section in the Office of Human Development of the U.S. Department of Health and Human Services, with a national advisory council. The federal Division of Maternal and Child Health also provides substantial support to the UAF program.

At the *state* level, each state has a state planning council as well as a state agency designated as responsible for administering the state developmental disabilities program; this may be located in any one of a variety of state agencies, such as health, mental retardation, mental health, vocational rehabilitation.

Definition

The definition of the term *developmental disability* is provided in Chapter 1.

Current Legislation

In September 1984, Congress enacted the Developmental Disabilities Act of 1984. The major parts of this new legislation are as follows:

1. It defines developmental disability, as provided in Chapter 1.

2. It sets the federal share of DD projects/services and activities at 75 percent, except if located in an urban or rural poverty area.

3. It requires an annual report from the state planning council of each state, and from the Secretary of the U.S. Department of Health and Human Services.

4. It contains new emphasis on steps to employ the handicapped.

5. It defines in some detail the rights of the DD individual for appropriate treatment, services, and habilitation in the least restrictive environment; public funds are not provided to any program that does not provide appropriate treatment, services, and rehabilitation, and does not meet minimal standards; the requirement that all programs for DD individuals meet standards.

6. It provides that each state must have a state plan and a state planning council.

7. It requires that each DD person who receives services under the program must have a habilitation plan in writing that has long-term goals, is developed jointly with the DD person's parents or representative, and is renewed annually.

8. It describes the protection and advocacy of individual rights.

9. It continues grants to UAFs to assist in the provision of interdisciplinary training, the conduct of service demonstration program, the conduct of an applied research programs, and the provision of service-related training to parents of DD persons.

10. It continues special projects grants for demonstration projects to increase and support the independence, productivity, and integration into the community of DD persons.

11. It supports a study of intermediate care facilities for DD persons.

12. Priority service areas consist of community living, child development, case management, and employment-related activities (services to increase independence, productivity, or integration of work settings, including employment preparation and training services leading from special education to employment and from sheltered work to supported or competitive employment.

Present Federal Authorization and Funding

The Developmental Disabilities Act of 1984, which was enacted in September 1984, established the following *authorization* levels:

	FY 1985	FY 1986	FY 1987
State grant programs	$50.25 M	$53.4 M	$56.5 M
Protection & advocacy systems	13.75	14.6	15.4
UAF programs	9.0	9.6	10.2
Special projects	2.7	2.9	3.1

Funding levels set for fiscal year 1985 are identical with the authorization levels for FY 1985 listed above.

UAFs

The UAF program was established to train interdisciplinary personnel; to provide care and services to DD individuals and their families; to demonstrate new techniques to diagnose, treat, educate, train, and care for the mentally retarded and other DD; to build improved linkages with state and local delivery systems; and to conduct applied research.

In 1984 there were 41 UAFs, including five satellite centers. Total federal funding from developmental disabilities funds in 1984 was $7.8 million, plus $5 million from the federal MCH Block Grant.

In 1980 a General Accounting Office review (1980) of the federally supported developmental disabilities program recommended that "the Commissioner of the Rehabilitation Services Administration establish goals, objectives, and performance standards for the University-Affiliated Facilities Program supported with developmental disabilities funds and periodically evaluate supported facilities".

VOCATIONAL REHABILITATION

Administration

The federal unit responsible for the program of vocational rehabilitation, the Rehabilitation Services Administration (RSA), is located in the Office of Human Development of the U.S. Department of Health and Human Services. At state level, there is an agency responsible for the administration of this program, existing either as a separate agency or as part of another state agency such as the state department of education.

Legislative Base

The basic legislation for the federal vocational rehabilitation program is the Rehabilitation Act of 1973, PL 93-112. This legislation sets forth as its purposes to (a) authorize programs to develop comprehensive and continuing state plans to meet the needs of funding vocational rehabilitation services to handicapped individuals; (b) evaluate the rehabilitation potential of handicapped individuals; (c) conduct a study to develop methods of providing rehabilitation services to meet the needs of handicapped individuals; (d) assist in construction and improvement of rehabilitation facilities; (e) develop new and innovative methods to apply, the most advanced medical technology, scientific achievement, and psychological and social knowledge to solve rehabilitation problems; (f) initiate and expand services for those underserved; (g) conduct studies and experiments on long neglected problem areas; (h) promote and expand employment opportunities; (i) establish client assistance pilot projects; (j) provide assistance to increase the number of personnel through training; (k) evaluate approaches to architectural and transportation barriers.

The legislation established the RSA in the U.S. Department of Health and Human Services. It also appropriated funds for federal grants to the states for the support of basic state vocational rehabilitation services. It required an individualized written rehabilitation program, with annual review, and provided funds for innovation and expansion grants, for research and training, and for construction of rehabilitation facilities. It established the National Center For Deaf-Blind Youths and Adults.

The Rehabilitation Act Amendments of 1984 (a) extends the state grant part of the Rehabilitation Act through fiscal year 1986; (b) extends all other programs of the act for 3 more years; (c) establishes a separate authority for the Helen Keller National Center for Deaf–Blind Youths and Adults; (d) establishes the National Council on the Handicapped as an independent agency; (e) requires the collection of individual client data for the annual report required of the RSA; (f) requires the development of standards for evaluation of existing independent living centers and projects with industry; (g) changes the client assistance program from a demonstration, discretionary program to a formal state grant program; (h) provides the director of the National Institute of Handicapped Research with authority to test new concepts and innovative ideas; (i) continues authorization for the Architectural and Transportation Barriers Compliance Board for 3 years; (j) extends the Developmental Disabilities Assistance and Bill of Rights Act.

Content

The vocational rehabilitation program is intended to provide disabled teenagers and adults with a variety of services to assist them to become independent and productive in both living and work. Federal and state funds are used to cover the costs of providing rehabilitation services, which include diagnosis, comprehensive evaluation, counseling, training, reader services for the blind, interpreter services for the deaf, and employment placement. They also assist with payment for medical and related services; prosthetic and orthotic devices; transportation to secure vocational rehabilitation services; maintenance during rehabilitation; tools, licenses, equipment, and supplies; vending stands for handicapped persons, including management and supervisory services; and assistance in the construction and establishment of rehabilitation facilities.

Funds are available for special projects—projects and demonstrations that hold promise of expanding and improving services for groups of mentally and physically handicapped individuals. These may include projects for client assistance, with industry, for migrant workers, and for the severely disabled.

Funds are available to provide independent living services for severely handicapped individuals to assist them to function more independently in family and community settings or to secure and maintain appropriate employment. Funds are used for attendant care, training in independent living skills, referral and assistance in housing and transportation, peer counseling, and advocacy.

Funds also are available to support training of personnel, to increase the number and improve the skills and personnel trained to provide vocational rehabilitation services to handicapped individuals.

Significance

The age at which handicapped teenagers are eligible for the official vocational rehabilitation program varies from state to state. The significance of this is to be aware of the need of timing and referral of handicapped teenagers for evaluation, counseling, education, training, and vocational placement. There is need for close working and cooperation between CC programs and other agencies serving handicapped teenagers and vocational rehabilitation agencies for the full rehabilitation of handicapped teenagers.

The RSA reported that for fiscal year 1980, the benefit/cost ratio of the federal–state vocational rehabilitation program is 10.4 to 1 (Office of Special Education and Rehabilitative Services, 1982, p. 6). This means that for every dollar spent on rehabilitation services, an estimated improvement of $10.40 in individual lifetime earnings will result.

Funding

The federal appropriation for fiscal year 1985 for the vocational rehabilitation program is as follows:

Program	Amount In Millions	Program	Amount In Millions
Basic state grants	$1,100.0	Evaluation	$ 2.0
Client assistance projects	6.3	Migrants/Indian tribes	1.7
Severely disabled	14.6	Helen Keller Center	4.2
Training	22.0	Nat'l. Council on the Handicapped	.75
Recreation	2.1	National Institute for Handicapped Research	
	27.0		39.0

Clients Served

Data on clients served in the vocational rehabilitation program in fiscal year 1982 (Office of Special Education and Rehabilitative Services, 1983, p. 3) are as follows:

1. Of the 958,537 persons receiving rehabilitation services, 571,542 (59.2 percent) were severely disabled. Severely disabled clients who were rehabilitated were 129,866 (57.2 percent) of the total 225,924 rehabilitated.

2. More than 9,504 blind and 13,735 visually impaired individuals were rehabilitated in FY 1981.

3. An estimated 18,736 persons with communication disabilities were rehabilitated.

4. There were 65 projects with industry serving 11,000 disabled persons, most of whom were severely disabled.

Unmet Needs

1. There is need to promote the closer working relationships and coordination between effforts of the vocational rehabilitation agency and services with those of the official SCCAs, developmental disability services, and special education.

2. Adolescents who are handicapped need to be referred for vocational assistance services in their early adolescent years.

3. Vocational experts need to be allocated in secondary schools that disabled adolescents attend, in order to provide vocational assistance readily.

4. Vocational agencies need to provide a high quality of medical care to their clients, similar to that provided by SCCAs.

HEAD START

Head Start is a federally funded program established by the Economic Opportunity Act in 1965 to provide a combination of socialization, education, health care, social service, and parent education to four-year-old children from low-socioeconomic-level, disadvantaged families. The purpose is to give them a "head start" in getting ready for entrance into school. The broad objective is to assist these children and their families in reaching their maximum potential and to break the cycle of deprivation and poverty.

The federal appropriation for Head Start for fiscal year 1985 was $1.05 billion, an increase of $80 million over fiscal year 1984. Funds are allocated to the states according to a formula based on the number of children on Aid to Families with Dependent Children (AFDC) (one-third) and the number of children under five years of age who live below the poverty line (two-thirds). Head Start serves 430,000 four-year-old children annually.

It was mandated in 1974 that Head Start accept and integrate handicapped children into its program, with a requirement that a minimum of 10 percent of the children in Head Start be handicapped. In 1983 it was reported that 12 percent of the children in Head Start were diagnosed as handicapped (Collins & Deloria, 1983); the majority are classified as mildly to moderately handicapped, although Head Start also serves a number of severely handicapped children. Handicapped children receive the full range of health and other Head Start services, as well as special education and other services targeted on their special needs.

For 1981–1982, it was estimated that there were 219,200 Head Start eligible handicapped children of preschool age (three to five years) in the United States (Head Start Bureau, 1984).

The number of handicapped children served by Head Start in 1981–82 was 49,991, accounting for 11.2 percent of the total enrollment in 1981–82. The diagnostic distribution of handicapped children in Head Start by primary handicapping conditions in 1981–82 was as follows:

Speech impaired	60%
Health impaired	10.7
Learning disabled	6.4
Mentally retarded	5.9
Physically handicapped	5.9
Emotionally disturbed	4.7
Hearing impaired	3.3
Visually impaired	2.6
Deaf	.3
Blind	.2

In 1982, 18.3 percent of the handicapped children enrolled in Head Start had multiple handicapping conditions; 16.6 percent required almost constant special education or related services; 50.9 percent required a fair amount; and 32.5 percent few or some of those services. In 1982, 98 percent of all Head Start programs had enrolled at least one handicapped child.

Services provided by Head Start to parents of handicapped children include counseling; referral to other agencies; visits to homes, hospitals, and the like; conferences with technical staff and other parent meetings; transportation; literature and special teaching equipment; workshops; medical assistance; and special classes.

REFERENCES

ASTHO Foundation. (1984). *Public health agencies 1982: Vol. 3. Services for mothers and children.* Kensington, Md: Association of State Territorial Health Officials Foundation.

Collins, R. C., & Deloria, D. (July-August, 1983). Head Start research: A new chapter. *Children Today,* 15–19.

General Accounting Office. (1980). *How federal developmental disabilities programs are working.* Report by the Comptroller General to the Subcommittee on the Handicapped, Senate Committee on Labor and Human Resources. Washington, DC: U.S. Government Printing Office.

General Accounting Office. (1984). *Maternal and Child Health Block Grant: Program changes emerging under state administration.* Report to the Congress of the United States by the Comptroller General. Washington, DC: U.S. Government Printing Office.

Head Start Bureau. (1984). *The status of handicapped children in Head Start programs.* Washington, DC: Office of Human Development Services Administration to Children, Youth, and Families.

Nelkin, V. (1983). *Six state collaborative projects.* Chapel Hill, NC: Technical Assistance Development Systems.

Office of Special Education and Rehabilitative Services, Department of Health and Human Services. (1982). *Programs for the handicapped.* Washington, DC: Author.

Office of Special Education and Rehabilitative Services, Department of Health and Human Services. (1983). *Programs for the handicapped.* Washington, DC: Author.

Chapter 5

VOLUNTARY HEALTH AGENCIES IN THE UNITED STATES

Leon Sternfeld

DEFINITION

A voluntary health agency has the following characteristics: (a) it is legally incorporated as a non-profit, tax-exempt entity with a written charter and by-laws; (b) the responsibility is vested in an autonomous board, which establishes policies, holds regularly scheduled meetings, collects funds for the support of the organization and its stated activities (from third-party payments and public contributions), and oversees the expenditure of funds for the conduct of the program; (c) it is administered by a (generally full-time paid) staff, which carries out the details of the program; (d) it includes in its program one or more of the following: direct services, information for health and education of the public, professional training, support for research, and advocacy (individual, group, system, and legal); and (e) it is concerned with a specific disease(s) or condition(s) (multiple sclerosis, cerebral palsy, muscular dystrophy, birth defects, cancer); disorders of organs and structures (locomotor-skeletal, heart, eyes, ears, teeth); and/or problems affecting a special population group (pregnant women, infants, children, the aged).

Excluded from the discussion in this chapter are official governmental health agencies; hospitals, dispensaries, clinics and outpatient departments; professional organizations of health and medical care personnel (medical, dental, nursing, physical therapy, public health, etc.); and the American Red Cross, which is a quasi-governmental agency chartered by Congress and functioning specifically during times of war and natural disasters.

71

DEVELOPMENT

The modern-day voluntary health agency in the United States began in 1892 with the establishment of the Pennsylvania Society for the Prevention of Tuberculosis. During the next 12 years 23 state and local anti-tuberculosis organizations were established, and these combined in 1904 to form the National Society for the Study and Prevention of Tuberculosis, better known in the middle of this century as the National Tuberculosis Association and currently as the American Lung Association. This organization has the distinction (among many) of developing "the most ingenious, effective fund-raising gimmick in the history of philanthropy" (Hood, 1973), the Christmas Seal, which has become as much a part of American tradition as Mother's Day and apple pie.

Between 1904 and 1922 the following national voluntary health agencies were organized: the American Cancer Society in 1912, the American Social Hygiene Association in 1914 (combining the Society for Social and Moral Prophylaxis, National League for the Protection of the Family, American Vigilance Committee, and the American Purity Alliance, which joined in 1916); the National Society for Crippled Children in 1921 (now called the Easter Seal Society); and the American Heart Association in 1922. A significant feature of these organizations (including the anti-tuberculosis societies) was the predominant organizing role played by physicians and other professionals. It is only a few decades since lay persons were involved in a meaningful way in determining policies and program activities.

During the hiatus from 1922 to 1945 (end of World war II) the major national voluntary health organization to come into being was the National Foundation for Infantile Paralysis, which was formally established in 1938 after four years of successful fund raising through the mechanism of President Franklin Delano Roosevelt's birthday balls each January 30. Some of the unique features of this organization are a much-beloved president of the United States as its founder and patron; a non-salaried president (for many years), Basil O'Connor, a close friend and law partner of Mr. Roosevelt, who was a genius at organization and who successfully pioneered mass fund-raising techniques; a definitive scientific objective—to eradicate poliomyelitis—which was successfully and fully achieved in the development of both killed (Salk) and live attenuated (Sabin) vaccines by 1955–1957 and the mass and maintenance immunization since then; establishing and supporting the Salk Institute at La Jolla, California, a unique complex of laboratories concentrating on cellular genetics and virology; and mobilization of the organization to work toward the prevention of birth defects (under the name of March of Dimes-Birth Defects Foundation).

In 1942 the National Health Council, which had been organized in 1921 by a group of health and professional agencies and had functioned as a "trade association," sponsored a 3-year study conducted by two experienced health professionals Selskar M. Gunn and Philip S. Platt and financed by a grant from the Rockefeller Foundation. The Gunn-Platt report (1945) was essentially the first in-depth study of U.S. voluntary health agencies as a group (including the American Red Cross). In tune with the sociopolitical tenor of the times, that of strong centralization (a direct result of the New Deal of the 1930s and the conduct of World War II), the report recommended that there be a strong central agency (viz., the National Health Council) to coordinate the various voluntary health agencies and to eliminate competition and duplication of appeals for funds. Predictably, the recommendations were not implemented, and the report was quietly filed and forgotten.

After 1945, the end of the war, there followed a rapid proliferation of voluntary health organizations. Among them are some of the major voluntary organizations concerned with the needs of handicapped children: United Cerebral Palsy Association in 1949, Association for Retarded Citizens in 1950, Epilepsy Foundation of America in 1968, National Society for Children and Adults with Autism in 1965 (these comprising organizations whose clientele are subsumed under the term *developmental disabilities* according to the federal definition in PL 91-157), Muscular Dystrophy Association in 1950, and Huntington's Disease Foundation of America in 1967. These oganizations, unlike the earlier ones, which were organized primarily by physicians, were established by parents of children with the various disabilities, whose needs, especially medical and health care and educational, were not being met under existing programs of governmental and voluntary agencies. (In 1946, a decade after the enactment of the Social Security Act, which included grants-in-aid to the states for services to "crippled children" under Title II, Part 2, children with cerebral palsy were not eligible for services in any state, and children with a birth defect such as club foot or cleft palate with mental retardation were ineligible in most states!) While new voluntary health organizations continue to be established as the needs of particular groups in the population become apparent (for example, AIDS Foundation), the wave seems to have crested toward a plateau considerably higher than that which existed at midcentury.

FUNCTIONS

The basic functions of voluntary health agencies include providing direct services not otherwise available, instituting needed training and educational activities, supporting research, and advocacy. The composition of this mix will vary from agency to agency, but all are included to some extent in each of the voluntary health agencies.

Direct Services

In providing direct services voluntary health agencies have frequently followed two pathways, that of setting up a demonstration service and that of surveying on a sample basis the needs of their clientele and their families. For example, many of the early tuberculosis screening activities were initiated by the National Tuberculosis Association and were then taken over by the official local and state health departments. The National Foundation for Infantile Paralysis and its local chapters provided hospital care for poliomyelitis patients and established respiratory treatment centers for those with bulbar polio. Easter Seal Society established a network of sheltered workshops, summer camps, and speech and hearing programs. United Cerebral Palsy and its affiliates have a network of developmental centers for infant development and for school-age children too severely involved for the local public school system (under the Education for All Handicapped Children Act, PL 94-142), work-training programs for adolescents and adults, and recreation and leisuretime services including adapted physical education and competitive sports.

Training

Voluntary health agencies have been in the forefront in developing and supporting training programs for professional and ancillary personnel. Usually this has been in the form of scholarships and fellowships for students enrolled in the curricula of established training centers. For many years scholarships were available, funded by the March of Dimes, for students to become enrolled in physical therapy curricula. United Cerebral Palsy (through its Research and Educational Foundation) funds a group of postspecialist clinical fellowships for physicians and dentists, as well as stipends for graduate students.

A unique contribution of voluntary health agencies, both in the provision of direct services and in training activities, has been the conceptual development and implementation in practice of the interdisciplinary process. Traditionally, physicians have been generally involved in solo practice or in some variation of such practice (e.g., partnerships) which is essentially unidisciplinary. With increased specialization of medicine and the rapid technological advances applied to medical practice in the latter half of the twentieth century, a multidisciplinary approach developed. This involves the primary care physician synthesizing the information and data obtained from other medical consultants from ancillary professional personnel such as nurses, social workers, and therapists, and from laboratory and radiology to determine the appropriate treatment and management plan. The interdisciplinary approach further integrates the needs of the individual and the family, and develops an integrated treatment and management plan for each individual client.

Closely related to the professional training activities of voluntary health agencies are the public information and health education materials that are prepared and disseminated widely. One may question how effective such efforts have been, but some of the voluntary health agencies have had an impact with these activities. Certainly, the American Cancer Society has imprinted on the public the "danger signs" and the need for breast self-examination, Pap smear, and mammography. The American Heart Association has been in the forefront of informing the public about appropriate nutrition to prevent atherosclerosis and hypertension, and the role of exercise and fitness in preserving normal cardiac function. Easter Seal, United Cerebral Palsy, Epilepsy Foundation of America, and others have been trying to inform the public about developmental disabilities, thereby modifying existing (pessimistic) attitudes about the abilities of such individuals.

Research

Some of the outstanding accomplishments of the voluntary health agencies have resulted from their support of specific areas of research. The elimination of poliomyelitis outbreaks is a direct result of the research activities funded by the March of Dimes (National Foundation), which culminated in the field immunization trials of 1954–55 with the Salk vaccine. Similar, though not quite as spectacular, accomplishments were the epidemiologic studies of the American Cancer Society relating smoking with respiratory cancers (and later other types of morbidity such as cardiovascular disease, prematurity, and peripheral vascular diseases) and the work supported by the American Heart Association in relating dietary factors (salt, cholesterol, and saturated fatty acids) to hypertension and atherosclerosis.

Generally, the agencies provide grants to investigators at established research centers. The mechanism is that of "peer review" following procedures developed by the National Institutes of Health (NIH), although considerably simplified in many instances. Occasionally, research is done intramurally, such as the epidemiologic studies of smoking referred to above. In the 1960s the Muscular Dystrophy Association maintained its own research center in close proximity to the Cornell Medical School–New York Hospital Center in Manhattan, but that was discontinued in favor of funding specific research proposals at a number of research centers.

The voluntary health agencies have staunchly supported NIH, and in some instances they have been instrumental in getting a new institute established. This happened in the case of the National Institute of Neurological and Communicative Disorders and Stroke (originally "and Blindness"), which was established in 1950 after a coalition of professional and voluntary health organizations interested in the neurosciences had campaigned with Congress and the White House. The agencies generally give strong support to NIH (as well as to the research and training activities of other federal agencies such as the Environmental Protection Agency, Veterans Administration, National Institute for Handicapped Research, etc.), and are in the forefront in urging each year that adequate appropriations be included in the federal budget. The agencies provide another type of support in helping to safe-guard the integrity and competence of the personnel in NIH, avoiding po-liticization as much as possible.

Inasmuch as biomedical and biotechnical research in the United States is in large part funded by federal dollars and also to some extent by com-mercial interests (pharmaceutical manufacturers, for example), is it neces-sary for voluntary health agencies to continue to expend funds for research instead of channeling such funds into the other functions, particularly direct services? No categorical answer can be given to this question. Generally, the research grants are made to investigators whose base of operation has been established and to some extent maintained by research grants from NIH. Both the administrators at NIH and research investigators in the field are of the opinion that the support of research by voluntary health agencies is not only significant but actually essential. The voluntary health agencies' re-search support is for very specific purposes and objectives (relating to the particular interests of the agency), can be made usually with less procedural red tape, and can involve somewhat more of a risk both as to the type of re-search (which may be somewhat tangential to the traditional route) and to the investigator (who may be academically qualified but has not yet developed a demonstrated research "track record"). From the agency standpoint a fur-ther advantage of sponsoring and supporting research is the goodwill that is engendered in the general public's attitude toward the agency.

During this decade of the 1980s it is likely that both training and re-search activities of the federal government will be curtailed, perhaps even severely. Therefore, these activities on the part of voluntary health agencies become more important. It is a recognized fact, however, that the efforts of all of the voluntary health agencies in toto cannot replace the loss sustained in the curtailed federal effort.

Advocacy

The advocacy function of the voluntary health agencies is, in the long run, perhaps the most significant function of all. Agencies have played the most important role in creating among the general population an awareness of a number of health problems and in modifying constructively the adverse attitudes of the public toward persons with such health problems (sometimes referred to as bringing those persons "out of the closet"). Some examples are tuberculosis, venereal (now called sexually transmitted) diseases, psychiatric problems generally, alcoholism, mental retardation, cancer, cerebral palsy, autism, epilepsy—and the list goes on and on.

Another important advocacy function is that of working with govern-ment agencies whose work related to that of the voluntary agency. The lat-ter is in a unique position to support the former in many ways, as well as to act, if necessary, in a monitoring role. Related to this is legislative advocacy that involves not only supporting favorable legislation (and also opposing harmful legislation) but actually introducing and sponsoring needed legislation. Three significant and far-reaching examples of federal legislation relating to handicapped children are the Developmental Disabilities Act and its renewals (Developmental Disabilities Services and Facilities Construction Act, PL 88-164 in 1963, PL 91-157 in 1970, and the Developmental Disabilities Assistance and Bill of Rights Act, PL 94-103 in 1975); the Education for All Handicapped Children Act (PL 94-142 in 1975); and antidiscrimination with regard to handicapping conditions in the Vocational Rehabilitation Act (PL 93-112, in 1973, Sec. 504).

Another example of an advocacy function that has achieved considerable widespread success has been that relating to the elimination of architectural and transportation barriers. Many cities now have curb cuts on their busy street corners, buses and other forms of transportation with lifts and kneeling devices, and ramps or other suitable modifications to permit access to public buildings (and many non-public ones also) as well as parks and other recreation areas. Federal, state, and local laws and regulations have been enacted to permit freer access generally to the disabled population. All of this is now more or less taken for granted, but it was the effort of some of the voluntary health agencies working for years, even decades, that has brought it about.

A number of agencies, particularly those involved with the various groups of handicapped children, are now working actively to have a variety of alternative living arrangements for handicapped persons, preferably in independent households or in small group residences. In addition, it is hoped that most handicapped persons can be gainfully employed at some time. These objectives seem far off at present; nevertheless, they are being pursued vigorously by many voluntary health agencies, and it is likely that they will be successful at some time in the future.

One additional type of advocacy is that which operates to assure that any agency, government, voluntary, or private (for profit), that provides direct services to handicapped persons and their families assure that these services (and the agency providing them) be of high quality and meet the standards that reflect "the state of the art." Currently, this is done, in part, by an accreditation process through two national voluntary accreditation groups established by various professional organizations and voluntary health agencies, the Council of Accreditation of Rehabilitation Facilities (CARF) and the Accreditation Council for Services for Mentally Retarded and Other Developmentally Disabled Persons (AC/MR-DD). Both councils have a manual of standards and a defined procedure that an agency applying for accreditation follows, including a self-survey prior to the survey carried out by surveyors of the councils. Essentially, the process is one of education of the staff, board, and clientele of an agency. Some voluntary health agencies (United Cerebral Palsy Association, Epilepsy Foundation of America) and several states (Maryland, Tennessee, California) require accreditation for affiliation or receipt of funds.

FUNDING

To maintain a voluntary health agency and enable it to carry out its functions, adequate funding is needed. Prior to the middle 1960s funds came for the most part from contributions from the public. Since 1965 when the Medicare and Medicaid programs were initiated, many of the voluntary health agencies, particularly those involved with direct services to the handicapped, have been receiving an increasing amount of third-party payments, much of it from government funds. Nevertheless, fund raising among the general public remains an important activity of voluntary health agencies, and this has aroused more adverse criticism than any other aspect of voluntary health agency functioning. Methods of fund raising include Christmas Seals (tuberculosis), Easter Seals (Easter Seal Society), Mothers' Marches (March of Dimes), Women's Crusade (Cancer Society), and the entire suffix family of "thons"—readathons, walkathons, bikeathons, telathons, radiothons, phonathons (United Cerebral Palsy, Multiple Sclerosis, March of Dimes, Easter Seal, Arthritis, etc.). Other special events include humanitarian award dinners, gambol nights, Mardi Gras, various society balls, theater parties, picnics, riverboat sails, door-to-door soliciting, mail appeals, and so on.

Some of the adverse criticisms of fund raising activities have been that it is raucous, in bad taste, an exploitation of the clientele, confusing to the general public, a distortion of priorities and needs, alarmist, and concerned more with achieving a high dollar value than with what the real purpose of the agency might be. All of these and many other criticisms are certainly valid. And yet the impulse of giving has a tradition of some 5,000 years.

One of many aspects of fund raising is the distribution of funds between the local chapters or divisions or affiliates and the state and national organization of each voluntary health agency. Some agencies are highly centralized (e.g., March of Dimes, Ameican Cancer Society, American Heart Association), but most are decentralized, federated agencies, where the local (and state) agencies are quite autonomous and support to a varying degree the national organization with which they are affiliated. Most of the agencies involved with handicapped children are in this latter category, as are all of the agencies in the so-called developmental disability group. Generally, the centralized agencies do not permit their local and/or state agencies to participate in the communities' United Way (a local community combined fund raising campaign). A number of the decentralized (federated) agencies may be member agencies of their local United Way, whereas others may be involved in independent fund raising.

Another aspect of fund raising by the voluntary health agencies that is definitely positive is the "educational" factor. Fund raising involves the efforts of an innumerable corps of volunteers who learn about the "cause" and in turn impart it to their families, friends, neighbors, and the public at large. Also, the technology of communication (radio, television, print) all impart an important message to the public. In years past, with regard to the handicapped population, much of this message tended to be sentimental and even deprecating to the handicapped person as well as fostering a dependent attitude; but currently handicapped persons are participating in fund-raising activities, monitoring those activities, and providing important suggestions for presenting a most positive image of the person with a handicap and that person's potential.

SUMMARY

Voluntarism has been a characteristic of the American people since the founding of the Republic, and before. This characteristic was sufficiently apparent that it received attention from De Tocqueville in his 19th-century classic *Democracy in America* as an important attribute of the American population quite different from the European peoples. Voluntarism involved with health causes is a more recent, 20th-century manifestation of the general characteristic of voluntarism, probably occurring with increased medical knowledge about disease etiology and control starting with the microbiologic era in the late 19th century.

The development and functioning of national voluntary health organizations during most of the 20th century have demonstrated the following positive values: (a) origins in commonly felt desires and needs; (b) attention and participation of outstanding citizens in the communities and the nation; (c) high standards of public responsibility and stewardship; (d) enlistment of a large number of volunteer workers who contribute their abilities, efforts, and time; (e) enlistment of wide support and goodwill from the general public; (f) freedom and independence not available to governmental agencies; and (g) a degree of adaptability that acts as a model for government agencies.

As the 20th century draws to a close, what is the future of voluntary health agencies? From the historical perspective it would seem that this movement will continue, particularly as there are many diseases yet to be understood and either prevented or controlled. Also, there are many unmet health needs in various segments of the population that will require the attention of existing health agencies and even the development of additional agencies. The major negative trend is the ideological political development in the 1980s of decentralizing the role of the federal government in many domestic affairs, with particular emphasis on "human services." Should the trend of de-emphasis be continued beyond the 1981–1988 administration, then the continuance of voluntary national health agencies may be endangered. However, political history in the United States shows that there have been pendulum-like swings a number of times, and one hopes this will occur again before the 20th century ends.

REFERENCES

Gunn, S. M., & Platt, P. S. (1945). *Voluntary health agencies: An interpretive study.* New York: Ronald Press.

Hood, R. R. (1973). *The role of national voluntary health organizations in supporting national health objectives.* New York: World Federation of Public Health Associations.

Chapter 6

ADVOCACY

Ernest Weinrich

Marginal man is the product of his society. He exists as such because his social status and role are clearly defined at the fringes of social organization. The status effectively isolates him from meaningful social participation. He, therefore, has little commitment to, or identity with, the generic goals of his society. The permanent problems of marginal groups, therefore, is their need for new social statuses and roles which will bring about their integration into the social life of the community accompanied by some personal feelings of achievement.
—George Fairweather, *Methods for Experimental Social Innovation* 1967

DEFINITION AND PURPOSE

Advocacy is the act or process of defending or maintaining a cause, the act or process of supporting a cause. Advocacy can be defined as a process that seeks to ensure to persons who are disabled their rights to appropriate services.

The above definition stresses assuring appropriate services. However, an additional important goal of advocacy relative to individuals who are disabled is that of ensuring an ever-improving quality of life. In effect, advocacy seeks to negate "marginal man" status for children, teenagers, and adults with disabilities.

Our society has always endeavored to provide for groups with special

81

needs, with greater or lesser success. Ever-increasing knowledge, medical and otherwise, has improved society's ability to assist children with disabilities to live satisfying lives and to enter society's mainstream. As a result, more and more programs have been established. A procedure was, and is, needed to assure that these opportunities and services be established and remain available, and that there be assistance to families to access the available services and to deal with the ever-increasing complexity of the delivery system. Advocacy processes have been developed and used for those purposes.

SOCIETAL FACTORS

Establishing and delivering appropriate services for children with disabilities, and concurrent and relevant advocacy roles and processes, are influenced by several societal factors. Three of these are historical factors, social attitudes, and family factors (impact of disability on the family).

Some Historical Factors

The initial step in developing appropriate services was to identify needs. This seemed to be relatively simple and direct. A group of parents with children with similar disabilities not receiving services brought themselves together into organizations so that appropriate opportunities for their children would be made available. Money was raised, and some service was started. Of course, medical service was the first need to be met, then education, recreation, and work. Next came social development and opportunities for children "not attending school."

At that time life appeared simple; a need was identified, organizations were organized, and if appropriate funds were available, a program was started. Then professionals became involved, and other persons became interested. Other needs were identified. Programs became sophisticated. Additional goals were set, leading to the present goal of improving the quality of life and mainstreaming individuals who are disabled into everyday societal activities. Government, at all levels, began to support and provide needed services. Services and programs became very complex, highly organized professionally administered; but as this all happened, it became more difficult to meet additional needs of individuals, including those leading to improved quality of life. Services became increasingly difficult to access, and organizations had to assist families, advocating in their behalf and, more recently, helping them to advocate effectively in behalf of their children with disabilities.

Social Attitudes

Social attitudes toward individuals who are handicapped are changing, but some damaging ones prevail. There still persists a feeling that "equality" equals sameness; and if people are different, they are therefore not equal and should not be rendered opportunities that will make them part of society. They are and in effect should remain "marginal."

Until rather recently society behaved as if it were abnormal to have people with handicaps as part of society. Indeed, the history was to place "disabled" people in institutions, away from the rest of society. This is gradually changing, but reluctantly. At a recent hearing to grant a variance so that a group home for persons who are retarded could be established in the community, neighborhood residents raised the following points: "Would not these people be more comfortable away from the tumult of everyday society?" "Will my children be safe? Will they be frightened?" "My property value will go down!"

Another attitude has it that a person with a disability is not a "whole" person. There are "parts" missing, and therefore some cannot make appropriate decisions. That attitude results in continuous paternalistic behavior toward them.

Apparently there is still prejudice stemming from lack of knowledge and fear because of that lack of knowledge. One important consequence stemming from this and other attitudes toward persons with disabilities and others with special needs is to decrease financial resources when the nation's economy has a downward trend, and in fact this has occurred in the past and is happening now. Nevertheless, things are changing and community group homes are being established; special parking spaces for the handicapped are prevalent, as are curb cuts, due to advocacy processes. PL 94-142 has been passed, "guaranteeing" a proper education in the least restrictive environment for children who are handicapped. An attempt was made to reduce this program and even eliminate it, but advocacy groups did not permit that to happen.

Family Factors: Impact on the Family

The changing family in our society impacts on everyone but has special significance where a family member is disabled; very often when one member is handicapped, there is a "handicapped family." Some things that have happened in the family:

> The mother, specifically in our ever-growing middle class, looks on childbirth and child rearing as an interim. The father is expected to take on a greater day-to-day role.

> The family that includes a child who is handicapped must deal with a specific deviant problem in a complex world.

> Emotionally, and in realistic terms, the child with a handicap and the parent (especially the mother) will become abnormally dependent on each other. How do you help a dependent person to want to become as independent as possible? This is particularly difficult when most of

those involved may think, or know, that he will be dependent in some measure all of his life.

Parents of children who are handicapped have to give up decisions that normally belong to parents.

Now consider the practical, everyday aspects: dressing, feeding, toileting, bringing the child to the treatment center, to school, back home, arranging for transportation and being a parent to the other children, as well as taking care of all of the household needs and doing all of the things with the child that the wonderful team says that a parent must do in order for that child to make as much progress as possible—a 26-hour day! And that doesn't include sleep and advocacy for the rights of the child with a handicap to sources and opportunities to improve his quality of life.

ADVOCACY FURTHER DEFINED

Generally, there are two types of advocacy: case and class. Case advocacy is engaged in either by an individual himself or in behalf of an individual by a professional, friend, or family member. Class advocacy is organized action in behalf of a group of individuals. Each category has several discrete processes, which are identified succinctly and appropriately in Table 6-1, prepared by Marie Moore when she was Coordinator of the federally funded five-year National UCPA Advocacy Project. For the words *developmentally disabled* one can also read "children with disabilities."

An additional word concerning community organization, an important advocacy process often engaged in by many persons without recognizing the need for conscious planning and procedure: Community organization is defined as processes by which a person or a group, by working with other groups and individuals, attempts to effect change in the community to reach certain specific goals to improve services and opportunities for an identified group of individuals. In community organization, as in all types of advocacy, goals and objectives need to be clearly defined and implementation steps definitively outlined. Responsibility, agency or person, should be identified so that it is clear who is responsible and what additional action is needed. Professional persons need to give as much conscious thinking to all advocacy processes as they give to practicing their professional disciplines.

Self-Advocacy

Self-advocacy, specifically identified in Table 6-1, needs special mention. Parents need to advocate in their own behalf and in behalf of their children, as do adults with disabilities. Indeed, the self-images of parents and consumers improve as they become more effective and successful in advo-

Table 6-1. Classifications of Types of Advocacy
for Developmental Disabilities[a]

System	Purpose	Governing Body
Case Advocacy		
Citizen advocacy	One-to-one relationship between a capable volunteer and a person who is developmentally disabled in which the volunteer advocate defends the rights and interests of the other and provides practical or emotional reinforcement for him	Citizen advocacy board, operated by a private association or agency
Ombudsman, private	One who acts as an advocate for an individual in receiving a grievance and investigating, interceding, or initiating action on his behalf	Advocacy council or committee, operated by a private organization or association
Ombudsman, public	Same as Ombudsman, private	As designated by law or executive or judicial order, e.g., a state or local human rights commission; an ombudsman may be assigned to an institutional service system
Legal advocate	One who represents a person in the litigation or legal negotiation process concerning rights, grievances, or appeals	None unless in a legal setting, e.g., a legal services attorney
Case manager/advocate, "personal" representative	A trained professional or volunteer who assists the individual in information referral, follow-along services as an advocate when there are barriers in the service delivery system	Public or private agencies
Protective service worker	One who has authority to investigate alleged abuses, etc., without the consent or request of a victim or to initiate action	Usually a public "protective" agency; may be a specially chartered protective organization, like the Society for the Protection of Children

[a]From Moore, M. L (May 1976). Advocacy systems. *AMICUS*. South Bend, IN: National Center for Law and the Handicapped, Notre Dame University. Used by permission of author.

**Table 6-1. Classifications of Types of Advocacy
for Developmental Disabilities**[a] (*continued*)

System	*Purpose*	*Governing Body*
Class advocacy		
Systems reforms and development	Using collective citizen action to mandate change to secure the rights of the developmentally disabled in areas such as human services, labor, transportation, housing, education, health care; includes but is not limited to legislative change or litigation	Non-profit advocacy organization
Community organizational advocacy	Using the community organization process to develop better communication among agencies serving the developmentally disabled; to assist in the development of cooperative or coalition efforts on behalf of the disabled by public and private providers of service and by consumers	Community planning groups; placement of consumers and consumer representatives in planning bodies; pressure groups of consumer advocates
Program development	Service modification and program expansion via negotiation to eliminate barriers and combine many resources	Voluntary professional or lay organizations working in cooperation with governmental and private agencies; state DD planning councils; other advisory bodies
Protective service system	An agency with authority to intervene in situations presenting actual or potential hazard to persons unable to protect themselves.	State government board or agency
Consumer action groups	Groups of parents or adults who are disabled that act as pressure groups or influencing groups and advocate for desired change	Independent organizations; groups associated with consumer representative organizations

cating in their own behalf. Therefore, training programs in self-advocacy for parents were established by agencies or parent groups, sometimes assisted by federal funds. Such programs conveyed to parents specific knowledge concerning their rights and those of their children, as well as about the advocacy role, so that they could effectively advocate in behalf of themselves and their children. Such training needs to continue. It would be very helpful if the training included how to deal effectively with the child's care or treatment team, how to be a more effective team member, and how to decrease adversarial functioning and feeling.

(In)Accessibility

In any discussion of advocacy the question of accessibility deserves emphasis, for it is not only the advocate's role to work for ever-increasing opportunities for children with disabilities but also to make certain that these services are accessible. There are at least four issues concerning accessibility: (a) to make certain that enough funds are available to serve all those who need the services; (b) to make certain that those who are delivering the service are as up to date as possible in the latest approaches and opportunities that will benefit children with disabilities and their families; (c) to assure that services are indeed accessible and that the primary concern of service deliverers is to see to it that services are properly delivered to the individual child; (d) to make the community and all of the resources (special and otherwise) physically accessible.

Conclusion

There is no question that advocacy activity has resulted in significant changes and opportunities for chidren with disabilities and their families. The Education for All Handicapped Children Act (PL-94-142) and the Independent Living Act are significant pieces of legislation not only mandating opportunities but expressing the change in societal attitude toward people with disabilities. The acceptance of the concept of the least restrictive alternative in planning and delivering service has been accomplished by advocates, singly and in concert.

As long as a society does not provide adequate opportunities for children with disabilities and their families, advocacy activities will be needed and engaged in by organizations, professionals, and consumers. Unfortunately, the burden will be greatest on the consumers, those who are in need of assistance so that they can adequately cope in our society. Consumers, professionals, volunteers, and organizations will have to gain better knowledge concerning advocacy processes, to change and improve, continuously and effectively, the service delivery system.

Chapter 7

LEGAL RIGHTS FOR THE HANDICAPPED

Sarah Rosenbaum
Barbara Milstein

For decades, people with disabilities in the United States were routinely excluded from access to basic public services, solely because of their handicaps. Congress, concerned over ensuring all individuals the opportunity to achieve self sufficiency and promote their integration into society, enacted Section 504 of the Rehabilitation Act of 1973.[1] Together with subsequent amendments designed in 1974[2] and 1978,[3] it was enacted "to prevent discrimination against all handicapped individuals regardless of their need for or ability to benefit from vocational rehabilitation services, in relation to federal assistance in employment, education, health services, or any other federally aided program" (U.S. Congress, 1973; 1974; 1978).

Section 504 provides that

> . . . no otherwise qualified handicapped individual . . . shall solely by reason of his handicap, be excluded from the participation in, be denied the benefits of, or be subjected to discrimination under any program or activity receiving Federal financial assistance or under any program or activity conducted by any Executive agency or by the United States Postal Service.

The language of Section 504 is virtually identical to Title VI of the Civil Rights Act of 1964 (prohibiting discrimination on the basis of race, color, and national origin) and Title IX of the Education Amendments of 1972 (prohibiting discrimination in education programs on the basis of sex). This explicit extension of civil rights protection afforded to other minorities and women reversed a long history of laws and policies that viewed people with disabilities as economically non-productive who required segregation and charity. Section 504 guarantees that disabled people have the right to participate fully in all aspects of society, with accommodations made where necessary to assure equal access and to make the opportunity to participate a meaningful one.

Under the law, *handicapped individuals* are persons with physical, mental, or emotional impairments that substantially limit one or more major life activity. The term *major life activities* refers to "functions such as caring for oneself, performing manual tasks, walking, hearing, speaking, breathing, learning and working" [45 CFR §84.3 (j) (2) (ii)].

Federally assisted programs include all those supported by federal grants or loans to states or other political subdivisions or to public or private agencies or other entities receiving federal financing assistance. (Smith, 1983).

Examples of federally assisted activities include all grant-in-aid or direct grant programs administered by the U.S. Department of Health and Human Services (HHS) (such as Medicaid,[4] the Title V Maternal and Child Health Grant Program,[5] or Title XX of the Social Security Act (the Social Services Block Grant).[6] Thus, any public or private hospital, school, or company, for example, that receives federal funding is prohibited from discriminating against its patients, teachers, and other employees on the basis of their disability.

Federally conducted programs are those funded directly by federal agencies or purchased through procurement contacts (Smith, 1983).[7] Examples of such programs include the Indian Health Service, Public Health Service hospitals, and the Supplemental Security Income program. All agencies that administer federally conducted or assisted programs are required to develop regulations specifically applying the requirements of Section 504 to programs within their jurisdiction.[8]

Nearly all of the federally assisted health and human service programs affecting children with disabilities fall within the jurisdiction of HHS.[9] This chapter will therefore examine HHS Section 504 regulations governing federally assisted programs, as well as court decisions interpreting key provisions of Section 504 as it affects federally assisted health and human services programs. As with any complex federal civil rights law, the meaning of key provisions of Section 504 have been extensively tested in court.

Who Are the "Otherwise Qualified" Handicapped Individuals Protected by the Act?

Section 504 does not prohibit all types of discrimination against the handicapped; it prohibits only discrimination against "otherwise qualified" handicapped persons. Regulations issued by HHS governing health and human services programs define qualified handicapped persons as those "who meet the essential eligibility requirements for the receipt of such services" [45 CFR §84.3(4)]. Thus, for example, if a child satisfies the general eligibility criteria under a state's Title XX–funded day-care program, the state and agency may not deny benefits solely because the child has a disabling condition. Similarly, if a state Title V crippled children's program defines its mission as, in general, one that provides care to children with disabling or chronic conditions, the program may not excuse a child simply because the child suffers from a mental, as opposed to physical, handicap.[10]

With respect to preschool, elementary, or secondary schooling, HHS 504 rules define qualified handicapped children to include children "(i) of an age during which non-handicapped children are provided such services, (ii) of any age during which it is mandatory under state law to provide such services to handicapped children, or (iii) to whom a state is required to provide a free appropriate public education under the Education for All Handicapped Children Act."

Whether or not a child is qualified to benefit from a healthy, educational, or recreational activity, and is therefore protected by Section 504, requires a careful evaluation of how the benefit is both structured and delivered. If the benefit—a swimming lesson, for example—is traditionally delivered to sighted children, the school may not refuse to admit a blind child into the swimming class simply because the swimming instructor is unfamiliar with teaching blind children. The school must modify the class in any of a variety of ways in order to permit the blind child to participate in the class.

On the other hand, if a school conducts a driver education class, Section 504 does not require the school to admit a blind child into the class. The child is not a qualified handicapped individual for purposes of this class because the child lacks sight, which is one of the skills basic to accomplishing the purpose of the class. Thus, the school is not required to lower or to modify its qualifying criteria if doing so would "fundamentally alter the nature of its program" (*Southeastern v. Davis*, 442 U.S. 398). Otherwise, 504 does require the acknowledgment that "discrimination against handicapped people cannot be eliminated if programs, activities and tasks are always structured in the ways that only people with 'normal' physical and mental abilities customarily undertake them" (U.S. Commission on Civil Rights, 1983).

What Actions Constitute Discrimination against Otherwise Qualified Handicapped Persons?

A broad array of actions can constitute discrimination against the handicapped. *Most important,* these actions do not have to be intentional; they may have the *effect* of discriminating and nonetheless constitute a violation of Section 504 (*Alexander v. Choate*, U.S. 105 S. Ct. 712, 1985).

HHS regulations describe in general certain actions that would constitute discrimination in federally assisted health and human services programs

(45 CFR §84.4). Recipients of financial assistance may not deny qualified persons the right to participate in or benefit from a benefit or service, an equal opportunity to participate in a benefit or service, or an equally effective aid or service. Recipients are also prohibited from providing qualified handicapped persons with separate services or benefits unless such action is necessary to provide such persons with equally effective services. Recipients may not significantly aid any grantee that discriminates. In general, a federal assistance recipient may in no way limit a qualified handicapped person in his or her enjoyment of any right, privilege or opportunity enjoyed by others.

Federal regulations also provide specific examples of actions by recipients of federal assistance that would constitute discrimination in the areas of education, health, welfare, and social services (45 CFR §84.52). Health, welfare and human service providers may not deny benefits or services to qualified handicapped persons, nor may they afford such persons a lesser opportunity to receive benefits or services. Such agencies also are prohibited from providing handicapped persons with less effective services or with services that have the effect of limiting participation.

The rules also provide that in determining the site or location of a facility, grantees may not select sites or locations that intentionally or effectively discriminate against handicapped persons. Thus, a hospital, for example, could not choose a site or location that was inaccessible to the handicapped.

Federal rules further provide that recipients that provide notices concerning benefits or services (such as welfare departments) or that provide written materials concerning waivers of rights or consent to treatment (such as hospitals) must "take such steps as are necessary to ensure that qualified handicapped persons, including those with impaired sensory or speaking skills, are not denied effective notice because of their handicap" (45 CFR §84.52).

Additionally, recipient hospitals must "establish a procedure for effective communication with persons with impaired hearing for the purpose of providing emergency health care" (45 CFR §84.52) and recipients that employ more than 15 people (such as hospitals or nursing homes) must "provide appropriate auxiliary aids to persons with impaired sensory, manual or speaking skills, where necessary to afford such persons an equal opportunity to benefit from the service in question" (45 CFR §84.52). Thus, for example, a nursing home employing more than 15 people would have to provide auxiliary aids to afford hearing-impaired patients an equal opportunity to benefit from the service. Even nursing homes (and all other recipients of federal funds) with fewer than 15 employees, however, must use auxiliary aids if doing so would not "significantly impair the ability of the recipient to provide its benefits or services" [28 CFR 42.503(f)].

Specific education protections under Section 504 cover numerous issues. For example, recipients of federal assistance that operate elementary or secondary education program must furnish a free and appropriate public education for qualified handicapped persons (45 CFR §84.33). An appropriate education is one that is designed to meet the individual needs of handicapped persons "as adequately as the needs of non-handicapped persons are met."

Moreover, educational agencies must, to the maximum extent appropriate, provide for the education of qualified handicapped children with persons who are not handicapped (45 CFR §84.34). All tests and other evaluation materials used to place persons who, because of handicaps, are believed to need special education must have been validated for the purpose for which they are used and must be administered by trained personnel in conformance with instructions (45 CFR §84.34). Tests must be tailored to measure specific areas of educational need and must not be designed simply to measure a single general intelligence quotient. Finally, the test must be administered so as to best ensure that, when administered to students with impaired sensory, manual, or speaking skills, their results accurately reflect the student's aptitude rather than his impaired senses (45 CFR §84.34).

Despite the numerous protections offered by the federal rules, many situations exist in which *disparate* treatment of the handicapped does not constitute *discriminatory* treatment. Unfortunately, this exception may tend to swallow the rule in critical human services situations.

Federal regulations specify that aid or benefits, to be equally effective, *need not* produce the identical results or achievements for handicapped persons. They must simply afford handicapped persons an equal opportunity to obtain the same results or benefits in the most integrated settings. Thus, for example, whereas a Medicaid agency cannot provide *fewer* covered days of hospital care per year to handicapped Medicaid beneficiaries, it can place arbitrary limits on the number of hospital days per year it will cover for *any* beneficiary. Even if the impact of such limits falls with disparate harshness on certain handicapped persons because of their greater need for hospital care, as long as the limit applies to all persons and is fiscally neutral, a limitation of this type does not constitute discrimination against the handicapped within the meaning of Section 504 (*Alexander v. Choate*, supra).

Today many state Medicaid programs place arbitrary but fiscally neutral limitations on coverage of benefits. Even though these limits often work a great hardship on the handicapped, they do not constitute discrimination under Section 504 merely because they render a program less effective for the handicapped than it is for the non-handicapped. As long as the benefits afforded to handicapped persons are the same as those afforded to the non-handicapped, arbitrary welfare restrictions would probably pass muster under current federal law.

One issue that raises the "disparate treatment versus discrimination" issue and has received widespread publicity is the so-called Baby Doe situation in which a decision is made to withhold medical treatment and/or supportive services from infants with medical conditions who also have certain disabilities.

In 1982, in response to a case involving the withholding of lifesaving corrective surgery, as well as food and water, from a Bloomington, Indiana, baby who suffered from Down syndrome, HHS promulgated regulations prohibiting hospitals receiving federal funds from failing to feed and care for handicapped infants. The rules were ultimately challenged on substantive grounds [AMA v. Heckler F.2d (1984)] and were set aside on the grounds that Congress did not intend Section 504 to reach medical decisions made in hospitals, even though such decisions may lead to the withholding of treatment on the basis of an infant's handicap. The Supreme Court will review this lower court decision in its 1985–86 term. In the meantime, numerous hospitals have now begun to establish bioethical panels to better ensure that the medical evidence on which the decision to withhold treatment is based is sound, and to offer a more controlled appropriate forum for this type of determination.

To What Activities Do the Protections Offered by Section 504 Apply?

Section 504 reaches any program or activity that is federally conducted or receives federal assistance. Grant-in-aid programs such as Medicaid and Medicare have been held specifically to constitute federal assistance for purposes of 504 [*United States v. Baylor University* 736 F.2d 1039 (5th Cir., 1984); *NAACP v. Wilmington Medical Center* 500 F.2d 1247 (3rd Cir., 1979)].

However, the requirements of Section 504 have been held to extend only so far as the federal assistance extends. Programs and activities that do not receive federal assistance are not bound by the law's requirements, even if they are part of a single institution that receives federal assistance for other programs and activities [*Grove City College v. Bell*, 465 U.S. 555, 104S. Ct. 1211 (1984)]. With respect to Medicare and Medicaid, however, courts have treated payments under those programs as permeating all departments of a hospital that are assisted by the programs (*U.S. v. Baylor Hospital*, supra). Thus, for example, it would be impossible for a hospital receiving Medicaid or Title V reimbursement for its pediatric inpatient services to claim that its pediatric department is exempt from the reach of Section 504. Courts also have ruled that complainants do not have to be beneficiaries of the Medicare or Medicaid program in order to invoke the protections of Section 504. Thus, a non-Medicaid–recipient deaf patient could challenge a Medicaid-funded hospital's refusal to provide her with an auxiliary aid. See *U.S. v. Baylor*, noted above.

What Remedies Exist for Violations of Section 504?

All recipients of federal financial assistance must submit assurances to their granting federal agencies that they will operate their programs in compliance with Section 504. Individuals who believe that they have been discriminated against may file a complaint with the civil rights division of the appropriate federal agency. If, on investigation, the agency finds that a recipient of federal assistance has been discriminated against in violation of Section 504, the agency may be required to take remedial action, including making accommodations to meet the needs of the handicapped.

In addition, the Supreme Court has held that private individuals may bypass federal and state agencies and bring their discrimination complaints directly to court [*Consolidated Rail Corp. v. Darrone*, 465 U.S. 624, 104 S.Ct. 1248 (1984)]. This case clarified the fact that complainants who could prove intentional discrimination were entitled to collect damages, and left the collection of damages in unintended discrimination cases up to individual courts. Finally, a more recent Supreme Court decision, *Scanlon v. Atascadero* decided that by the Court in June 1985, reaffirmed the right of individuals to sue for discrimination, but raised questions about the individual's ability to sue in federal, rather than state court.

NOTES

[1] PL 93-112, 87 Stat. 394. Section 504 of the act was codified at 29 USC§794.

[2] PL 93-516. The purpose of the 1974 amendments was to expand the definition of "handicapped individual" which, in the original act, had been based on impaired employability. The 1974 amendments clarified that "handicapped individuals" were to include persons with physical or mental impairments that substantially limited one or more major life activities, regardless of their employability.

[3] PL 95-602, 92 Stat. 2982. The 1978 amendments expounded the scope of the 1973 protections to cover not only federally assisted activities but also federally conducted activities (such as the postal services or Public Health Service hospitals).

[4] 42 USC §1396, et seq., providing grants to states for the purpose of providing medical assistance payments on behalf of certain individuals.

[5] 42 USC §401, et seq., providing grants to states for the purpose of providing cash assistance to families with dependent children.

[6] 42 USC §300a, providing direct grants for the provision of voluntary family planning services, especially to low-income persons.

[7] At the same time Congress enacted §504, it also enacted §503, which prohibits discrimination against the handicapped under federal contract programs. Originally the Department of Labor was given jurisdiction to enforce §503, and the Department of Health, Education and Welfare was given coordination responsibility for §504. Since 1981, however, §504 coordination responsibilities have rested with the Department of Justice.

[8] The Department of Health, Education and Welfare (HEW) was the first agency to publish rules for federally assisted programs, in May 1977. The HEW rule was adopted for use by other federal agencies in 1978. In 1981 the Department of Justice, which in 1980 had been given responsibility for reviewing and approving all §504 rules, reissued the original model regulation for federally assisted programs. No substantive changes were made. In 1983 the Department of Justice issued to other federal agencies (but did not formally publish) a prototype regulation rule for implementation of §504 as it applies to federally conducted programs. No agency has yet issued final rules covering federally conducted programs within its jurisdiction.

[9]Prior to 1980 educational programs such as the Education for all Handicapped Children Act (PL 94-142) were administered by the Department (at that time known as the Department of Health, Education and Welfare). After the Department of Education was created, jurisdiction over the act, as well as other federally assisted educational programs, was placed in the new Department.

[10]A different question is whether a Title V program can extend coverage only to children suffering from specific types of crippling conditions, thereby discriminating *among* the handicapped on the basis of their particular condition. Under federal law, it is not illegal to exclude non-handicapped persons from the benefits of a program limited by federal statute or executive order to handicapped persons, nor is it illegal to exclude a specific class of handicapped persons from a program limited by federal statute or executive order to a different class of handicapped persons. An example of such a permissible excluding entity would be the federally financed Galaudet College for the Deaf in Washington, DC [45 CFR §84.4(c)]. However, the Maternal and Child Health Block Grant Act (42 CFR §701 et seq.), unlike its predecessor, the Title V Maternal and Child Health and Crippled Children's program, contains no definition of "crippled child." Prior to 1981 the old law defined a crippled child as "an individual under the age of 21 who has an organic disease, defect or condition which may hinder the achievement of normal growth and development" [42 CFR §714 (1980)]. In 1981, as part of the Omnibus Budget and Reconciliation Act, Congress eliminated this definition from the statute entirely and, in addition, amended the law expressly to apply §504 (as well as other federal civil rights laws) to the program [42 CFR §708 (1982)]. These two Congressional actions, taken together, indicate Congress's intent to eliminate the exception afforded to crippled children's agencies under 45 CFR §84.4(c) and to require those agencies to serve handicapped children without regard to the basis of their handicap.

REFERENCES

Smith, M. (1983). *Section 504 of the Rehabilitation Act: Statutory provisions, legislative history, and status of regulations.* Congressional Research Service, Report No. 83-207 EPW. Washington, DC: US Government Printing Office.

U.S. Commission on Civil Rights. (1983). *Accommodating the spectrum of individual abilities.* Washington, DC.: U.S. Government Printing Office.

U.S. Congress. (1974). Senate Report 93-1270, 93rd Congress, 2d session: Washington, DC: U.S. Government Printing Office.

Part III

SERVICES IN THE CARE OF HANDICAPPED CHILDREN AND YOUTH

Chapter 8

EARLY IDENTIFICATION

Kathryn E. Barnard
Diane L. Magyary

Early identification of children with handicapping conditions is a long-sought-after ideal. Reaching this goal demands defining conditions that are handicapping. Two diametrically opposed concepts need to be considered: first, the concept of risk, and second, the concept of optimality.

It is common to speak of children being at risk, generally meaning a child has biological or environmental conditions that could result in physical, mental or emotional problems. On the other hand, the use of optimality was suggested first by Prechtl (1967) as a solution to the failure of previous attempts to define risk. Prechtl developed an optimality scoring for pregnancy, labor, and delivery. This list contained 41 conditions, all of which needed to be present for an optimal pregnancy and infant outcome. Prechtl's idea was not a reversal of complications but rather the most favorable conditions. It followed that optimal pregnancies, with all factors present, had no or very few complications (Prechtl, 1980, 1983).

RISK FACTORS

The majority of early identification schemas are currently based on risk factors (Stangler, Haber, & Routh, 1980; Brazelton & Lester, 1983; Barnard & Douglas, 1974; Frankenburg, 1983). In the neonatal period "established risk" refers to conditions such as Down syndrome, hydrocephaly, spina bifida, congenital anomalies, and central nervous system dysfunction. Most handicapping conditions related to established risk are identified at birth or within the first three months. The newborn examination, as well as historical family and pregnancy information, are used to make these diagnoses. Since at least 97 percent of all U.S. births take place in hospitals, the surveillance for such risk conditions is excellent. In addition, testing for metabolic conditions such as phenylketonuria takes place during this early period. In all instances whatever treatment is appropriate is offered. This includes surgical or medical treatment and supportive guidance for the parents and family.

Furthermore, it is now an accepted part of medical practice to do prenatal diagnosis for detecting severe fetal anomalies in the middle trimester (Barry, Walker, & Dumars, 1985). Thee to five percent of all infants are born with significant birth defects or genetic disorders, only a few of which are detectable prenatally. It is advisable for couples to consider prenatal diagnosis when the mother is thirty-five or older, the father is fifty-five or older, and/or there is a family history of chromosome rearrangement, congenital malformation, autosomal dominant or recessive disorders, X-linked conditions, exposure to teratogenic agents, previous infertility, or study results that suggest fetal abnormality.

"Biological risk" refers to those conditions that propose a possible insult to the central nervous system. These include prematurity, low birth weight, abnormal motor tone, delay in achieving gross or fine motor milestones, abnormal neurological signs, and early feeding difficulties. It is especially for this group of infants that good tracking systems are important. Most authorities agree it is impossible to predict the outcome of infants with biological risk factors from any simple screening procedure or development task. It is through careful observation and testing over time that a pattern establishes normal, as opposed to abnormal, function. In a follow-up study of preterm infants (Magyary, Barnard, & Hammond, 1983) we found most motor abnormalities were diagnosed during the first year, whereas disorders of mental performance and communication were not clearly established until the later preschool years.

The final risk category is environmental risk. This refers to the potential for delayed development because of limiting early environmental experiences such as problematic family situations; parenting alterations due to low education, income, or age; developmental disability of the parents; parental substance abuse; or history of child abuse and neglect. It is estimated that 75 percent of all cases of mental retardation are of cultural-familial type in which the IQs range from 50 to 75 (Frankenburg, 1983). Research indicates that a limiting environment is one in which infants and young children have little positive interaction with their parents or others, where there is limited contingent responsiveness and few instances of adult-mediated play with or without objects. Because the infant's emerging attention and activity are not responded to, the infant rapidly extinguishes the tendency to explore. A cycle of failure begins where the early parenting deficit promotes an infant who either withdraws or becomes ineffectively overactive.

The identification of children at environmental risk is not adequate. This population has typically been followed through programs of public health nursing home visits, well-child clinics, and WIC (special supplemental food program for women, infants and children) when resources are available. The activities of Head Start, Child Find, and the like reach only about 10 to 15 percent of children who fall in this category. Furthermore, the parents may not be receptive to professional surveillance; and these children and their families get lost until risk becomes dysfunction. More adequately financed programs of maternal and child health could remedy the situation.

Many contempory research studies demonstrate that the cycle of failure can be broken (Barnard, Booth, Mitchell, & Telzrow, 1983, 1986; Bromwich, 1977; Olds, 1982) Parents can be taught and motivated to provide an optimal environment. Infants can be handled in a way that maximizes their alertness and responsiveness. We have developed a profile of optimality that we use to guide both early identification and intervention with these environmentally at-risk infants and families. Table 8-1 outlines the parent, family and infant characteristics we assess and use to guide intervention. The bottom line is that infants can't wait. More health care and educational programming is needed for environmentally at-risk families to improve parenting and likewise to supplement infant experiences with positive interaction and stimulation. Infants in mutiproblem families do not escape the environmental risk of their families without optimal conditions of positive, contingent interaction and stimulation (Barnard, Booth, Mitchell, & Telzrow, 1986).

SOCIETAL TRENDS: STRUCTURE, TIMING AND METHOD OF EARLY IDENTIFICATION

Within the past decade, more formal recognition has been given to society's responsibility to facilitate the earlier than usual diagnosis and treatment of handicapped children. There is a shift from depending on exams at school entry to continuous monitoring from birth. Historically, two federally mandated projects have contributed to the advancement of early health and developmental identification programs. First, the Early and Periodic Screening, Diagnosis and Treatment Program under Medicaid (EPSDT) provided federal monies for the development of statewide case-finding programs aimed at early recognition and treatment of illness and handicapping conditions. Second, with the passage of the federal Education for All Handicapped Children Act (Public Law 94-142), states were required to identify, locate, and evaluate yearly all handicapped children; This was commonly referred to as the Child Find System. In addition, all handicapped children three to twenty-one years old are guaranteed a free, appropriate public education at no cost to their parents.

To date, the development, implementation, and effectiveness of these

Table 8-1. Optimal Parent-Infant Profile[a]

	Prenatal	Newborn	1 Month	4 Months	8 Months	12 Months
Mother's psychosocial assets	Is pleased about pregnancy	←--------------------------- Is satisfied with marriage ---------------------------→				
	Has someone to share concerns with	←-------------------- Has positive feelings about motherhood --------------------→				
	Has enough physical & emotional help	←--------------- Is satisfied with father's involvement in child care ---------------→				
	Planned the pregnancy	←---------------- Has positive experiences with motherhood ----------------→				
	Little disruption in plans	←----------------------- Has adequate help in home -----------------------→				
Father involvement	Pleased about pregnancy	←------------------------------- Living with family -------------------------------→				
	Gives physical & emotional help	←------------------- Moderate or high participation in child care -------------------→				
	Shares mother's concerns			←--------------- Participates in teaching child ---------------→		
		←---------------- Is concerned about child's welfare and development ----------------→				
Life change		←------------------------------------ Low ------------------------------------→				

[a]The timing for specific entries is determined by the age of most importance and by the age at which the dimension was measured in tl.is study.

AP, antepartum; PP, postpartum.

Previously published in *Nursing Child Assessment II*, June 1979, publication No. HRA-7925.

Parents' developmental expectations	Realistic about when infant sees, hears, is aware, etc. AP classes	← Recognize increasing social responsiveness →	← Expect increasing child mobility, curiosity, and independence →
Mother's health	No perinatal complications. Recommended AP & PP care	← Few health problems →	
Infant's health	No perinatal complications	← Normal growth pattern → ← Minimal illness → ← Few accidents, nine serious → ← Recommended well-child care →	
Infant behavior	Alert for good interaction Smooth, coordinated motor behavior Habituates to repetitive stimuli Cuddly Consolable	Responds with looking, movement or makes sounds Attends to mother's presence, especially voice Socially modulated behavior	Initiates behavioral interactions more frequently More verbal Increased mobility such as crawling More exploratory behavior Uses movement, looking, listening for a purpose

← Moderate motor activity →
← Low irritability, predominantly good mood →
← Attends to specific stimuli →

Table 8-1. Optimal Parent-Infant Profile[a] (continued)

	Prenatal	Newborn	1 Month	4 Months	8 Months	12 Months
Infant sleep–activity patterns			Sleeps about 14 hours per day	Decreased crying	Begins to have night awakenings again, but frequency not problematic to parents ←-----	
			Has at least 4 feedings per day			
				Regularity of night sleep ←-------------------------→		
				Infant can adapt to changes in his daily routine ←---------------------→		
Mother–infant interaction				Mother is comfortable during interaction ←------------------------→		
				Mother facilitates learning ←---------------------→		
				Mother encourages exploration of toys and objects ←-----------------→		
				Mother provides positive feedback ←---------------→		
				Mother does not use forcing controlling techniques ←----------------→		
			Infant demonstrates readiness to learn and involvement ←-------------------------→			
			Mutuality and adaptation of mother and infant behaviors in routine caretaking activities such as feeding ←------------------------------------→			
				Infant becomes more adaptive ←----------------→		

Stimulation in the home environment

(not measured) ←----→ High emotional & verbal responsivity to child

" ←----→ Low restriction & punishment

" ←----→ Temporal environment organized

" ←----→ Appropriate play materials provided

" ←----→ High maternal involvement with child

early-identification programs have varied widely from state to state. Continued interdisciplinary input is needed to further develop, refine, and evaluate cost-effective quality programs. These programs must be designed to reflect the greater recognition given to three principles of development. First, children's health and development status needs to be defined from a holistic perspective that involves different but equally important and interrelated physiological as well as psychological-social components. Second, children reciprocally interact with their environment, each influencing and producing changes in the other. The degree of directional influence varies depending on the child's status and environmental factors. Third, the health and development of children within an environmental context are dynamic and thus subject to fluctuation and change over time. In consideration of these three principles, accurate and early identification will evolve only from tracking systems characterized to be comprehensive in their focus, continuous in their reevaluations, and accessible to all children. Only then will early identification be implemented at an opportune time to improve outcomes.

An early-identification program based on a *comprehensive* focus includes appraisal of the child's physical and developmental health status as well as the child's environmental context. Monitoring of defined health and environmental parameters varies depending on the child's age. Prior to school age, the protocol for physical appraisal should include a set of standardized procedures for evaluating physical health status such as history data base, growth measurements, physical examination, immunizations and tuberculin testing, dental screening, sensory vision and hearing screening, blood pressure measure at three years of age and thereafter, laboratory procedures and diagnostic tests as indicated. In addition, developmental appraisal includes standardized procedures to evaluate age-appropriate competencies in the domains of perceptual-neuromotor coordination, attention capacity, cognition, social-emotional status, speech, language, and self-help skills. Environmental appraisal should also be included in early identification programs; however, standarized formal procedures are less frequently used compared with physical and developmental appraisal procedures. Parental factors beyond the domains of parental age, educational level, and socioeconomic status need to be considered. Home environmental issues are also important. For example, screening for increased lead absorption may be appropriate for certain housing conditions and epidemiological evidence of lead poisoning. Safety environmental features also should be appraised.

Once the content focus of an early-identification program has been defined comprehensively, the schedule of visits for *continuous monitoring* needs to be established. The optimal number of reevaluation visits for all children prior to school entrance is impossible to establish and is subject to revision, depending on the latest research, the population being served, and each child's own health and environmental status. The latest *Standards of Child Health Care* (American Academy of Pediatrics, 1977) serve as a general guideline to be used by health professionals who provide preventative care and monitoring services to essentially well infants and children. The suggested frequency of health supervision visits during the infancy period includes a minimum of five visits during the first year and three visits during the second year. During the preschool period visits should be made at least three times: at about two years of age, three years of age, and again at five or six years of age.

It is important to note that the content and frequency of health appraisal visits may vary, depending on risk factors related to the child, family, and the broader environmental context. Identified factors may include the presence or possibility of perinatal disorders, congenital defects or familial disease; recurrent episodes of acute illnesses; chronic health problems; abnormal developmental patterns; parents with particular needs or with first-borns; and disadvantaged social or economic environment. Genetic screening may be advised for families and subpopulations with a high incidence of a particular genetic condition. Past experiences highlight the need to couple genetic screening programs with well-planned public educational programs and genetic counseling, especially when nonroutine genetic screening is being considered (Nora & Fraser, 1981).

Comprehensive and continuous monitoring becomes an especially important issue for high-risk populations. Magyary, Barnard and Hammond (1983) found that high-risk children were usually noted for concern because of complex health conditions involving two or more physical and/or developmental areas, as well as environmental issues. In addition, especially during the early years of infancy and toddlerhood, the patterns of development fluctuated across visits; thus, a single evaluation did not necessarily depict the child's health and development status. What was important were the patterns that emerged from continuous monitoring over time.

The economics of implementing a comprehensive and continuous monitoring system begs to be addressed if early-identification programs are to be *accessible to all children.* As a means to meet the criteria of a comprehensive and continuous developmental screening program that is cost-effective, Frankenburg (1983) has proposed a two-stage developmental screening process that varies depending on the population being served. The first-stage screening process is designed to err in terms of over-referrals rather than under-referrals. The procedures are very quick, simple, and economical and usually consist of a parent questionnaire or a prescreening test. If the first-stage screening results are nonsuspect, then future rescreening continues to occur at the first-stage level until findings become suspect. At that time, the second-stage screening procedures are implemented, which are usually longer, more complex, and costlier, as well as more valid in decreasing false positives and false negatives. Positive or suspect second-stage screening results need to be followed by in-depth diagnostic procedures.

Although standards have been suggested as guidelines for comprehensive and continuous evaluation of a child's physical and developmental health status, not all children receive care according to the standards. Reasons for this may vary from parents' lack of easy access to early-identification programs or health care systems to health professionals' not having the skills or taking the time to complete a careful, comprehensive child evaluation (Frankenburg, 1983; Kovar, 1981). The practice of not relying on formal and routine pediatric evaluations often results in children who start school at a less than optimal state of health and development. As Frankenburg (1983) indicated, the failure of health professionals to identify delayed children during the first few years of life has prompted other professionals (e.g., in school systems) to seek alternative methods of delivering accessible early-identification programs. Child Find programs are being implemented wherever access to children may occur, especially for children who are not seen on a regular basis within a defined health care system. Early-identification protocols are being implemented within day-care centers, preschools, hospital emergency rooms, and public health departments' immunization and WIC programs.

A growing concern expressed by professionals is that the development and implementation of early-identification programs may be fragmentally carried out by a variety of service systems. The coordination of services is essential and may require statewide and local planning to avoid duplication or omission of services. Community-based support through public education is another vital ingredient contributing to the success of early identification programs. The base of this support broadens as professionals educate parents and lay persons who work with children (e.g., day-care personnel) to assume some degree of responsibility in monitoring development and implementing specified first-stage screening procedures, e.g., questionnaires.

Finally, screening programs are useful only if they are coordinated with diagnostic and intervention programs. Given the dynamic nature of health and development, treatment needs to be implemented at the most effective time for optimizing a child's successful beginnings in school. Comprehensive, continuous, and accessible early-identification programs (birth to six years) provide the basis for promoting a preventive and optimal orientation toward health and development.

REFERENCES

American Academy of Pediatrics. (1977). *Standards of child health care* (3rd ed.). Evanston, IL: American Academy of Pediatrics.

Barnard, K. E., Booth, C. L., Mitchell, S. K., & Telzrow, R. (1983). *Newborn nursing models* (Final Report). Seattle, WA: University of Washington, Division of Nursing, Bureau of Health Resources Administration, Department of Health and Human Services, NCAST.

Barnard, K. E., Booth, C. L., Mitchell, S. K., & Telzrow, R. (1986). Newborn nursing models: A test of early intervention to high-risk infants and families. In E. D. Hibbs (Ed.), *Infancy in prevention.* New York: International Universities Press.

Barnard, K. E. & Douglas, H. B. (Eds.) (1974). *Child health assessment part 1: A literature review.* DHEW Pub. No. (HRA) 75-30, Stock no. 174-00082, Washington, DC: US Government Printing Office.

Barnard, K. E., Eyres, S. K., Lobo, M., & Snyder, C. (1983). An ecological paradigm for assessment and intervention. In T. B. Brazelton & B. M. Lester (Eds.), *New approaches to developmental screening of infants* (pp. 199–218). New York: Elsevier.

Barnard, K. E., Hammond, M. A., Mitchell, S. K., Booth, C. L., Spietz, A., Snyder, C., & Elsas, T. (1985). Caring for high-risk infants and their families. In M. Green (Ed.), *The psychosocial aspects of the family: The new pediatrics* (pp. 245–266) Lexington, MA: Lexington Books.

Barry, L. R., Walker, A. P., & Dumars, K. W. (1985). Prenatal diagnosis: The state of the art. In *Developmental handicaps: Prevention and treatment.* Silver Spring, MD: American Association of University Affiliated Programs for Persons with Developmental Disabilities.

Brazelton, T. B., & Lester, B. M. (1983). *Approaches to developmental screening of infants.* New York: Elsevier.

Bromwich, R. M. (1977). Stimulation in the first year of life? A perspective on infant development. *Young Children, 32*(2), 71–82.

Frankenburg, W. K. (1983). Developmental assessment: Infant and preschool developmental screening. In M. D. Levine, W. B. Carey, A. C. Crocker, & R. T. Gross (Eds.), *Developmental behavioral pediatrics* (pp. 927–937). Philadelphia: W. B. Saunders Co.

Kovar, M. G. (1981). *Better health for our children: A national strategy.* The report of the select panel for the promotion of child health (Vol. III, statistical profile, DHHS #79-55071). Washington, DC: U. S. Department of Health and Human Services, Public Health Service.

Magyary, D. L., Barnard, K. E., & Hammond, M. A. (1983). *Premature infant refocus follow-up, maternal and child health special project* (Final Report). Washington, DC: Department of Health and Human Services, Public Health Service.

Nora, J. J., & Fraser, F. C. (1981). *Medical genetics: Principles and practice.* Philadelphia: Lea & Febiger.

Olds, D. L. (1982). The prenatal early infancy project: An ecological approach to prevention of developmental disabilities. In J. Belsky (Ed.), *In the beginning: Readings on infancy.* New York: Columbia University Press.

Prechtl, H. F. R. (1967). Neurological sequelae of prenatal and perinatal complications. *British Medical Journal, 4,* 763–767.

Prechtl, H. F. R. (1980). The optimality concept. *Early Human Development, 4,* 201–205.

Prechtl, H. F. R. (1983). Risk factors and the significance of early neurological assessment. In T. B. Brazelton & B. M. Lester (Eds.), *New approaches to developmental screening in infants* (pp. 125–135). New York: Elsevier.

Stangler, S. R., Haber, C. J., & Routh, D. K. (1980). *Screening growth and development of preschool children: A guide for test selection.* New York: McGraw-Hill.

Chapter 9

SCREENING FOR DEVELOPMENTAL DISABILITIES[1]

Kenneth W. Dumars
Deborah Duran-Flores
Carol Foster
Stanley Stills

Developmental disabilities (DD) are estimated to produce severe impairments in just over 1 percent of the population (State Council on Developmental Disabilites, 1982). Many studies have shown improved outcomes for children with or at risk for DD who are identified and provided treatment at very early stages (Weikart, 1984). Since pediatricians and family practitioners are among the few professionals who, as a group, see almost all infants and young children, they play a major role in the early identification of children with DD by the use of screening.

Purpose of Screening for DD

Screening is the application of a simple accurate method for determining which children in the population are likely to be in need of special services in order to develop optimally. Screening procedures should not be viewed as diagnostic; they simply divide the population into those who need diagnostic work and those who are not at risk for the condition. Diagnosis determines the extent and, in some cases, the cause of the disorder. (Cross & Goin, 1977).

[1] A longer version of this chapter appears in the *Western Journal of Medicine*, 1985, *143*, 349–356.

CHARACTERISTICS OF SCREENING PROGRAMS

Screening procedures should be

1. Less costly in time, materials and other resources than the diagnostic procedures.
2. Simple. Screening tests adequate for detection should be inexpensive, easily replicated, and capable of being conducted by a health, educational, or psychological assistant. An extremely difficult or painful procedure cannot be justified for every child when only 1 out of 10,000 may have the condition.
3. Comprehensive. For instance, a screening program for DD also should screen for biomedical conditions such as sickle-cell disease, psychological problems such as attention deficit disorder, and sociocultural problems such as child abuse.
4. Effective in prevention or amelioration of DD. Screening is appropriate whenever age of onset and duration of process aggravate or worsen the outcome. The screening test should be accompanied by a minimum of false positives and false negatives. False negatives (failing to refer individuals who do have the condition) should be avoided for conditions that are potentially devastating, such as those identified in biochemical newborn screening.
5. Cost-effective. Relatively costly procedures for extremely rare disorders need to be considered carefully. The cost of lead screening on the East Coast (see Table 9-1) has been considered a worthwhile investment because of the incidence of lead poisoning there. It is unclear if this is an appropriate activity in many western states because young children's access to lead is extremely limited.

Screening tests imply surveillance of a large at-risk population together with availability of accurate diagnostic capabilities accompanied by effective intervention modalities or strategies. There are situations where screening occurs best within a limited population. For example, Tay–Sach's and sickle-cell diseases occur in fairly circumscribed groups. A crucial decision is when the screening program should be applied. For example, screening for phenylketonuria (PKU), galactosemia, and hypothyroidism during the newborn period identifies those at risk during the early period, when treatment is most effective, rather than, for example, screening at the preschool ages. Referrals for further testing and intervention can follow. On the other hand, screening for Huntington's disease—using the latest technology, which will soon be available—during the newborn or early years is inappropriate, for

Table 9-1. Regional Percentages of Children Screened for Lead Poisoning who Required Pediatric Management, October 1, 1980 through September 30, 1981

Region	Total Screenings	Total Requiring Pediatric Management	Percentage
I (CT, MA, RI—6 programs)	51,282	1,622	3.16
II (NJ, NY—14 programs)	171,728	8,786	5.11
III (DE, MD, PA, VA, Washington, DC—12	84,195	3,722	4.42
programs	47,631	614	1.28
IV (GA, KY, SC, TN—4 programs)	108,430	5,087	4.69
V (IL, IN, MI, OH, WI—15 programs)	48,944	571	1.16
VI (AR, LA, TX—4 programs)	19,487	1,481	7.62
VII (IO, MO, NE—5 programs)	4,033	9	0.22
IX (CA—2 programs)			

we have nothing to offer those who may be identified as carriers and thus ultimately affected.

Screening for development must be a collaborative venture between those testing the child and the child's guardian, usually his parent. A child who generally functions within normal limits may score in the questionable range for reasons of ill health, emotional stress, culture, or language barriers.

RECOMMENDATIONS FOR THE PHYSICIAN'S ROLE IN SCREENING

The physician who has regular contact with the family has an especially important role in screening for and preventing the occurrence of a developmentally disabling condition. The physician's role at three stages—preconceptual, prenatal, and postnatal—will be described.

Preconceptual

The health of a newborn is to some extent related to the state of the mother's health. Certain safeguards for the newborn infant can be undertaken by the mother. Optimally, the mother should be in good health prior to and during her pregnancy. Table 9-2 lists the situations that increase a mother's risk for complications, including the birth of a handicapped infant.

Certain disorders, such as hyperextension, diabetes, and heart or renal disease, increase the risk for complications. Optimally, prior to pregnancy all mothers should receive the rubella vaccine and/or have serologic evidence of rubella immunity. The presence of genetic disorders and maternal age influence the risks of delivering a handicapped infant. It is useful to know the

Table 9-2: High-Risk Obstetrical Patients

Socioeconomic
　Age less than 18 or greater than 34
　Parity 0 or greater than 4
　Marital status unwed
　Under 125% of poverty level
　Educational status less than 12 years
　Poor conditions for home delivery
Nutritional
　Weight falling outside of standard weight range
　Hb less than 10 g
Past pregnancy performance
　Difficult labor, prolonged labor (over 24 hours)
　Previous cesarean section
　History of postpartum hemorrhage
Past pregnancy outcome
　Fetal death (infant greater than 500 g; 1 lb, 2 oz)
　Neonatal death (infant greater than 500 g; 1 lb, 2 oz)
　Major congenital anomaly (incompatible with extrauterine life)
　Low birth weight (less than 5½ lb)
　Three consecutive abortions (less than 500 g)
　Damaged infant (especially neurological defects)
Medical or obstetric complication, present pregnancy, including but not limited
　to
　Preeclampsia—eclampsia
　HVD
　Diabetes
　Heart disease
　Rh sensitization
　Sickle-cell anemia
　Hemoglobinopathies
　Renal disease
　Mental retardation as evidenced by one of the following:
　　Previous enrollment in a special education class
　　Evaluation by Vocational Rehabilitation
　　Evaluation by Department of Mental Retardation
　　Evaluation by a licensed or state certified psychologist
　　Substantial evidence of inability to manage daily self-care
　Mental illness as evidenced by one of the following:
　　Diagnosis from psychiatrist
　　Evaluation by mental health center
　　Evaluation by psychiatric hospital

blood and Rh type of the mother; if the mother is blood type O and/or Rh-negative, the father should be tested. In selected populations it is advisable for couples to have reproductive testing for sickle-cell disease (in Black populations), thalassemia (Asian and Mediterranean population groups), and Tay–Sachs disease (in Jewish populations).

Prenatal

Wilson (1977) has listed genetic and environmental causes of developmental defects, as shown in Table 9-3. A note of caution regarding the

**Table 9-3: Causes of Developmental Defects in Humans—
Estimates Based on Surveys and Case Reports in the Medical Literature**

Known genetic transmission		20%
Chromosomal aberration		3–5%
Environmental causes		
Ionizing radiations,		<1%
therapeutic	Nuclear	
Infections		2–3%
Rubella virus	Varicella virus	
Cytomegalovirus	Toxoplasma	
Herpesvirus hominis	Syphilis	
Maternal metabolic imbalance		1–2%
Endemic cretinism	Phenylketonuria	
Diabetes	Virilizing tumors	
Drugs and environmental chemicals		4–5%
Androgenic hormone	Anticonvulsants	
Folic antagonists	Oral hypoglycemics (?)	
Thalidomide	Few neurotropic/anorectics(?)	
Oral anticoagulants	Organic mercury	
Maternal alcoholism		
Combinations and interactions		?
Unknown		65–75%

Source: Wilson, 1977.

interpretation of this table is necessary, however. A developmental defect differs from a developmental disability. For example, cleft lip/cleft palate is a developmental defect but frequently occurs without associated developmental disability.

As part of preconceptional or prenatal care, one should obtain a brief pedigree, inquiring specifically about fetal loss, malformation, mental retardation, short stature, myopathies and neuropathies, and common disorders such as cystic fibrosis, Huntington's disease, and other late-onset disorders. Based on this information and/or parental age, families with the following characteristics must be notified about the availability of prenatal diagnosis for genetic disorders:

1. The mother will be thirty-five or older or the father will be fifty-five or older at the time of the child's birth.

2. Either parent has had a previous child with Down syndrome or another chromosomal abnormality.

3. There is a history of a relative with a proved potentially heritable chromosomal anomaly or mental retardation.

4. The couple has had a history of two or more miscarriages or infertility.

5. Either parent carries a balanced chromosome rearrangement (inversion or translocation).

6. There is a history of congenital malformation in either parent or in a previous child.

7. There is a family history of neural tube defect (i.e., spina bifida or anencephaly).[2]

8. Both members of the couple are carriers for an autosomal recessive disorder (e.g., Tay–Sachs disease, sickle-cell disease, thalassemia, or PKU).

9. The mother is a known or possible carrier for an X-linked condition, e.g., Duchenne's muscular dystrophy, hemophilia A, or X-linked mental retardation.

10. Either parent is affected with or has been shown to carry the gene for an autosomal dominant condition, e.g., achondroplasia, Marfan's syndrome, tuberous sclerosis, neurofibromatosis.

11. The mother is an insulin-dependent diabetic, requires medication for epilepsy, or has a history of other potential teratogenic exposure (e.g., rubella, X-ray, or certain drug use during pregnancy).

12. The parents are consanguineous (blood-related).

13. There is reason to suspect fetal abnormality on the basis of other studies (ultrasound, maternal serum alpha-fetoprotein, Rh titer).

The environmental risks listed in Table 9-3 are self-evident. These authors cannot emphasize enough the importance of maintaining adequate medical records, especially those related to environmental mechanisms. In light of our present knowledge, environmental agents are responsible for but a small segment of developmental defects and an even smaller segment of DD. However, the practitioner must be cautious in prescribing drugs during pregnancy. For a litigious American public, lack of absolute proof that an agent causes a defect is not an adequate safeguard when a physician is faced with a lawsuit in front of a lay jury. We need only cite the enormous settlements awarded to patients and families who have a history of Bendectin use during pregnancy or paternal exposure to Agent Orange. These pending settlements occurred despite the fact that neither of these two agents are clearly identified as being embryotoxic. Nonetheless, clear record keeping is

[2] On April 7, 1986 California instituted a statewide screening program for neural tube defects utilizing maternal serum alphafetoprotein (AFP). This will be voluntary and will be carried out at 15–16 weeks gestation. The blood sample will be drawn in private offices and clinics and then forwarded to central laboratories. This will identify, in the tested mothers, 80 percent of the conceptuses affected with neural tube defects. The other 20 percent will not be detected as the sac on the back is covered with normal skin and will not t allow the escape of AFP containing cerebrospinal fluid from the fetus reaching the amniotic fluid and ultimately the maternal serum.

essential in documenting the need for any drug, along with adequate information given to patients.

Maternal substance abuse, particularly alcohol, is a significant contributing agent to the occurrence of developmental disabilities in offspring. It is estimated that fetal alcohol syndrome (FAS) is the third most common cause of DD, with a frequency of 1:1,000 to 1:2,000 of live born infants (Smith, Jones, & Hanson, 1976), just a bit less than the incidence of Down syndrome.

Though recreational and street drugs have not been demonstrated to be embryotoxic, the addicting drugs, such as heroin, methadone, and the like, certainly produce addiction in the newborn and endanger the infant's survival. Cigarette smoking probably does not cause DD. Infants born to mothers who smoke, however, are often of low birth weight, with its attendant risks.

Postnatal

The physician is the most likely professional to detect early developmental problems. Table 9-4 presents recommendations for specific screening tests and their timing from birth through adolescence. Tables 9-5 and 9-6 provide further information on factors to include screening. The physician, or assistant, should be familiar with these procedures, schedule them on routine visits, and monitor each child's development longitudinally.

If the results from any of these procedures indicate a questionable status, the physician should either apply the appropriate diagnostic procedures or refer to the appropriate agency. The decision for referral is dependent on the state and how services are provided. In general, the physician should have colleagues in physical therapy, occupational therapy, social work, nutrition, dentistry, ophthalmology, audiology, speech and language, education, and psychology who can cooperate in diagnosis and the development of intervention strategies.

Another important role the physician provides is communication with the family. By treating screening as part of routine pediatric care, the physician will be communicating with the family on the child's development and will be orienting them toward prevention efforts. As the child grows, parents and physician will discuss motor development, the child's response to parents, and use of language. Parents are excellent observers of their children (Blacher-Dixon & Simeonsson, 1981), and discussion with them can augment the physician's perception of the child. In addition, discussions on development will make the need for further testing more understandable in those infrequent instances when it is necessary.

A related responsibility of the physician is preparing parents for the diagnostic testing and possible intervention. Parents should be informed of what to expect, how long it will take, if pain is involved, what information will be obtained, and so on. A few minutes of discussion on a procedure such as the

Table 9-4

	Age of Person Being Screened														
Screening Procedure	Birth	1–2 Mos	3–4 Mos	5–6 Mos	7–9 Mos	10–12 Mos	13–17 Mos	18–23 Mos	2 Yrs	3 Yrs	4–5 Yrs	6–8 Yrs	9–12 Yrs	13–16 Yrs	17–20 Yrs
Interval until next exam	*1 mo*	*1 mo*	*2 mo*	*2 mo*	*3 mo*	*2 mo*	*5 mo*	*6 mo*	*1 yr*	*1 yr*	*2 yr*	*3 yr*	*4 yr*	*4 yr*	*none*
History & Physical Examination															
Developmental history and assessment															
Infant/child indicators of high-risk status	X														
Dubowitz & Dubowitz (1981) or comparable newborn evaluation	X														
Evaluation of motor development (Paine, 1960, Fig. 7)	X	X	X	X	X										
PDQ—DSST (Frankenburg et al., 1976, 1981)					X			X				X			
Dental assessment															
Nutritional assessment															
Health education	X	X	X	X	X	X	X	X	X	X	X	X	X	X	X
Vision screening															
Snellen/Equivalent Visual Acuity Test									X[2]	X	X	X	X	X	X
Clinical observation	X	X	X	X	X	X	X	X	X	X	X	X	X	X	X
Hearing Screening															
Audiometric										X	X	X	X	X	X
Nonaudiometric		X	X	X	X	X	X	X	X	X					
Laboratory Tests															
Hematocrit or hemoglobin					X						X		X	X	X

Screening Procedure	Birth	1-2 Mos	3-4 Mos	5-6 Mos	7-9 Mos	10-12 Mos	13-17 Mos	18-23 Mos	2 Yrs	3 Yrs	4-5 Yrs	6-8 Yrs	9-12 Yrs	13-16 Yrs	17-20 Yrs
Interval until next exam	1 mo	2 mo	2 mo	3 mo	2 mo	5 mo	6 mo	1 yr	1 yr	2 yr	3 yr	4 yr	4 yr	none	
Urine dipstick or urinalysis											X	X	X	X	X
Newborn screening	X														
Free erythrocyte protoporphyrin (FEP)					May be done only if health history warrants.										

Source: Screening schedule originally from California Child Health Disability Prevention Program and modified by the authors.

**Table 9-5. Post-natal variables Related to an Infant
Being at Risk for Developmental Disabilities**

Medical factors
    Prematurity (less than or equal to 32 wks)
    Postmaturity (greater than or equal to 44 wks)
    Low birth weight (less than or equal to 1,500 g)
    Small for gestational age (Lubchenco Scale)
    Assisted ventilation with persistent respiratory instability (including recurrent apnea)
    Prolonged hypoxemia
    Prolonged hypoglycemia, hypocalcemia
    Hyperbilirubinemia (greater than or equal to 15 mg)
    Seizures or transient neurological signs (+ or −) in first 5 days of life
    CNS bleeds (grades 2–4)
    Confirmed correlating infections of the CNS (meningitis, encephalitis, etc.)
    Multiple congenital anomalies requiring specialized services
    History of maternal chemical exposure (alcohol, hydantoin, warfarin)
    Abnormal neurological exam in premature infant:
        Not significant if:
            Atypical tone
            Asymmetry
            Startles and/or tremors
        but *Yes,* significant if combined with
            Lack or inconsistent visual pursuit
            Decreased popliteal angle
            Decreased mobility
Clinical/behavioral factors
    Persistent feeding problems (mechanical)
    Persistent inability to self-calm
    Erratic sleep–wake patterns
    Persistent tonal problems
    Continued evidence of delay in one or more developmental areas
Social/environmental factors
    Poor maternal–infant attachment
    Prior family history of abuse/neglect (parents, other siblings)
    Neonatal addiction or maternal history of substance abuse
    Mother's medical or mental condition of a nature to require professional supervision and support to assure necessary child care (e.g., severe CP, mental retardation, depression, alcohol, etc.)
    Maternal age is less than or equal to 16[a]
    Lack of or inadequate use of support systems (e.g., church, parents, etc.)[a]
    Opinion of an interdisciplinary team, such as hospital discharge planning team, that the infant is at high risk of becoming developmentally disabled

[a]May not be used as a single criterion.
Source: Office of Maternal and Child Health, 1982.

auditory evoked potential can greatly reduce apprehension and promote the physician's rapport with the family.

School

    The physician's involvement with the educational system is important because of the federally mandated screening program. The federal mandate

Table 9-6. Normal Ages of Appearance and Disappearance of Neurologic Signs Peculiar to Infancy

Response	Age at Which Normally Appears	Age at Which Normally No Longer Obtainable
Spontaneous stepping	Birth	2–6 weeks
Positive supporting (neonatal type)	Birth	3–6 weeks
Crossed extension (allongement croisée)	Birth	1–2 months
Trunk incurvation	Birth	1–2 months
Moro's reflex	Birth	1–3 months
Redressement du tronc	Birth	Variable
Leg flexion in vertical suspension	Birth	4 months
Rooting	Birth	3–4 months awake, 7 months asleep
Palmar grasp	Birth	6 months
Adductor spread of knee jerk	Birth	7 months
Plantar grasp	Birth	9–10 months
Tonic neck patterns (imposable)	2 months	5 months
Landau's reflex	3 months	12–24 months
Neck righting reflex (imposable)	4–6 months	12–24 months
Positive supporting (weight bearing)	6 months	(persists)
Parachute reaction	8–9 months	Variable

relating to pediatric screening is labeled EPSDT (early and periodic screening, diagnosis, and treatment). It is designed as an ongoing federally funded source of medical checkups and care for all persons, birth to twenty-one years of age, enrolled in a state Medicaid program.

The EPSDT screening model promotes an interest in identifying recognizable pediatric disorders that interfere with health and development. The screening periodicity chart (see Table 9-4) indicates the schedule for obtaining relevant screening information at each of the age levels from birth to twenty-one years. Developmental data can be gotten through simple techniques and communication skills.

The Denver Developmental Screening (DDST-R) (Frankenberg, van Doornick, & Liddell, 1976; 1981) is the standard tool used by pediatric nurse practitioners and physicians to assess development in children ages birth through six years. Beyond six years of age, medical tests, clinical observations, home–school psychosocial adaptation, and knowledgeable judgment are the health professional's tools of developmental assessment. The newly revised DDST-R is less time-consuming than earlier versions. Specifically, 12 items or less are all that are necessary to obtain a result on children up to six years old. Even more simply, a prescreening developmental questionnaire (Frankenberg et al., 1976) can be given to parents to complete in a few minutes.

Most of the children identified after age six are referred by teachers, parents, nurses, and classroom aides, relatively few from physicians at present. A typical "child study team" might be the first level of response to a referral. Following a carefully delineated set of procedures, an interdisciplinary team will review a child's level of performance and determine potential eligibility for special education services and, if appropriate, also develop an individual education plan (IEP). Physicians may be asked to participate in these decisions.

The physician can request an assessment of the child's performance and eligibility for "special services" by contacting a county office of education, local school district office, or school principal. The physician should look with sensitivity and scrutiny at a child's developmental history and current status and should engage the child *and* the parents in obtaining information in order to document physical and behavioral elements of each young patient. A team approach can guard against such problems and ensure that providers, parents, and children are given the opportunity for each child to maximize developmental potential.

MEASURES OF EFFECTIVENESS

The evaluation of any major social program such as screening for DD represents a complex but important issue.

One measure of effectiveness can be found in ascertaining the cost of various conditions to the state or to the family. All states except two have mandatory screening for phenylketonuria PKU, which affects approximately 1 in 17,000 births. In California, about 20 to 25 cases are detected each year (Cunningham, 1983). Since 1966, when the program began, there has not been a single admission to the state hospital system. There is a direct relationship between the length of time that a child is untreated and the decrease in intellectual functioning (Berry, O'Grady, & Perlmutter, 1979; Williamson, Koch, & Azen, 1981). The conservative cost–benefit analysis shows that approximately $7.00 is saved for every dollar spent (Cunningham, 1983). Estimates of how much a child with DD costs above a child without this condition are available. For example, according to the California State Council on Developmental Disabilities (1982), it costs $360 per month to keep a child of three years at home. The cost varies with size of family, age of child, and gross income. If the child has a developmental disability and is placed out of the home, the cost can be as high as $6,000 per month (Department of Developmental Services, 1984).

The effects of screening and early intervention also have been documented through cost analyses. Children who receive two years of preschool saved more than seven times the cost of the preschool for their public education as compared to a matched control group (Weikart, 1980). Wood (1981) did an analysis of costs and found that the cost of education for 940 multiply handicapped children was dependent on the age at which intervention was started. The cost was $37,273 for children who began programs at birth, compared to $45,816 for those who started at age six.

The human impact is even more important than the financial aspects. The High/Scope Education Research Foundation has demonstrated that children in Head Start experience changes that are evident even after 12 years of public school. These children were more likely to finish high school, get a job, enroll in postsecondary education, and score well on tests of functional competence than their matched peers who had not attended Head Start (Weikart, 1980). They were less likely to require special education, be arrested, be on welfare, or become pregnant during teen years. Other studies have shown changes in intelligence (Kirk, 1958), ability to adapt to regular education (Horton, 1978), and ability to be self-supporting (Skeels, 1966; Skeels & Dye, 1939).

Another area where early intervention has proved to be quite effective is in the follow-up programs for high-risk infants from neonatal intensive care units (NICUs). In California, where these projects have been conducted on a pilot basis, it has been found that there are significant reductions in child abuse, in the length of the original hospitalization, and in the rate of rehospitalization (California Department of Developmental Services, 1984).

SUMMARY

The physician's continued contact with children presents an excellent opportunity to screen for a variety of developmental problems that may place the child at risk for DD or learning problems. The physician's referrals to and continuing contact with other professionals and the family can augment the continuity of care. Communication with the family and relevant agencies may prevent the occurrence of these developmental problems or at least may ameliorate their effect.

REFERENCES

Berry, H. K., O'Grady, D. J., & Perlmutter, L. J. (1979). Intellectual development and academic achievement of children treated early for phenylketonuria. *Developmental Medicine and Child Neurology, 21,* 311–320.

Blacher-Dixon, J., & Simeonsson, R. J. (1981). Consistency and correspondence of mothers' and teachers' assessments of young handicapped children. *Journal of Diseases of Early Childhood, 3,* 64–71.

California Department of Developmental Services. (1984). *Prevention—California's future. A plan for the prevention of developmental disabilities and birth defects.* Sacramento, CA: Author.

Centers For Disease Control. (March 12, 1982). *Monthly Morbidity and Mortality Weekly Report, 31,* 119.

Cross, L., & Goin, K. (Eds.). (1977). *Identifying handicapped children: A guide to casefinding, screening, diagnosis, assessment & evaluation.* New York: Walker.

Cunningham, G. C. (1983). *Genetic Disease Branch activities.* Sacramento, CA: California Department of Health Services, Genetic Disease Branch, Community Health Services Division.

Dubowitz, L., & Dubowitz, V. (1981). The neurological assessment of the preterm and fullterm newborn infant. In *Clinics in developmental medicine* (Vol. 1). London: William Heinemann.

Frankenberg, W. K., Van Doornick, W. D., & Liddell, T. N. (1976). The Denver pre-screening developmental questionnaire (PDQ). *Pediatrics, 57,* 744–753.

Frankenberg, W. K., van Doornick, W. D., & Liddell, T. N. (1981). The newly abbreviated and revised Denver Developmental Screening Test. *Journal of Pediatrics, 99,* 995–999.

Horton, K. B. (1978). Early intervention for hearing-impaired infants and young children. In T. D. Tjossem (Ed.), *Intervention strategies for high-risk infants and young children.* Baltimore: University Park Press.

Kirk, S. A. (1958). *Early education of the mentally retarded.* Urbana, IL: University of Illinois Press.

Office of Maternal and Child Health. (1982). *Report of the Association of Regional Center Agencies Prevention Task Force.* Sacramento, CA: Author.

Shorter, J. Executive Director, California State Council on Developmental Disabilities. August 1984. Personal communication.

Skeels, H. M. (1966). Adult status of children with contrasting early life experiences. *Monographs of the Society for Research in Child Development*, No. 3. Chicago: University of Chicago.

Skeels, H. M., & Dye, H. B. (1939). A study of differential stimulation on mentally retarded children. *Proceedings and Addresses AAMD, 44*(1), 114–136.

Smith, D. W., Jones, K. L., & Hanson, J. W. (1976). Perspectives on the cause and frequency of fetal alcohol syndrome. *Annals of the New York Academy of Sciences, 273,* 140–145.

State Council on Developmental Disabilities. (1982). *California developmental disabilities state plan 1984–1986: Part I. Foundation for services to Californians with developmental disabilities.* Sacramento, CA: Author.

Weikart, D. P. (December, 1980). *Effects of the Perry preschool program on youths through age 15.* Paper presented at the Conference of the Handicapped Children's Early Education Program, Washington, DC.

Weikart, D. P. (September 1984). Press release available from High Scope Educational Research Foundation, Ypsilanti, MI.

Williamson, M. L., Koch, R., & Azen, C. (1981). Correlates of intelligence test results in treated phenylketonuric children. *Pediatrics, 68,* 162–167.

Wilson, J. G. (1977). Embryotoxicity of drugs in man. In J. G. Wilson & F. C. Fraser (Eds.), *Handbook of teratology: General principles and etiology* (Vol. 1, pp. 309–355). New York: Plenum Press.

Wood, M. (1981). Cost of services. In J. Swanson & G. Woodruff (Eds.), *Early intervention for children with special needs and their families: Findings and recommendations.* Monmouth, OR: Western States Technical Assistance Resource (WESTAR).

Chapter 10

EVALUATION, DIAGNOSIS, TREATMENT, AND HABILITATION

Bruce K. Shapiro
Renee C. Wachtel
Frederick B. Palmer
Arnold J. Capute

Diagnosis, treatment, and habilitation are essential components in the care of handicapped children. Although arising from a medical model, these components are applicable to nonmedical disciplines as well. Evaluation necessitates the recognition of a problem, referral to an appropriate resource, and delineation of the degree of impairment and likely disability. Diagnosis represents the interpretation of the evaluative process. Treatment and habilitation aim to ameliorate the effects of the handicap and prevent secondary complications. Finally, it is important to recognize that even "static" handicaps change, and therefore optimal care requires periodical reassessment by repeating the process of evaluation and diagnosis with ongoing modification of treatment and habilitation.

EVALUATION

Recognition and Referral

The first phase of the evaluative process is the recognition of a problem. However, there are few data that assess the mechanisms by which children with handicaps are referred. Three broad mechanisms of identification can be delineated: (a) screening of asymptomatic populations, (b) developmental surveillance of "at risk" populations, and (c) parental concern.

126

Screening is based on the premise that most handicapped children do not come from "risk" populations. Screening is applied to "normal" populations, but because the prevalence of screened conditions is low, misclassification is a major limitation of screening efforts. Surveillance of the development of risk populations, e.g., very low birth weight infants, presumes that effective identification procedures exits; it is labor-intensive and has a low yield because most children do not develop the condition that they are at risk of having. Anecdotal impressions suggest that parents usually are the first to bring a problem to the attention of a professional. Of 738 children initially evaluated at the Kennedy Institute for a possible developmental disability, only 4 were referred because of failed screening tests (Lock, Shapiro, & Capute, 1985). This is further supported by studies showing the limited amount of time pediatricians spend in developmental surveillance (Resinger & Bires, 1980) and the types of disorders missed by well-child care (Haggerty, 1985).

In contrast to the low yield of screening, it is our experience that by the time a mother has decided that her child is suspect, she has usually obtained "backyard" or "over the fence" consultation (spouse, aunts, neighbors, grandparents), controlled for race, sex, socioeconomic status, and genetic effects (through comparison with neighborhood children, siblings, and cousins), and allowed for moderating influences (such as prematurity, transient delays that would be outgrown, and intercurrent illness). The mother (or any family member) who feels that a child is suspect should be heeded! Statistically significant correlations have been shown between parental estimate of function and mental age derived from standard IQ testing (Schulman & Stern, 1959).

Developmental failure is the prime reason for referral. The parent has recognized that the child is not meeting the expectations that are appropriate to his age. During the first six months of life, referral is primarily for physical stigmata, unresolved neonatal problems, or disturbances of autonomic function (breathing, sleeping, or feeding). Abnormalities in motor development are the focus of referral concerns during the next year (six to eighteen months of age). Disorders of spoken language are prominent reasons for referral during the preschool, whereas disorders of written language (reading) predominate during school years. Neurobehavioral disturbance (such as hyperactivity) is usually not delineated from normal infant behavior until three years of age and continues to be a major reason for referral both alone and in combination with other developmental concerns throughout childhood.

As would be expected, referral sources mirror the provision of services in the community. Infants are referred primarily from health care resources. School-age children come from schools and social agencies, whereas preschoolers are not in any clear service delivery system and therefore come from a variety of sources, including health, social services, and education (through Child Find or programs mandated by PL 94-142 to identify handicapped infants). Older schoolchildren begin to be referred from social and legal agencies in addition to schools.

Delineating the Problem

Once a problem has been identified, the task is to define the dysfunction. Although it is important to evaluate the presenting symptoms, the possibility of additional handicaps must be considered. Neurologic dysfunction in children is usually diffuse, and although not identified on referral, multiple areas of dysfunction are the rule (Capute & Palmer, 1980). For example, to evaluate an infant with motor delays and find mild spastic diplegia but overlook moderate mental retardation will result in incomplete treatment and habilitation because appropriate goals cannot be set.

In addition to the spectrum of neurological dysfunction and its additional, associated handicaps, there is a temporal continuum wherein mild delays that are non-handicapping prove to be markers of other neurologic dysfunctions (Capute, Shapiro, Palmer, 1981; Nelson & Ellenberg, 1982). The temporal continuum is a reflection of our limited abilities fully to assess certain areas of development at early ages and is based on the premise that the various aspects of development are related to each other. A typical pattern seen is the child who presents with delay in coming to sit (12 months), walks later than 15 months, is not talking in two-word sentences until 30 months, and is felt to be clumsy and "immature" (synonymous with significant lag) in nursery school coupled with difficulty in learning to read in first grade. If evaluated in temporal proximity to his walking (e.g., at 18 months), such a child may be deemed a "late bloomer," and people would be relieved that this child did not have cerebral palsy. By failing to realize that the motor delay was only part of a more generalized spectrum of developmental dysfunction, intervention would be delayed until the child demonstrated school failure.

Ultimately the results of an evaluation must enable one to answer six questions:

1. What is the diagnosis? (What is the nature and degree of this handicap?)
2. Are there additional handicaps?
3. What are the current needs?
4. What are the long-term goals?
5. What treatments are currently appropriate?
6. Is there a likelihood that later children will be affected?

In order to answer these questions satisfactorily, an evaluation of the child's abilities is indicated. The details of such an evaluation are beyond the scope of this review but have been discussed elsewhere (Accardo & Capute, 1979; Capute & Biehl, 1973).

Inquiry related to genetic conditions or moderating factors, such as chronic disease states or metabolic/progressive neurologic processes, is dictated by history and general physical examination. Assessment of special senses reveals developmentally significant problems with vision and hearing. Evaluating the child's abilities in language (spoken and written), problem solving, and social/adaptive and motor domains permits the delineation of a developmental profile with patterns of strength and deficit. Although gross motor delay may be a clinical marker for the need for a more general assessment, the addition of language assessment might improve the diagnostic accuracy of developmental disability. Contrasting the rates of development in the major domains yields developmental diagnosis.

Developmental diagnoses permit answering the questions about the nature of the handicap and the presence of other associated deficits. Viewing the developmental profile's pattern of strength and deficit in terms of the diagnoses determines the degree of handicap, allows delineation of current needs and treatment, and sets long-term goals.

Because of the wide range of abilities (both strengths and weaknesses) subsumed by functional evaluation, no single discipline is able fully to assess all areas. The multidisciplinary approach is the most common method of evaluation of children with developmental failure. In this approach various disciplines evaluate the child and make independent recommendations. Unless someone assumes the role of coordinator, there is no resolution of differences, and the parents may be faced with conflicting information and unrealistic, or at least unprioritized, treatment recommendations. By contrast, the interdisciplinary approach focuses on a comprehensive program for the child, with each discipline bringing its expertise to effect a coordinated approach to the child's and family's problems. The interdisciplinary approach has been criticized as being time-consuming, rigid, expensive, and, because multiple disciplines are responsible for the treatment program, diffuse. These criticisms do not take into account the long-term costs in time, dollars, and energy that are associated with an incomplete habilitation program. Although the differences between multidisciplinary and interdisciplinary approaches are not insignificant, in practice good multidisciplinary teams have someone perform coordination tasks.

DIAGNOSIS

Diagnosis is the culmination of the evaluative process. Diagnosis has been dismissed as being irrelevant; we would strongly disagree.

A full developmental diagnosis permits the establishment of a developmental profile with reasonable goals. It is not possible to interpret functional abilities in the absence of diagnosis. For example, the child with language delay may be hearing-impaired, have a central communicative disorder, or be mentally retarded. In the deaf child, language therapy without aural rehabilitation would be useless, and family, child, and therapist would be frustrated.

The provision of services depends on the establishment of a diagnosis. Many states mandate diagnostic categories for provision of special education services under PL 94-142. For example, academic underachievement alone is not sufficient to obtain additional assistance in school. If there is a substantial difference between cognitive potential and achievement and the diagnosis of specific learning disability made, then appropriate educational services can be provided.

Diagnosis permits prognostication. Although no two children are exactly comparable, grouping children with similar diagnoses permits general statements about the natural history, associated dysfunctions, goals, and long-term outcomes of the diagnosed condition. Additionally, those children who do not perform as expected would serve as a basis for further investigation, e.g., children who were thought to be mildly retarded but did not show adequate academic progress and were found to have a superimposed learning disability (perceptual/processing disability).

Lack of a diagnosis precludes genetic counseling. The inheritance of most developmental disorders is unclear; however, there are syndromes that have known patterns of Mendelian inheritance. Informing the parents of their risk of recurrence requires a definite diagnosis to be established.

Although we feel that diagnosis is important, diagnosis alone is not sufficient for treatment and habilitation. It is impossible to develop a comprehensive treatment program based on diagnosis in the absence of a developmental profile. Developmental diagnosis is based on the most obvious manifestations and, even allowing for multiple diagnoses, does not adequately describe abilities that may be important for treatment and habilitation. For example, of two children who had full-scale IQs of 60, one had only a slight degree of variability ("scatter") on testing; the other had a marked amount but with the same summary scores. Although both were mildly retarded, it is likely that the long-term outcome for both children will not be the same. The first child will likely function consistently as mildly retarded in social and academic areas. In contrast, the second child's testing suggests additional processing/perceptual dysfunction, which may preclude the development of academic abilities to the mildly retarded level. However, the latter child may function as mildly retarded in non-academic areas. This may be considered a learning disability profile in a child with mental retardation and be seen as an explanation for the relative academic underachievement. Because of the diffuse nature of neurologic dysfunction, the wide variance within diagnostic categories, and multiple diagnoses, it can be said that *there is no "garden variety" of developmental disorder.*

TREATMENT AND HABILITATION

Perhaps the most controversial aspects of the care of the developmentally disabled are treatment and habilitation. Therapy, treatment, management, habilitation, and rehabilitation are used interchangeably to describe interventions to improve the lives and function of developmentally disabled children. Treatment refers to interventions designed to ameliorate or improve the diagnosed condition. Habilitation is a comprehensive program designed to facilitate a child's development, with the long-term goal of maximizing function. The goals of habilitation are (a) to treat the diagnosed conditions and (b) to prevent the development of secondary handicaps. In contrast to habilitation, rehabilitation focuses on skills previously acquired.

Although the goals of habilitation are clear, the efficacy of the treatment is not. Early treatment has been shown to be effective in a limited number of conditions (hypothyroidism, phenylketonuria, branched chain ketoaciduria, and galactosemia). However, even in those conditions where disability can be prevented, cure is not the result. In the majority of developmental disabilities, other than those few related to biochemical defects, treatment is based on the premise that peripheral stimulation can result in positive alteration of the central nervous system. This has been shown to be true in lower life forms, but proof is lacking for humans.

Although proof of therapeutic efficacy is lacking, treatment is mandated by law (PL 94-142, The Education for All Handicapped Children Act). This has made the objective evaluation of efficacy difficult. "We could not participate in a controlled trial of therapeutic efficacy because we did not think it was ethical to withhold therapy" is a common refrain. We would suggest that the ethics of providing untested therapy should be questioned.

Others have suggested that therapy serves to maintain a child's developmental rate, or prevent the appearance of secondary handicaps such as behavioral disturbance or scoliosis. However, interventions designed to prevent secondary handicaps are not always delineated from treatment of the primary disorder. This has led to a rather nonspecific approach to the habilitation of handicapped children. The lack of specificity of approach is worsened when the goals are not clear. (In rehabilitation one is able to set premorbid function as the goal, but in habilitation establishment of functional outcomes is precluded by a lack of valid methods of prediction.) Despite reservations about the lack of specificity of treatment of developmental disorders, two factors consistently are shown to influence outcome: the therapist and the family. Indeed in some interventions, the therapist and family factors are as important as the type of therapy.

Therapy that is applied to a child with an incomplete developmental profile can have adverse effects. Overstimulation at a level that is inappropriate to the child can result in behavioral disturbance. Trying to treat each aspect of neurologic dysfunction in a fragmentary approach usually leads to parental "burnout." Maintenance of family function is a major tenet of habilitation and may necessitate relieving the parents of the responsibility of being the primary therapist.

REEVALUATIONS

There is a need to repeat the process of evaluation and diagnosis. The reasons for reevaluations are (a) to determine if the original habilitation program is still appropriate, (b) to review the evaluative data with the parents and assist them in understanding the information, and (c) to modify habilitative recommendations. Developmental disabilities are static neurological disorders, but the peripheral manifestations change with time. The child may no longer require active intervention from a therapist, or a new therapy (such as special education) needs to be added to the program. There are no absolute rules concerning the frequency of reevaluation, but factors that seem related to the need for reevaluation include age of the child, nature of the handicap, the specific findings on the current evaluation, family function, and community resources.

The developmental status of young children is more likely to change. Consequently, reevaluations are performed more frequently in young children and less frequently as the child gets older. However, as the child ages there is a need to provide new information that may have been unnecessary or unavailable earlier. Initially, the focus is on the diagnosis and on restoring confidence in the parents' ability to parent. Later the focus shifts to the habilitative program/school and questions of programmatic adequacy. With the onset of puberty come questions of sexuality and shortly thereafter questions concerning after-school life adjustment (vocation, living arrangements, parental mortality).

Children with uneven (deviant) cognitive profiles or those with findings that require direct intervention also may need revaluation. Examples of specific findings that mandate reevaluation may be the appearance of behavioral disturbances or an impending hip subluxation in a child with spastic diplegia. Some children with metabolic dysfunction may need frequent reevaluations as would children with unstable baseline functioning.

Factors relating to the child's external environment, e.g., family and community resources, also influence the need for reevaluation. Some families are able to advocate effectively for their children and have a satisfactory arrangement for service delivery. Other families are disorganized or unable effectively to obtain services for their child in the community. Reevaluation will provide the family with current information about their child's needs and the pros and cons of the available therapeutic options.

SUMMARY

Diagnosis, treatment, and habilitation are the foundations on which care is given to developmentally disabled children. A full profile of the child's functional abilities, coupled with a complete developmental diagnosis, permits the establishment of a treatment program with appropriate short-term and long-term goals that not only address the primary diagnoses but also address prevention of secondary handicaps. Revaluation offers the opportunity to ensure that recommendations are still valid, that the habilitation program is modified to reflect current needs, and that information is reviewed with the parents so that they might be better advocates for their child.

REFERENCES

Accardo, P. J., & Capute, A. J. (1979). *The pediatrician and the developmentally delayed child.* Baltimore: University Park Press.

Capute, A. J., & Biehl, R. F. (1973). Functional developmental evaluation: Prerequisites to habilitation. *Pediatric Clinics of North America, 20,* 3.

Capute, A. J., & Palmer, F. B. (1980). A pediatric overview of the spectrum of developmental disabilities. *Journal of Developmental and Behavioral Pediatrics, 1,* 66.

Capute, A. J., Shapiro, B. K., & Palmer, F. B. (1981). Spectrum of developmental disabilities: Continuation of motor dysfunction. *Orthopedic Clinics of North America, 12,* 3.

Haggerty, R. J. (1985). The Rand health insurance experiment. *Pediatrics, 75,* 969.

Nelson, K. B., & Ellenberg, J. H. (1982). Children who "outgrew" cerebral palsy. *Pediatrics, 69,* 529.

Lock, T. M., Shapiro, B. K., & Capute, A. J. (1985). Factors affecting referral of the developmentally disabled. *Developmental Medicine and Child Neurology, 27,* 119.

Resinger, K. S., & Bires, J. A. (1980). Anticipatory guidance in pediatric practice. *Pediatrics, 66,* 889.

Schulman, J., & Stern, S. (1959). Parents' estimate of the intelligence of retarded children. *American Journal of Mental Deficiency, 63,* 696.

Chapter 11

NUTRITION SERVICES FOR CHILDREN WITH HANDCIAPS

Marion Taylor Baer

Nutrition services are an essential component of any health delivery system. They are especially important in the prevention of handicaps, as well as in the treatment and/or habilitation of children with chronic illness or other handicapping condition.

Primary prevention is not the major focus of this chapter. However, the reader should be aware that research findings suggest that improved nutrition would greatly lower the incidence of low birth weight (Edozien, Switzer, & Bryan, 1979; Kennedy, Gershoff, Reed, & Austin, 1982), which is the single most important risk factor for the subsequent development of a handicapping condition in an infant (National Academy of Science, 1979). Other studies, in both humans and animal models, indicate that micronutrient deficiencies, either dietary or resulting from drug–nutrient interaction, may be responsible for more environmentally caused birth defects (Bergmann, Makosch, & Tews, 1980; Cavdar, Arcasoy, Baycu, & Himmetoglu, 1980; Flynn et al., 1981; Hambidge, Neldner, & Walravens, 1975; Hurley, 1980; Laurence, Campbell, & Nansi, 1983), as well as subtle learning disabilities (Golub, Gershwin, Hurley, Cheung, & Hendrickx, 1985; Oski, Honig, & Helu, 1983), than has been previously recognized.

Dietary treatment, as a form of secondary prevention, also can attenuate the devastating effects of hereditary metabolic disorders. Phenylketonuria (PKU), for example, which used to result in severe mental retardation if untreated, can now be treated by dietary means. If the treatment is instituted early in life, the child's growth and development are nearly normal (Dobson, Williamson, Azen, & Koch, 1977; Pennington & von Doorninck, 1985). Diet is also the key in the treatment of chronic illnesses such as diabetes and cystic fibrosis.

Nutrition is also important for tertiary prevention (habilitation), or the minimalization of the potentially debilitating effects of an existing handicapping condition. A well-nourished child has a greater chance of remaining healthy and of reaching his potential development both physically and intellectually. This is true of all children, but is especially so for the child with a disability. In addition to the nutritional risks facing normal children, disabled youngsters also may have risk occasioned by structural anomalies, neuromuscular dysfunction, mental retardation, behavioral abnormalities, or any combination thereof. In addition, the medical condition itself, or the drugs required to control it, may alter nutrient needs or interfere with nutrient absorption and/or utilization.

The recognition of the importance of nutrition services has grown steadily in the last 50 years (Caldwell, 1982). This increased national concern has been reflected in legislation mandating their inclusion, for example, as part of comprehensive services to children with handicaps under the various provisions of Title V of the Social Security Act. However, despite these facts, not all children at risk have routine access to nutritional care. For this reason, an effort is currently under way nationwide to ensure that nutrition services are available to all children with handicapping conditions. The approaches to service delivery that have thus far been developed vary according to the resources and constraints of the states and localities. Examples of these approaches can be found in recent publications (Baer, 1982; Kozlowski, 1980) that have resulted from the interdisciplinary efforts of professionals across the country who are interested in promoting the health and welfare of children with handicaps. The purpose of this chapter is (a) to outline the commonalities involved in developing a system for nutrition service delivery, and (b) to briefly describe the content of those services.

DEVELOPING NUTRITION SERVICES FOR CHILDREN WITH HANDICAPPING CONDITIONS

Needs Assessment

Nutrition needs. The first step in developing comprehensive nutrition services is to ascertain what services currently exist and to what degree they are meeting the needs of the children to be served. These needs vary from very complex problems requiring highly specialized interdisciplinary assessment and care (American Dietetic Association, 1981; Howard, 1981; Palmer & Ekvall, 1978; Smith et al., 1982; Wodarski, 1985; Worthington, Pipes, & Trahms, 1978) to relatively simple questions in the area of normal nutrition, food purchasing and storage, or information relative to the client's eligibility for government-sponsored food distribution and/or nutrition education programs.

In conducting a needs assessment, one of the goals is to determine the prevalence of nutrition problems as well as factors suggesting high nutritional risk within the population. If there has been no coordinated system of service delivery (including data collection) to date, this information may need to be inferred from the types of disorders seen. Table 11-1 presents a list of problem areas most often associated with certain diagnostic classes. The problem areas are divided arbitrarily into those related directly to the child and his condition and those related to the caregiver(s).

Once an estimate of the patient service need has been established, programmatic considerations must be addressed. These include nutrition-program-management needs as well as service-delivery potential within the existing financial constraints of the overall program. Here, information based on the assessment of existing nutrition services and resources can be matched to the estimated needs, to identify gaps as well as overlaps in the existing system.

Existing services.   A wide spectrum of services is necessary to meet identified nutrition needs. To assess the adequacy of existing services, the following questions are helpful:

1. Do the children served receive nutrition screening as an integral part of the total health screening?

2. Do children identified as being at risk during the screening receive further nutrition assesssment?

3. Is nutrition intervention (counseling, education, therapeutic diets, etc.), if indicated, included in the individualized service plan? Is it implemented?

4. Is there specialized nutritional support for children with severe neuromotor dysfunction (e.g. special feeding equipment) or inborn errors of metabolism (e.g., special dietary products)?

5. Do children with nutrition problems receive periodic monitoring of the resolution of those problems? Are children not at nutrition risk regularly rescreened?

6. For which nutrition problems are there established policies and procedures for nutritional care, and to what extent are they being implemented?

7. For which problems have standards for nutritional care been elaborated and to what extent are they being monitored?

8. Is there coordination and referral among individuals and agencies at all care levels? Are there gaps in service delivery; is there duplication of services?

Existing resources.   Resources available to support nutrition services may be found within the Crippled Children's (CC) program. However, it is also necessary to assess what may be available to CC clients through other sources—both public agencies and within the private sector—to avoid costly duplication of service. Relevant questions follow:

1. Are funds available for nutrition services in (a) the CC Program; (b) other agency programs—e.g., maternal and child health, developmental disabilities services?

2. Are nutrition services reimbursable through (a) Medicaid, Medicare; (b) private insurance companies?

3. Are personnel available for (a) nutrition screening; (b) nutrition assessment and intervention; (c) coordination of nutrition services, monitoring and quality assurance and data gathering?

4. Is/are there adequate space, supplies, equipment?

5. Where can personnel obtain specialized training, if necessary?

Goals, Objectives, and Activities

Nutritional goals and objectives should be developed from the results of the needs assessment activities and integrated into the overall service delivery system. Broad goals may be broken down into specific and measurable objectives, with a given time frame, which can then be effectively evaluated.

Setting Priorities

Given the probability that the demands of the total program will exceed its resources, priorities must be set as a matter of policy. Again, these vary from state to state as individual programs determine how best to serve the maximum number of children within their overall service delivery system.

Utilization of Resources

Once the goals and objectives have been decided on and prioritized, steps can begin toward the utilization of identified community resources to implement the program. This may involve redirecting or augmenting the efforts of service providers within the agency and/or establishing linkages with, and arranging for financing for, service providers in other agencies.

Nutrition personnel.   In order to provide efficient and effective nutrition services, a public health nutrition director/administrator who functions in a coordinating role at the state level is desirable. Depending on the needs of the state, he may be full-time with CCS or be designated by another agency (e.g., MCH) to assume these responsibilities. This person should be trained

Table 11-1. Frequently Reported Nutrition Problems and Factors Contributing to High Nutritional Risk of Children with Handicapping Conditions

Diagnostic Classes of Conditions/Diseases[a]	Percentage of Children with Conditions/Diseases[a]	Examples of frequently reported nutrition problems and factors contributing to high nutrition risk
I. Infective and parasitic diseases	0.8	1,9
II. Neoplasm	1.2	1,2,7,10,12,14,15
III. Allergic, endocrine system, and nutritional diseases (eg. asthma, PKU, rickets, diabetes, etc.)	1.6	1,2,3,4,6,9,11,12,14,15
IV. Diseases of blood and blood-forming organs (eg. sickle cell anemia, etc.)	0.6	2,4,7,10,12,14
V. Mental, psychoneurotics and personality (eg. Down Syndrome, etc.)	4.7	1,3,5,8,10,11,12,13,14
VI. Disorders of nervous system and sense organs (eg. cerebral palsy, epilepsy, hearing impairment, etc.)	26.3	1,2,3,4,5,7,8,10,11,12,13,14
VII. Diseases of circulatory system	2.3	1,2,3,7,11,12,13,14
VIII. Diseases of respiratory system	1.2	1,6,7,10,12,14
IX. Diseases of digestive system (eg. cystic fibrosis, etc.)	3.2	1,2,4,5,9,12,13,14,15
X. Diseases of genito-urinary tract (nephritis, nephrosis, etc.)	1.1	2,10,14,15
XIII. Diseases of bone and organs of movement (eg. muscular dystrophy, scoliosis, etc.)	20.7	1,5,8,11,12,14
XIV. Congenital malformations (eg. cleft plate and lip, spina bifida, circulatory system, etc.)	18.9	1,3,4,5,8,11,12,13,14
XV. Certain diseases of early infancy (eg. brain injury, etc.)	1.3	1,8,10,11,12,13,14
XVI. Accidents, poisonings and violence (eg. amputations, burns, etc.)	2.8	1,2,8,11,14

Nutrition Problems and Factors Contributing to High Nutritional Risk

A. Directly Child-Related

1. Altered energy needs/caloric intake
2. Altered nutrient needs
3. Condition of oral cavity hampers food intake and/or indicates nutrition problems
4. Nutrient deficiencies
5. Constipation/diarrhea
6. Food allergies
7. Poor appetite
8. Delayed feeding skill development/ mechanical feeding problems
9. Malabsorption
10. Nutrient-drug interactions
11. Maladaptive behaviors

B. Indirectly Child-Related; Directly Caregiver-Related

12. Lack of nutrition knowledge/vulnerability to misinformation
13. Inappropriate feeding practices
14. Reluctance to control food intake
15. Difficulty in understanding and/or implementing diet instructions

[a]Children who received Physician services under Crippled Childrens Program FY76

Taken from: Baer, M. T. (Ed.), 1982

and experienced in working with children who have handicapping conditions, as well as in program development, in order to best assist in program planning, development, implementation, and evaluation (Kaufman, 1982).

In addition to the state-level public health nutritionist, others may have a similar function in designated geographic regions, especially in a large state, and/or in one with a decentralized health delivery structure. These individuals in other situations may serve in a consultant role working with other agency staff; supervise nutritionists, dietitians, or paraprofessionals providing direct service; or even provide some direct service themselves.

Service delivery personnel are nutritionists with at least a bachelor's degree and who are registered dietitians (RD). They may be assisted by nutrition or dietetic technicians, trained (AA degrees) to work under their supervision (Kaufman, 1982).

Other members of the health care team.   The discussion of personnel involved in the nutritional care of children with handicaps has thus far focused on nutritionists. However, the complex problems presented by these conditions most often require an interdisciplinary approach to their solution. A child may have any combination of medical (physicians), oral structural (dentists, hygienists), neuromuscular (physical therapists, occupational therapists, speech pathologists), or behavioral (psychologists, behavioral specialists) problems that interfere with the intake or utilization of nutrients. Input from these disciplines, as well as from nurses and social workers who can assess the family and community resources, must often form an integral part of the nutrition assessment. Furthermore, it often may be a clinician from another discipline who is most appropriate to implement the care plan decided on by the team. The nutritionist then becomes a consultant to the primary therapist. By the same token, when nutrition personnel are limited, some other member of the health care team must assume responsibility for assuring the routine use of nutrition screening procedures and, when indicated, referral mechanisms.

Other community nutrition services.   Although many states do not yet have a coordinated system for the delivery of nutrition services, with full-time CCS nutritionists at both the state and local levels, there are many potential resources within the community at both levels. If the agency is not yet in a position to employ full-time nutritionists, several types of assistance may be useful in both planning and implementing the delivery of nutrition services. However, it will probably be necessary to assign responsibility for the nutrition component to another member of the agency staff in order to assure effectiveness. Following are suggested resources:

1.   To assist with nutrition program planning and development, evaluation and training, the agency may request consultation

in the form of interagency cooperation or contracts from nutritionists in the following positions:

public health nutrition directors/consultants in state and local health agencies; nutritionists in programs serving children with handicapping conditions, such as University-Affiliated Programs, Pediatric Pulmonary Centers, Diagnostic and Evaluation Clinics, Regional Centers for the Developmentally Disabled, etc.;

public health nutrition educators in university settings.

2. To provide direct nutrition services, the agency may establish contracts with the following:

nutritionists in programs serving children with handicapping conditions (see above);

nutritionists in private practice who have received specialized training, in a University-Affiliated Program, for example;

nutritionists and dietitians working in local child health programs, such as public health departments, hospitals, WIC, EPSDT, Head Start (these professionals may require some in-service training depending on background and experience).

3. To provide specialized therapeutic nutritional management (metabolic disorders, for example), the following professionals would be qualified:

nutritionists in programs serving children with handicapping conditions;

pediatric dietitians in university-affiliated teaching hospitals.

4. To provide food assistance:
WIC and CSFP;

food stamp program;

school feeding and child-nutrition programs;

emergency food assistance through various community programs.

5. To provide assistance with meal planning and food purchasing, storage, and preparation:
Cooperative Extension home economists;

Expanded Food & Nutrition Education Program (EFNEP) aides for low-income families;

nutrition or dietetic technicians and community aides.

In addition, policy decisions have to be made regarding specific nutrition services to be reimbursed, under what conditions, and at what level (in-depth assessment, counseling, specialized dietary management, e.g., metabolic disorders; specific formulas, foods, feeding equipment to be reimbursed; standards for providers.

Implementation Plan

Once resources have been identified, needed inter- and/or intra-agency agreements are in place, and appropriate policies established, a plan for implementation of the delivery of nutrition services can be developed. The plan is sequential, with an overall timetable specifying target completion dates for each objective which may include the following:

1. Staff training.
2. Development of a nutrition screening protocol and establishment of clear criteria for referral.
3. Development of a nutrition assessment protocol.
4. Design of a system for recording and retrieving data relative to nutrition, in order to monitor progress.
5. Development of a system of evaluation to measure effectiveness, efficiency, and productivity.

DELIVERY OF NUTRITION SERVICES

Although there is no one prescription for the organization or financing of nutrition services, the components of a nutrition service delivery system are more universal. They can be divided into indirect services, or program management functions, and direct service delivery.

Each state, based on its needs, resources, and the existing CCS program structure, must develop its own approach to the delivery of nutrition services.

Program Management Functions

In most settings, for purposes of efficiency, it is desirable that program management be carried out, or at least coordinated, at the state level. However, the method of translating the following functions into activities may again be variable:

1. Writing the nutrition component of the overall service delivery plan.
2. Identifying resources (individuals or agencies) for referrals and serving as a liaison between them in order to avoid duplication of efforts and gaps in services, and providing consultation and technical assistance as needed.
3. Developing statewide standards for nutrition screening, criteria for referral for individual assessment, assessment protocol and guidelines for nutrition care.

4. Providing workshops or other educational programs (in conjunction with University-Affiliated Programs, whose mandate is training in this area) and/or printed materials for direct service providers of all disciplines.

5. Providing field experience for public health nutrition students.

6. Advocating for the nutrition needs of children with handicapping conditions, both within the agency and within the nutrition profession.

7. Evaluating program effectiveness.

8. Assessing needs for applied research.

Direct Service Delivery

The nutritionist, or dietitian, providing direct nutrition services to children with handicapping conditions is responsible for screening, in-depth assessment, development of a nutrition care plan, provision of care, rescreening or reassessment, and evaluation (Fomon, 1976; Smith, 1976). In some cases, such as screening and provision of nutritional care, another professional may actually be carrying out the protocol. However, the nutritionist is trained to design, evaluate, and integrate the various components of an assessment, and should be involved in developing the care plan as well.

Screening and assessment. The components of a nutrition screening and assessment protocol are summarized in Table 11-2. There are five major approaches to assessment of nutritional status in children. It is beyond the scope of this chapter to present them in detail. However, they are briefly described below.

Anthropometric. Growth is the best indicator of a child's nutritional status. Therefore, careful measurements of height and weight, using appropriate and well-calibrated instruments, are essential. Measurements over time are especially helpful for children with handicapping conditions in order to determine whether the often substandard height is likely to be due to nutritional, as opposed to non-nutritional (normal growth *rate*), factors.

Estimation of body composition using a combination of skinfold measurements and arm circumference further defines body weight. A child may be underweight for height but still have adequate fat stores, especially if lean body mass is reduced because of an underlying medical problem. The converse also may be true; a child may be overweight if well-muscled but not overfat.

Table 11-2. Guides for Nutritional Screening, Referral and Assessment of Children with Handicapping Conditions[a]

I. Anthropometric

Purpose: To collect data related to growth and body composition

A. Screening
1. Weight[b]
   a. Conditions: no shoes, light clothing
   b. Suggested standard: NCHS Growth Charts
2. Height
   a. Conditions: recumbent length[c]
   b. Suggested standard: NCHS Growth Charts

B. Referral

Growth deviations

C. Assessment

In addition to screening data
1. Skin fold triceps and subscapular desirable
   a. Conditions: obtain duplicate readings
   b. Suggested standard: Fomon
2. Arm circumference[d]
   a. Conditions: obtain duplicate readings
   b. Suggested standard: Gurney and Jelliffe nomogram
3.
4.

D. Equipment specification and maintenance
1. Calibrated weight scale (balance-type)
2. Measuring board (stadiometer) for measuring recumbent length or vertical surface with leveler for measuring standing height
3. Narrow flexible steel or plastic coated tape measure for measuring arm circumference
4. Calibrated calipers

II. Clinical

Purpose: To observe clinical signs of chronic or subacute disease

A. Screening

Review of past and present records of medical and dental examinations for signs suggestive of poor nutritional status

B. Referral

Specific nutritional disorders or inborn errors of metabolism

C. Assessment
1. In depth collection of health history with special attention to areas of nutritional risk, e.g.
   a. Prenatal pattern and total amount of maternal weight gain, complications of pregnancy, etc.
   b. Postnatal client or family history of diabetes, coronary heart disease, infections, anemia, constipation, diarrhea, hyperactivity, food intolerances, pica, inborn errors of metabolism, malabsorption syndromes, etc.
2. Observation
   (1) General appearance
   (2) Speech
   (3) Oral hygiene

D. Suggested standards
1. Fomon
2. Christakis
3. Goldsmith

III. Biochemical

Purpose: To obtain objective data related to present nutrition status or recent dietary intake

A. Screening
1. Hemoglobin or Hematocrit

B. Referral

Does not meet accepted standard.

C. Assessment

The following as needed:
1. Complete blood count
2. Routine urinalysis including microscopic
3. Serum total protein and albumin
4. Fasting blood glucose
5. Serum urea nitrogen
6. Transferrin saturation
7. Quantitative urinary and plasma amino acid screening[e]
8. Organic acids
9. Other tests to respond to special conditions or problem

Condition/Problem	Test[e]
a. anticonvulsants	folic acid, ascorbic acid, calcium, vitamin D, alkaline phosphatase, phosphorus, vitamin B_6
b. Prader-Willi Syndrome	glucose tolerance test
c. pica	lead, hemoglobin

D. Suggested standards
1. Fomon
2. Christakis
3. State or local health agencies
4. Center for Disease Control

IV. Dietary

Purpose: To determine a usual dietary pattern and/or nutrient intake

A. Screening
1. Twenty-four hour recall using food models and/or measures and food frequency with verbal questioning
2. Feeding history questionnaire to include parents concerns regarding nutrition status

B. Referral
1. Evidence from screening questionnaires of deficiencies of one or more nutrients
2. Family income
3. Response to parents or other professionals concerns
4. Requires special diet
5. Bizarre food habits

C. Assessment
1. Three-day dietary intake kept by parent
   (a) Verbal instruction in dietary record keeping
   (b) Kept during two week days and weekend day
   (c) Dietary supplements and/or medications included
   (d) Occurrences affecting validity recorded, i.e., illness or holidays
   (e) Quantity, preparation and brand names of food included
   (f) Where, when and with whom client eats included
2. Activity record (as needed)
3. Pertinent historical information related to feeding
4. Present influences on dietary intake
5. Other

Certain conditions (i.e., inborn errors of metabolism or syndromes) may require further dietary investigation necessitating more detailed data collection

D. Suggested standards
1. Recommended Dietary Allowances
2. Fomon
3. FAO

V. Behavioral and Feeding Skill Development

Purpose: To determine the influence of level of feeding development and behavior on nutritional status

A. Screening

Questionnaire including
1. Parental perception of feeding skills and behavior
2. Professional perception of feeding skills and behavior

B. Referral
1. Mechanical feeding problems
2. Feeding skills below mental age
3. Feeding behavior problems

C. Assessment
1. Review of past history and interview to determine feeding skill development and present level of functioning
2. Observations[f]
   (a) Physical
      1. Oral structure and function including primitive reflexes, sucking, swallowing, biting, chewing, occlusion and caries
      2. Neuromuscular development including gross and fine motor skills, head and trunk control, eye-hand coordination and position for feeding
   (b) Behavioral
      1. Parent (care-giver)-child interaction
      2. Reinforcement patterns (positive and negative)
      3. Environmental influences
      4. Child-examiner interact

D. Suggested standards
1. Gesell and Amatruda
2. Vineland Social Maturity Scale

---

[a]Adaptation of Guides for Nutritional Assessment of the Mentally Retarded and Developmentally Disabled, MA Harvey Smith (Ed.) 1976

[b]Measurement to be made by well-trained, motivated personnel

[c]Standards for recumbent length for normal children are available only up to 2 years of age; however, this method yields more accurate measurement of physically handicapped children over 2 years, especially when they are unable to stand without support

[d]Screening with multiple Guthrie tests and/or thin layer chromatography or hematography alone

[e]Professional judgement is warranted and a current search of literature should be done to determine appropriateness of tests before they are used

[f]Observations both at home and outside home with and without primary care-giver and/or conjoint professional assessments are valuable

Taken from Baer, M. T. (Ed.), 1982.

Clinical.   Clinical indications of possible nutritional disorders include signs apparent on medical examination of the child, such as abnormal skin or hair conditions. These are rare because they appear only after a prolonged period of nutrient deficiency. They are often quite non-specific as well and must be substantiated by dietary or biochemical data. The dental examination also may provide information relative to the child's nutritional status, such as extensive dental caries, resulting perhaps from bedtime bottles or overuse of sweets.

Review of medical records from a nutritionist's point of view would include a search for a history of anemia, recurrent infections, chronic constipation or diarrhea, food intolerances or allergies, pica, and the like. Other relevant historical information: prenatal maternal weight gain, birth weight, early feeding problems and practices, growth pattern, laboratory data.

Biochemical.   Laboratory assessment of nutritional status, most commonly using fasting serum (or plasma), red or white blood cells, or urine samples (casual or 24-hour), can be used to estimate nutrient stores, or preferably the functional capacity of nutrient-dependent enzymes, to determine the effects of chronic medications such as anti-convulsants or of pica. Biochemical methods also are used to diagnose genetic disorders of metabolism that can be treated by diet, such as PKU.

Dietary.   Analysis of a child's dietary pattern can predict and prevent nutrient deficiencies. It may range from a simple screening, by food groups, of a 24-hour dietary recall to a computer-facilitated nutrient analysis of a record kept for 3 or more days. Other information pertinent to this analysis includes: child's level of activity; dietary supplements and/or medications; how, where, when, and with whom the child eats; bizarre food habits or inappropriate feeding behaviors; and the cultural/economic constraints on the family's diet as a whole.

Feeding skill development.   Children with handicapping conditions often exhibit a significant delay in the development of feeding skills. This may be due to neuromuscular dysfunction, resulting in the persistence of primitive reflexes, or to muscle incoordination, which makes positioning, chewing, or hand-to-mouth movement difficult. It also may be due to cognitive delays in a neurologically intact child, leading to infantilization by his caregivers. Assessment of the child's developmental level with respect to these skills, and the child–feeder interaction if there are behavior problems, is essential to developing an intervention strategy and may require interdisciplinary observation of an actual feeding session.

Developing a nutrition care plan.   A nutrition care plan is developed from the integration and interpretation of the results of the five components of the assessment. It is also influenced by input from other members of the health care team, as well as from the parents and/or teacher of the child, as the overall individual service plan is formulated. The nutritionist also builds guidelines into the plan for monitoring progress in achieving the goals, both short and long term, that the team has prioritized.

Providing nutrition care.   The role of the nutritionist/dietitian in providing follow-up may range from direct service delivery, even serving as case manager, to serving as a consultant to the case manager, to assisting in finding another resource for direct service. In any situation the monitoring function must be operative.

Rescreening/reassessment.   Children in high-risk categories must be rescreened periodically for nutrition problems, even if none are identified at first. Those for whom intervention is indicated also must be reassessed at regular intervals to evaluate the success, or lack thereof, of the strategies decided on during the development of the individual service plan.

Evaluation.   Standards must be set for measuring the efficacy of the intervention strategies so that nutrition care may be made consistent from one clinic to another and so that uniform data may be collected for purposes of quality assurance and determination of cost-effectiveness. Nutrition data should be classified according to diagnosis; nutrition problem codes for use in identifying and reporting problems of children are available (Commission on Professional and Hospital Activities, 1978; USDHEW, 1977).

EVALUATION

Methods for ensuring program quality and evaluating the effectiveness of the program should be developed as an integral part of the implementation plan, both at the program management and the service delivery levels (Baer, 1982; Peck, 1975; USDHEW, 1978). Criteria used have traditionally related to structure, process, and outcome USDHHS, 1981).

Structural criteria relate to the personnel, equipment, and facilities required to carry out the program. Evaluation in this area includes adequacy of staff in terms of both availability and qualifications (USDHEW, 1971); appropriateness of equipment, such as that needed for accurate anthropometric measurements or as effective educational materials; and space, both in offices and in clinics.

Process criteria evolve from the written policies and protocols developed at the program management level during the planning phase. They relate to established activities and procedures used by nutrition care providers at the service delivery level; and as part of the program evaluation, it must be documented that they are actually being carried out as specified.

Outcome criteria are the measurable results of the nutrition intervention, based on anthropometric, biochemical, clinical, and dietary data. Ideally, nutrition data collection forms are designed from the beginning to answer the specific questions related to evaluation and based on criteria established as a result of the planning process. For example, if during the needs assessment a large percentage of the children seen in myelomeningocele clinics are found to be overweight, and this is seen as a priority area because of the already limited mobility of such children, an outcome criterion might be a reduction in that percentage as a result of nutrition intervention. Additional and desirable dimensions in evaluating outcome criteria are cost-efficiency and cost-effectiveness studies that provide information leading toward better utilization of resources.

The goal of the evaluation process is to be able, on a regular and ongoing basis, to reassess existing nutrition services. Where goals and objectives are not being met, these criteria should provide needed clues as to why, so that procedures and activities can be altered accordingly. As goals and objectives are achieved, new priorities can be set and resources redirected toward meeting those needs.

UNMET NEEDS

Although there has been much progress in the last 25 years in recognizing and responding to the nutrition problems of children with handicapping conditions, this is still an underdeveloped area of research, both basic and applied. More data also are needed relative to the benefits of nutrition intervention in order to document its cost-effectiveness.

One of the problems resulting from the lack of a body of information about the nutritional needs of this population has been a lack of trained specialists. Many of those at the forefront of the profession pioneered as nutritionists in Title V–funded Child Development Centers and University-Affiliated Programs. The latter are now helping to form a new generation of leaders in the field through long-term pre-service training. As research leads to increased knowledge, in-service and continuing education for professionals in all the health fields will remain an indispensable adjunct to this basic training.

Unmet service needs, however, are of paramount importance at this time. The potential for the delivery of nutrition services, in terms of both the newly emerging knowledge base and the numbers of well-prepared professionals, far outstrips what exists at present. Much of the reason for this appears to be a combination of financial constraints and a lack of awareness on the part of planners/administrators. It is to be hoped that creative and coordinated planning and programming in the future will help to overcome the present gap between nutrition needs and nutrition services so that all children with handicapping conditions may benefit.

REFERENCES

American Dietetic Association. (1981). Infant and child nutrition: Concerns regarding the developmentally disabled. *Journal of the American Dietetic Association, 78,* 443.

Baer, M. T. (Ed.). (1982). *Nutrition services for children with handicaps: A manual for state Title V programs.* Los Angeles: Children's Hospital of Los Angeles, Center for Child Development and Developmental Disorders.

Bergmann, K. E., Makosch, G., & Tews, K. H. (1980). Abnormalities of hair zinc concentration in mothers of newborn infants with spina bifida. *American Journal of Clinical Nutrition, 33,* 2145.

Caldwell, M. (1982). Nutrition services for the handicapped child. *Public Health Reports, 97,* 483.

Cavdar, A. O., Arcasoy, A., Baycu, T., & Himmetoglu, O. (1980). Zinc deficiency and anencephaly in Turkey. *Teratology, 22,* 141.

Commission on Professional and Hospital Activities (1978). *International classifications of diseases* (9th rev.): *Clinical Modifications* (Vol. 1, ICD-9-OM). Ann Arbor, MI: Edward Brothers.

Dobson, J. C., Williamson, M. L., Azen, C., & Koch, R. (1977). Intellectual assessment of 111 four-year-old children with phenylketonuria. *Pediatrics, 60,* 822–827.

Edozien, J. C., Switzer, B. R., & Bryan, R. B. (1979). Medical evaluation of the special supplemental food program for women, infants and children. *American Journal of Clinical Nutrition, 32,* 677.

Flynn, A., Martier, S. S., Sokol, R. J., Miller, S. I., Golden, N. L., & Del Villano, B. C. (1981). Zinc status of pregnant alcoholic women: A determinant of fetal outcome. *Lancet, 1,* 572.

Fomon, S. J. (1976). *Nutritional disorders of children: Screening, follow-up, prevention.* Rockville, MD: U.S. Department of Health, Education and Welfare.

Golub, M. S., Gershwin, M. E, Hurley, L. S., Cheung, A., & Hendrickx, A. G. (1985). Effects of marginal dietary zinc deprivation on development of rhesus monkey infants. *Federation Proceedings, 44,* 932.

Hambidge, K. M., Neldner, K. H., & Walravens, P. A. (1975). Zinc, acrodermatitis, enteropathica and congenital malformations. *Lancet, 1,* 577.

Howard, R. B. (1981). Nutritional support of the developmentally disabled child. In R. M. Suskind (Ed.), *Textbook of pediatric nutrition.* New York: Raven Press.

Hurley, L. S. (1980). *Developmental nutrition.* Englewood Cliffs, NJ: Prentice-Hall.

Kaufman, M. (Ed.). (1982). *Personnel in public health nutrition for the 1980's.* McLean, VA: Association of State and Territorial Health Organizations Foundation.

Kennedy, E. T., Gershoff, S., Reed, R., & Austin, J. E. (1982). Evaluation of the effect of WIC supplemental feeding on birth weight. *Journal of the American Dietetic Association, 80,* 220.

Kozlowski, B. W. (Ed.). (1980). *Meeting nutrition service needs of clients of Crippled Children's Services and supplemental security income disabled children's programs.* Columbus, OH: Ohio State University, The Nisonger Center.

Laurence, K. M., Campbell, H., & Nansi, E. J. (1983). The role of improvement in the maternal diet and preconceptual folic acid supplementation in the prevention of neural tube defects. In J. Dobbing (Ed.), *Prevention of spina bifida and other neural tube defects.* London: Academic Press.

National Academy of Science. (1979). *Healthy people: The Surgeon General's report on health promotion and disease prevention.* Washington, DC: U.S. Government Printing Office.

Oski, F. A., Honig, A. S., & Helu, B. (1983). Effect of iron therapy on behavior performance in non-anemic, iron-deficient infants. *Pediatrics, 71,* 877.

Palmer, S., Ekvall, S. (Eds.). (1978). *Pediatric nutrition in developmental disorders.* Springfield, IL: Charles C. Thomas.

Peck, E. (1975). *Program planning and evaluation in maternal and child nutrition* (Final Report of HSMHA-MCH Project No. 339). Berkeley, CA: University of California, School of Public Health.

Pennington, B. F., & van Doorninck, W. J. (1985). Neuropsychological deficits in early treated phenylketonuric children. *American Journal of Mental Deficiencies, 89,* 467.

Smith, M. H. (Ed.). (1976). *Guides for nutrition assessment of the mentally retarded and the developmentally disabled.* Memphis, TN: University of Tennessee, Child Development Center.

Smith, M. H., Connolly, B., McFadden, S., Nicrosi, C. R., Nuckolls, L. J., Russell, F. F., & Wilson, W. M. (1982). *Feeding management of a child with a handicap: A guide for professionals.* Memphis, TN: University of Tennessee, Child Development Center.

U.S. Department of Health, Education and Welfare. (1971). *Guide class specifications for nutritionist positions in state and local public health programs.* Rockville, MD: U.S. Government Printing Office.

U.S. Department of Health, Education and Welfare. (1977). *Nutrition problem classification for children and youth* (HSA Publication No. 77-5200). Rockville, MD: U.S. Government Printing Office.

U.S. Department of Health, Education and Welfare. (1978). *Guide for developing nutrition services in community health programs* (HSA Publication No. 78-5103). Rockville, MD: U.S. Government Printing Office.

U.S. Department of Health and Human Services. (1981). *Preliminary guide to quality assurance in ambulatory nutrition care* (HSA Publication No. 81-51174). Rockville, MD: U.S. Government Printing Office.

Wodarski, L. A. (1985). Nutrition intervention in developmental disabilities: An interdisciplinary approach. *Journal of the American Dietetic Association, 85,* 218.

Worthington, B., Pipes, P., & Trahms, C. (1978). The pediatric nutritionist. In E. Allen, V. Holm, & R. L. Schiefelbusch (Eds.), *Early intervention: A team approach.* Baltimore: University Park Press.

Chapter 12

ORAL HEALTH CARE FOR THE
HANDICAPPED CHILD

Martin J. Davis
Heidi L. Hills

All children are entitled to quality oral health care. For no group of children is this more essential than for those who are handicapped. The optimal approach to providing the special child with all needed care is through a team approach, which coordinates the various health care providers. Complete oral health care is a critical aspect of each child's individualized program.

The basic philosophy of oral health care is one of prevention. The handicapped child is vulnerable to at least the same levels of oral disease and its recurrence as is the child without such conditions. Additionally, certain handicapping or medically compromising conditions may of themselves manifest oral health problems. The treatment subsequently necessary for both routine and related problems may be more difficult with the special child. Hence, the need to prevent caries (decay) and periodontal (gum) disease is more pressing for the handicapped child.

The rationale for ensuring that the handicapped child has adequate oral health care is based on three essential needs. The first is the need for the child to have freedom from pain, infection, and treatable pathology. In particular, for the disabled child who may have concomitant problems such as cardiovascular disease, there must be no source of systemic infection from badly decayed teeth or inflamed gingiva (gums).

Second, even the young child with a handicapping condition often has difficulty with his self-image. The perception of self is exquisitely related to the oral-facial complex; most people conceive of the psychological "self" as residing behind the face. If an esthetic problem involving the oral structures is present, the reactions of others to this appearance can be particularly damaging to the psyche of a handicapped individual. If children are aware of substantial problems in this area, seriously negative effects may ensue during the development of self-image; the confidence with which they present themselves to the world may be affected negatively.

The third area of need is the basic consideration for quality of life. The handicapped child is frequently engaged in a complex milieu of treatments and therapies and is being shuttled back and forth between various health care providers. It is most inappropriate for this child to have oral health care placed in a low-priority position or to have difficulty in finding quality care. It is the right of all children to have sound oral health care; for children with special needs this care is essential to prevent the addition of further burdens to their lives.

All too often the "emergency only" approach is applied, resulting in an insidious pattern of sequential unplanned extractions of diseased teeth or intermittent, temporary treatments to relieve discomfort. Such fractionated dentistry results only in a further handicapped child. It is inexcusable for such children to experience dental emergencies because inappropriate oral health care had been continually deferred while other medical problems were addressed. Given the complexities of the lives of handicapped children, we must ensure that their care is timely and preventive in nature. Regular, quality oral health care with a preventive philosophy is the only approach to avoid painful emergencies.

Certain specific measures should be included in a comprehensive prevention-oriented oral health care plan as part of the team care effort. It is important to ensure that in addition to regular access to an appropriately trained dentist, particular attention is paid to oral hygiene and nutrition. Most parents and guardians are aware that the more refined sugar or sucrose a diet contains, the more likely the child will experience an increased decay and gingival disease rate. Nonetheless, many special children in institutions or even residing with their parents have diets high in sucrose-containing foods. This may be the result of numerous factors, including rewards from the caretaker for appropriate behavior or as reinforcement for "productive" activities. In more complex situations, such high-sucrose diets may be part of a system of bribes, the result of unresolved parental guilt, or a manifestation of lack of discipline in supervising the child's diet. The relationship between increased dietary sucrose and increased oral disease is well documented in numerous classical studies.

It has recently become clear that increasing the amount of fiber in the diet can be beneficial even for those children who continue to have relatively high sucrose intakes. High-fiber diets serve to aid oral hygiene. Fibrous foods help remove other "sticky" foods—retained foods that support the bacteria that produce the acids that cause decay. Children with neuromuscular problems, such as cerebral palsy, often have difficulty chewing and swallowing food, leading to accumulations of food on and around the teeth for prolonged periods. For these children, it is essential that the diet consist of non-adherent, low-sucrose foods.

Another key area of prevention for these children is adequate oral hygiene. The thorough daily removal of the bacterial plaques that form on all children's teeth is critical in decreasing the decay and periodontal disease rate. Children motivated to participate in their own oral care should be encouraged to do so. The handicapped child, like any young child, may not have the manual dexterity necessary to attain personally an appropriate level of oral hygiene. It is critical that the parent or caretaker assist with or perform the brushing and flossing to eliminate plaque effectively. In addition, the adult must help the child receive professional regular removal of any hard deposits that may form on the teeth.

The dentist can advise the family whether it is appropriate for the child to assume the primary role in plaque removal and can teach appropriate "second-party" oral hygiene techniques. There are numerous devices and aids available for the more able child to assist in attaining acceptable levels of oral hygiene. Special handles may be attached to brushes to allow a better grip. The electric toothbrush can be a significant aid. Dental floss holders, water irrigators, and other types of appliances for plaque removal are available widely. If these cannot be obtained through local pharmacies, dentists in the area are a source for assistive devices.

Fluoridated water or, in its absence, drops or tablets form systemic dietary fluoride supplements; vitamin–fluoride combinations are particularly effective agents in reducing decay rates. Fluoride is incorporated into developing teeth and makes the enamel more decay-resistant. A second type of fluoride that can be used for teeth that have already erupted into the mouth is called topical fluoride. Fluoride toothpaste, fluoride mouth rinses (for children who can reliably expectorate the rinse after use), and professional topical fluoride treatments are absorbed into the outer tooth surface and "strengthen" the enamel. Finally, fluorides can even halt or reverse early decay. For children with high caries levels, daily fluoride gel applications via custom-made fluoride trays are beneficial.

Fluoride is most effective in combating decay on the smooth "in-between" surfaces of teeth. A relatively recent caries-prevention technique for the posterior biting surfaces is the application of pit and fissure sealant coatings. These thin, well-retained films of hard plastic are bonded directly over the small grooves on the biting surfaces of a child's tooth and thereby prevent entry of both bacteria and food particles into the grooves. At this time, more than 50 percent of the cavities in the mouths of children in the United States occurs in these grooved surfaces. By applying sealants to the biting surfaces, they also can be protected. This technique is limited in that it requires a relatively cooperative patient; it can only be provided by an oral health care professional. It is nonetheless a significant and important preventive aid, especially for the handicapped child. Sealants should be considered in each child's total oral health care program.

In addition to preventive measures, the early identification of developing problems is important. Early identification and treatment is the purpose of regular examination of the handicapped child. If the child's previous dental history has been one of high disease rates, examinations should be more frequent than the classical 6-month interval. A 3-month interval permits better observation; any developing problem can be identified and addressed as early as possible.

A particular area of concern for early recognition and treatment is guidance of the growth of the developing dentition. Many orthodontic or misalignment problems of the teeth may be prevented or intercepted if identified at their inception. Such conditions, if allowed to progress untreated, eventually may require tooth loss or may result in more extensive and expensive care needs.

Certain handicapping conditions may help to cause orthodontic problems. Conditions that have a neurological basis or affect the airway may make the child unusually prone to developing faulty bite relationships (malocclusions). When the functions of various muscle groups are altered as a result of a neurological or handicapping condition, the development of the normal anatomy of the orofacial complex may be hindered. In turn, appropriate alignment, spacing, and function of the teeth may be negatively affected.

Cerebral palsy is a classic example of a condition in which there may be altered muscle function that creates problems. These include poor lip closure, resulting in the drooling of saliva and skin irritation of the lips and chin. Further, because of the hypertonicity or increased contraction of muscle groups associated with the neck, face, and tongue, the development of the dental arches may be substantially altered. Such alteration can be identified and corrected in many patients.

Another example of an orthodontic manifestation of a handicapping condition is the inherent lack of mid-face growth seen in the patient with Down syndrome. Additionally, the tongue may be relatively larger than usual. Since the Down patient often has a degree of mental retardation compounding the difficulties of appropriate oral hygiene, such patients may indeed have a particular need for dental attention.

Children with cranio-facial syndromes often present with cleft palates and other more complex anomalies. They may develop severe caries or peridontal or orthodontic problems that are related to the cleft or the altered growth patterns. If these children also are affected by mental retardation, the oral hygiene difficulties compound the direct effects of the disorder. Children with systemic medical disorders such as blood dyscrasias and immunity disorders often develop oral manifestations such as ulcerations, early tooth loss, malocclusions, and periodontal problems. These children also require intensive preventive care and should be provided with early identification and treatment of problems as they occur.

For some children, orthodontic correction or prosthetic (tooth replacement) treatment is not possible. If an acceptable level of oral hygiene is not maintained, or if the child is not able to understand the goals of treatment and cooperatively wear appliances, more damage than benefit may result. Parents, concerned about attaining a "normal" appearance for their child, may have unrealistic expectations of what can be accomplished dentally. An appropriately trained and experienced dentist with experience in management of the handicapped child can best assess appropriate treatment options for each individual.

Many of the more common or related manifestations of specific disorders, conditions, or treatments are listed in tables 12-1 and 12-2. Please refer to these tables for more detailed information.

Most experienced dentists who work with children with handicapping conditions attempt to provide needed care in as normal or routine a manner as possible. Care is taken that the child does not feel unwanted or that they are a burden to the practitioner. Additionally, all appropriate services can be provided to the child by these highly trained individuals in an efficient and organized manner. This "normalization" of care is critical to enable the child to receive the care to which he is entitled.

For a dentist to be effective in addressing the routine and special needs of these children, a certain amount of training in addition to the usual four years of dental school is indicated. Educational programs such as the two-year residency in pediatric dentistry ensure that those who obtain this training have had extensive experience in addressing the issues presented by the handicapped child. Foremost among these skills is the ability to assist the parent or caretaker in learning the appropriate methods of good oral hygiene and to create an awareness in that individual of the need for regular oral health care. It is insufficient merely to present this information to the responsible individual; it must be presented in a form in which it is comprehended and appropriately learned. If this is not done, the result is that no benefit ensues to the child.

The dentist who has had supervised educational experiences in working with the special child has increased abilities in several areas. Such dentists are better prepared to deliver the care the child needs. They are more aware of concomitant and potential problems associated with handicapping conditions. Additionally, such dentists are more aware of the needs for unrestricted physical access to the office through appropriate office design, including ramps on stairs and carefully designed waiting areas and treatment rooms. Further, he is familiar with the team approach, and as a member of a hospital staff, he will be more able to communicate with physicians, therapists, and other members of the child's total health care team.

These communication skills produce appropriate referrals through the network of specialists. Additionally, experienced dentists will have access to a major teaching hospital or treatment center in the event unusual care is needed. The result is that the child is not "bounced" between various individuals who do not have the indicated levels of experience. The child and parent do not "burn out" by receiving ineffective and frustrating health care.

Table 12-1. Oral Effects of Disorders

Disorder	Bone	Teeth	Soft Tissue	Special Considerations
Cardiovascular Disease				
Cyanotic heart disease (*uncorrected*: tetralogy of Fallot, transposition of great vessels, pulmonary stenosis, pulmonary atresia)	—	Teeth may have bluish-white discoloration May have delayed eruption of teeth May have defects of enamel formation	May have bluish/purplish lips, fissured tongue, bright bluish-red gums, inflamed enlarged gums	Antibiotics required for dental care to protect against life-threatening cardiac infection Anxiety reduction may be accomplished through reassurance and pharmacologic means to avoid undue stress Some types of dental treatment may be contraindicated because of risk of infection; in such cases, the affected teeth should be extracted
Acyanotic heart disease (ventricular septal defect, atrial septal defect, patent ductus arteriosus; uncorrected: coarctation of the aorta, aortic valve stenosis)	—	—	—	Some types of dental treatment may be contraindicated because of risk of infection; in such cases, the affected teeth should be extracted
Diseases of blood and immune system				
Anemia				
Sickle-cell anemia	—	Enamel may be poorly formed	May have higher incidence of gum disease	Preventive dental care is paramount to avoid infections that may trigger a "crisis" Frequent periodic examinations are necessary If oral infection occurs, prompt treatment is imperative Antibiotics may be needed for some dental care to prevent overwhelming infection; general anesthetics are avoided whenever possible

Disorder	Bone	Teeth	Soft Tissue	Special Considerations
Thalassemia	Enlargement of upper jaw with associated malalignment of teeth	Spaced teeth because of jaw enlargement	Pale oral tissue	May require antibiotics before and after some types of dental treatment General anesthetics are avoided whenever possible
Cyclic neutropenia	Loss of bone supporting roots of teeth	Early loss of teeth (primary and permanent)	Severe inflammation of gums Oral ulcers	Prone to oral infection
Bleeding disorders (including hemophilia)	—	May have oozing after natural loss of primary tooth/teeth	Prone to hemorrhage from oral trauma	Excellent oral hygiene and optimal fluoride use will minimize dental disease and treatments that may cause bleeding May need factor replacement and medication [epsilon-amino-caproic acid (EACA)] for dental treatment, especially extractions or oral surgery
Leukemia	—	—	Bleeding gums Oral ulcers (see also chemotherapeutic drugs) Prone to fungal infections	During acute phase dental treatment avoided (except emergency care) All decayed teeth, gum disease, etc., should be treated when patient in remission Meticulous oral hygiene should be practiced to avoid gum irritation (exception: when platelet count lower than 75,000, clean teeth with soft swab only) Avoid strong commercial mouthwashes Avoid oral irrigating device (example: Water Pik)

Table 12-1. Oral Effects of Disorders (continued)

Disorder	Bone	Teeth	Soft Tissue	Special Considerations
Diseases in bone Eosinophilic granuloma	May have early loss of bony support of teeth	May have early loosening of teeth with exposed roots	May have ulcers of gums around exposed root with associated pain May have swollen red, bleeding gums	See also chemotherapy and radiation therapy effects
Osteogenesis imperfecta	Fragile jaw bones	May also have dentinogenesis imperfecta: discolored primary and permanent teeth (bluish-amber translucence); teeth wear down quickly	—	Extractions should be avoided due to fragile jaw bones Extensive dental care needed for dentinogenesis imperfecta: teeth usually require crowns Antibiotics may be required for dental appointments if cardiac complications
Neurofibromatosis	Facial distortion related to tumors in facial and jaw bones May cause malocclusion	—	May have enlargement of tongue due to tumor growth	—
Renal disease Chronic renal failure	Retarded bone growth may lead to malocclusion	May have malformed, discolored, or rough teeth if renal failure occurs during development of teeth (under age 6).	May have facial puffiness May have gum inflammation especially with poor oral hygiene	Frequent routine dental visits for examination and preventive services will minimize need for complicated procedures Tests may be needed before surgical procedures Fluoride preparations should be avoided

Disorder	Bone	Teeth	Soft Tissue	Special Considerations
Dialysis	—	May have loose teeth May have high rate of decay due to high-carbohydrate diet	—	May require antibiotics for dental treatments Best time for dental care is 1 day after dialysis More frequent dental cleanings (oral prophylaxis) are needed Anticoagulant status must be assessed before any surgery is performed to avoid bleeding problems Fluoride preparations should be avoided
Kidney transplant	—	—	—	Prone to oral infection due to immunosuppressive drugs being taken Vigilant preventive dental care and meticulous oral hygiene needed Antibiotics needed before and after dental treatment to avoid life-threatening infection
Syndromes Cleidocranial dysostosis	Upper jaw small and overdeveloped lower jaw with resulting malocclusion	Overretained primary teeth Delayed eruption of teeth Extra teeth common	—	Primary teeth are usually not extracted because permanent teeth may fail to erupt With significant mental retardation, pharmacologic management may be necessary for patient to accept needed dental treatment

Table 12-1. Oral Effects of Disorders (*continued*)

Disorder	Bone	Teeth	Soft Tissue	Special Considerations
Down syndrome	Lack of development of bones of middle 1/3 of the face: short, broad nose, small upper jaw, and high arched palate with resulting malocclusion. Prone to early loss of bone supporting the roots of teeth, especially lower incisors	Eruption of teeth (both primary and permanent) is often delayed. Incisors may be abnormally shaped. Missing teeth are common. May also have extra teeth. Loss of teeth from gum disease may occur as early as late adolescence	May have large tongue with fissures on surface. High prevalence of gum diseases leading to early loss of teeth. Lips may be fissured and chronically chapped or cracked	Meticulous oral hygiene (which may need to be provided by parent or aide) will reduce severity of gum disease. Cardiovascular condition may indicate need for antibiotics for dental treatment to prevent serious complications. With significant mental retardation, pharmacologic management may be necessary for patient to accept needed dental treatment. Extensive gum surgery not indicated as the gum disease is part of a general systemic problem and will progress
Ectodermal dysplasia	—	Fewer teeth develop. Teeth are often malformed (conical shape)	Protuberant lips	Dentures or partial dentures can be made to assist in eating, speaking, and for improved appearance, even in young children.
Papillon–Lefevre	Early loss of bone supporting teeth	Early loss of primary and permanent teeth	Inflamed gums until teeth are lost	—
Other craniofacial syndromes	Variable	Variable	Variable	Orthodontic and/or surgical management of deformity as indicated. Periodontal therapy as indicated on an individual basis

Disorder	Bone	Teeth	Soft Tissue	Special Considerations
Cleft palate	Concave facial profile Malocclusion related to bony clefts	Uneven alignment of teeth especially in cleft area Teeth may be missing or misshapen, especially in cleft area Extra teeth may be present Eruption of teeth may be delayed	Gum inflammation around cleft	—
Miscellaneous				
Juvenile diabetes mellitus	—	Uncontrolled diabetics show increased decay rates	May have enlarged gums May have dry mouth Poorly controlled or uncontrolled diabetics have increased incidence of gum disease/infection	Regular preventive care at frequent intervals is important to avoid serious infection Antibiotics may be required for some dental procedures, especially if diabetes is poorly controlled. Dental appointments should be scheduled to minimize interference with regular mealtimes See also medication effects (Table 12-2)
Juvenile rheumatoid arthritis	May have difficulty opening mouth wide or soreness ("earache") if temporomandibular joint ("jaw joint") is involved If severe involvement of temporomandibular, deficient	Increased incidence of decay if restricted jaw opening limits oral hygiene	Increased incidence of gum disease if restricted jaw opening limits oral hygiene	

Table 12-1. Oral Effects of Disorders (*continued*)

Disorder	Bone	Teeth	Soft Tissue	Special Considerations
	growth of the lower jaw may occur requiring orthodontic and surgical management			
Seizure disorders	—	Surface of teeth may have markings At higher risk for traumatic injuries to teeth, especially upper incisors	—	Sedatives may be used in anxious patient to reduce anxiety and related seizure activity Mouth props are useful in guarding against sudden mouth closing in patients with poorly controlled seizures See specific drug effects (Table 12-2)
Cerebral palsy	May have a malocclusion related to poor muscle control and mouth breathing Facial bones may be asymmetrical depending on posture of patient	High incidence of gum disease related to poor oral hygiene and mouth breathing Teeth may have defective enamel (especially primary teeth) Teeth may be worn down from chronic tooth grinding (bruxism)	May have chapped lips from drooling Difficulty swallowing causes feeding problems	Food often remains on teeth because of swallowing problems, a low-sucrose diet is imperative Patient is usually unable to manage thorough oral hygiene on his own: an electric toothbrush may help Uncontrollable movements may be managed with reassurance, mouth props, physical restraint, and/or pharmacologic methods

Disorder	Bone	Teeth	Soft Tissue	Special Considerations
Respiratory diseases				
Asthma	—	—	Chronic mouth breathing causes increased gum disease	Psychological and pharmacologic techniques may be used to lessen anxiety regarding dental procedures to reduce anxiety-related asthmatic episodes If patient uses inhaler to control asthma, it should be brought to dental appointments See medication (Table 12-2) effects if patient is taking corticosteroids
Cystic fibrosis	—	Discoloration of teeth may occur following multiple exposures to some antibiotics (especially tetracyclines)	Gum inflammation is common due to chronic mouth-breathing	—

Table 12-2. Oral Effects of Treatments of Disorders

Agent	Bone	Teeth	Soft Tissue	Special Considerations
Drug				
Aspirin (chronic, high-dose, *chewable* or *liquid*)	—	Increased decay rate	—	Platelet function must be assessed before any surgical procedure
Cyclosporine	—	—	Enlargement of gums	—
Corticosteroids (long-term)	—	—	—	An increase in steroid dose may be required before and for a short time after dental treatment Patient may require antibiotics before and after dental treatment to prevent infection
Depakene (valproic acid)	—	—	—	Blood tests may be necessary before oral surgery or tooth extraction
Chemotherapeutic regimens	—	—	Oral ulcerations Bleeding gums Sore, smooth tongue	Poor resistance to infection Viral and fungal infections common May require antibiotics prior to and after dental treatment May require a mild surface anesthetic for sore areas Whenever possible, dental treatment should be provided in periods of remission
Dilantin (diphenylhydantoin sodium)	—	May have delayed eruption of teeth May have maligned teeth due to gum overgrowth	May have moderate to severe overgrowth of gums (about 50% of patients)	Gum enlargement often requires surgery Meticulous oral hygiene will reduce occurrence of gum overgrowth; appliances are sometimes used to control gum enlargement

Agent	Bone	Teeth	Soft Tissue	Special Considerations
Gold salts	—	—	Sore, irritated oral tissues	Blood tests may be necessary before oral surgery
Tegretol (carbamazepine)	—	—	—	—
Miscellaneous	—	—	—	Any sucrose-containing liquid or chewable tablet medication will promote decay of teeth if used on a long-term basis; patients requiring these medications for long term use should have their teeth cleaned immediately after each dose.
Other				
Radiation therapy (involving neck and jaw area)	—	More prone to rapid decay if salivary gland function is affected; Developing teeth may be destroyed by therapeutic radiation and fewer teeth may erupt	Dry mouth due to poor nonexistent salivary gland function; Sore mouth	Artificial saliva is available to help with dry mouth problems; Special trays can be made to apply fluoride to the decay-prone teeth; Badly decayed teeth should be extracted at least 10 days before radiation therapy to allow for bone to heal properly.

An additional area of importance in the training of the dentist who treats the handicapped child is behavior management. Many handicapped children have seen "too many white coats" and have developed high anxiety levels associated with any aspect of health care. This anxiety may prevent the delivery of care. The pediatric dentist, the hospital-trained general practitioner, or individuals who have received fellowship training have attained facility in the appropriate management of the behavior of the special child. In addition to traditional methods for addressing these children in a reassuring and forthright manner, these professionals have training and are skilled in the more complex approaches to behavior management. Modulation of the voice, familiarization of the child with the equipment involved, application of appropriate behavioral psychology, and a general understanding brought by the highly trained professional to the treatment setting are all important techniques for ensuring that care can be rendered for the child in need. The use of anti-anxiety techniques such as nitrous oxide/oxygen psychosedation and other pharmacologic agents increases the receptivity of these children to oral health care.

For the severely involved child, who is not capable of understanding the experience, pharmacologic approaches such as oral or injectable sedation and, where unavoidable, general anesthesia in the hospital operating room can be utilized more safely by these individuals. Appropriate training in this broad spectrum of skills provides the health care benefits to which the special child is entitled.

There are also training programs supported by various foundations to help train oral health care providers in these special areas. For example, the United Cerebral Palsy Foundation supports postdoctoral fellowships for dentists to spend an additional year of active learning and research in cerebral palsy and related conditions, with particular emphasis on the oral health care aspects of this disorder. The Robert Wood Johnson Foundation has supported training grants in schools and continues to provide funding for related projects to train general practitioners in managing the handicapped patient.

The current efforts of many dental schools in this area resulted from the support of these foundations. At this time, most dental schools provide some education regarding the special patient during the four-year doctoral curriculum. Additionally, the departments of pediatric dentistry in those schools provide specific information about care of the handicapped child. The parent or guardian of a child with a handicapping condition should feel no compunction in asking the prospective oral health care provider if he has experience in working with such children or if he would suggest another individual or setting for the child to receive appropriate care.

It may be difficult to identify individuals or centers where the special child can have access to appropriate, high-quality dental care. Certain national organizations can be useful in helping to obtain referrals. These organizations and their addresses are listed in Table 12-3. Most metropolitan

Table 12-3. Organizations Providing Information for the Handicapped

American Academy of Dentistry for the Handicapped
211 East Chicago Avenue
Chicago, IL 60611

American Academy of Pediatric Dentistry
211 East Chicago Avenue
Suite 1036
Chicago, IL 60611

American Association of Dental Schools
1625 Massachusetts Avenue, NW
Washington, DC 20036

American Society of Dentistry for Children
211 East Chicago Avenue
Suite 920
Chicago, IL 60611

Epilepsy Foundation of America
733 Fifteenth Street, NW
Washington, DC 20012

March of Dimes
622 Third Avenue
New York, NY 10007

Robert Wood Johnson Foundation
P.O. Box 2316
Princeton, NJ 08540

United Cerebral Palsy
66 East 34th Street
New York, NY 10016

areas will have at least one medical center with trained personnel and needed equipment to approach even the most severely handicapped child's needs. These programs may be either privately or government-supported and can usually be found by calling appropriate state agencies or through the general information office of the medical center. Additionally, if the child is enrolled in a special school or educational program, individuals involved at those sites are frequently aware of professional offices or centers where children can have access to quality care.

Sites exist and more are being developed where a child may be placed for a short period of time, i.e., three to six months, for intensive, rehabilitative medical and dental treatment. For instance, Blythedale Chidren's Hospital, located near New York City, provides dental care to all children admitted to receive appropriate medical, supportive, and rehabilitative services. A school, which is part of the local public school system, is in the center, thereby addressing the child's educational needs during the stay at the hospital. This center is similar to others that are being developed throughout the country as children with handicapping conditions are being assisted in attaining more normal, productive lives.

In summary, the child with handicapping conditions has a right to competent, appropriately delivered oral health care. The emphasis of this health care must be on prevention; these children, in addition to having the same oral disease patterns as the rest of the pediatric population, may have problems resulting from their handicapping condition. Identifying and reaching the practitioner with appropriate training is a critical issue for such children. The individual who will care for the child, in addition to being properly trained and experienced, should be part of a health care team that addresses the needs of the whole child. Children with handicapping conditions merit our special attention to guarantee that their quality of life can be as positive and as normal as possible.

Chapter 13

OCCUPATIONAL THERAPY

Marie L. Moore

Evaluation and analysis of occupational performance and behaviors are major responsibilities of occupational therapists. Within the bodies of knowledge utilized by occupational therapists are elements of biological, behavioral, and social sciences, with focus on adaptation to environmental demands. Specific adaptations of interest to occupational therapists are related to processes of self-maintenance, productivity, and leisure activity. Mosey (1981) defines occupational behaviors and performance as "ability to perform life tasks to meet own needs and be a contributing member of the community."

Human development throughout the life span is an essential component of knowledge for measuring performance of life tasks or daily living skills. Beginning with the neonate, occupational therapists provide essential services for improving or normalizing performance.

Farber and Williams (1982) describe primary occupations of the neonate associated with self-maintenance—rest, feeding, and elimination of metabolic waste products. Communication by crying is a developing skill for communicating psychologic needs for self-maintenance. The presence of an upper neuron lesion disrupts the self-maintenance process and becomes life-threatening unless there is intervention through the use of appropriate scientifically based procedures.

As the neonate develops into later stages of infancy, childhood, and adolescence, the emphasis expands to work and play as well as self-maintenance. Occupational therapists consider the development of skills necessary within the concept of temporal adaptation, which is defined as "the integration of an entire spectrum of activities, the organization of which supports health on an ongoing daily life basis" (Reed, 1984).

ROLES AND CONTRIBUTIONS

Occupational therapists serving children, youth, and their families have several roles. Many occupational therapists provide direct services described as a process of assessment, program planning, intervention or program implementation, reevaluation, discharge, and follow-up. Many other occupational therapists serve in the primary role of consultant, using the process of assessment; program recommendations; training of parents, teachers, and other significant persons in the life of the child; and monitoring the progress of status of the child (Clark & Allen, 1985). A smaller number of occupational therapists assume roles of educators or researchers in those specialty areas associated with disabling conditions common among children and youth. Roles and contributions of occupational therapists are usually related to length of experience and level of education.

In the areas of practice, education, and research there has been an increase in contributions made by occupational therapists relative to specific problems found from infancy through adolescence. Theories related to mastery in the performance of life tasks/occupations have been explored and refined. Habilitation processes are based on adaptations of purposeful behaviors and activities (Reed, 1984).

Among the pioneers of practice models frequently used in occupational therapy are A. Jean Ayers (sensory integration), Margaret S. Rood (sensorimotor), Lela A. Llorens (facilitating growth and development), Anne Cronin Mosey (adaptive performance), and Mary Reilly (occupational behavior). These models have been further synthesized by Barbara Banus (the neurobehavioral model) and Gilfoyle and Grady (the spatial–temporal adaptation model) (Reed, 1984). These models have a basis in neurosciences and psychosocial sciences that examine five skill-component areas required for performance of life tasks—neuromotor, sensory-integrative, cognitive, emotional, and social functions.

There are two levels of occupational therapy personnel who provide services—the occupational therapist, registered (OTR) and the certified occupational therapy assistant (COTA). The OTR is a graduate of an accredited professional education program, and the COTA is a graduate of an accredited technical education program. Both are required to pass national certification examinations prior to practicing within the profession. The role of the OTR is that of an independent practitioner who provides direct services to clients through evaluation, planning, implementation and administration of programs, and supervision of personnel. The COTA works under the direct supervision of the OTR or in consultation/collaboration with an OTR in providing direct services. In addition, the OTR may provide indirect services, including consultation, academic/continuing education, and research (Reed & Sanderson, 1983).

A case illustrative of the roles of occupational therapy personnel in direct service may involve an adolescent girl who has bladder and bowel control but is dependent on others for toileting. This problem has social/emotional as well as physical implications when she wishes to participate in activities with her normal peer group in the community. The OTR's assessment of areas of function and dysfunction in toileting is a first step in solving problems. The COTA may follow up with specific training for the client and also train selected peers to assist the client (Moore, 1983).

SOURCES OF CONTENT OF OCCUPATIONAL THERAPY SERVICES FOR CHILDREN AND YOUTH

Occupational therapy services for children and youth have been established within pediatric practice of the medical model of health care. As occupational therapists have moved from the traditional medical model to a biopsychosocial model, from the hospital to the education setting, from the residential institution to community-based programs and private practice, the scope of practice has expanded. Occupational therapy services include prevention, early identification, remediation (treatment), referral and health maintenance (Ramm, 1983).

The advent of PL 94-142 (the Education for All Handicapped Children Act) and the refinements of third-party purchase of service contracts (public and private) have brought forth significant documents that define occupational therapy processes and procedures in a number of settings. Three comprehensive publications are listed below:

1. *Training: Occupational Therapy Educational Management in Schools (TOTEMS).* Eight competency-based educational program modules developed by the American Occupational Therapy Association, Inc., Division of Professional Development; supported by the U.S. Department of Education, Office of Special Education and Rehabilitation Services Grant #G007801499. Edited by E. M. Gilfoyle (1979–1980).

2. *Occupational and Physical Therapy Services School Based Programs Organizational Manual 1982–1983.* A procedural manual developed by the Psychological Services Division of Harris County (Texas) Department of Education (McKee et al., 1982–1983).

3. *Occupational Therapy for Children.* A textbook edited by Pat Nuse Clark and Anne Stevens Allen, published by the C. V.

Mosby Company, 1985. Contributions of 22 occupational therapists describing the practice of pediatric occupational therapy.

There is a broad number of occupational therapy and related assessment tools for evaluating the function of neonates up through the adolescent years. Lists, samples, descriptions and sources of specific tools are found in Banus, Kent, Northon, Sukiennicki, and Becker (1979), Farber (1982), Hopkins and Smith (1983), and Clark and Allen (1985). Occupational therapy pioneers in the area of assessment include Mary Fiorentino (1972), Nancy Takata (1969), and A. Jean Ayers (1972). Assessment of adaptive behaviors and performance in the areas of sensory integration, gross/fine motor maturation, reflex integration and physical capacities are made, and diagnostic indicators are given for evaluating performance in feeding (oral motor) behaviors; independent function in eating, dressing, grooming and hygiene; performance of education-related sensorimotor activities; performance of vocation-related sensorimotor activities; emotional/social behaviors; and use of non-verbal communication devices requiring selected motor responses.

WHERE OCCUPATIONAL THERAPISTS ARE EMPLOYED

The report *Occupational Therapy Manpower: A Plan for Progress* (Ad Hoc Commission, 1985), based on a 1982 survey, includes the following:

Thirty-three percent (33%) of the occupational therapists registered and 17.5 percent of the certified occupational therapy assistants work exclusively with patients/clients under the age of twenty (20). This is an increase of both practitioners, from previous surveys but a greater increase among COTA's than OTR's due to the former having increased number of positions in school systems. School systems employ 18.3 percent of the OTR's and 11.3 percent of the COTA's. Among occupational therapy personnel working with diagnostic groups associated with childhood and youth the breakdown is as follows:

Health Problem	OTRs	COTAs
Cerebral palsy	12.6%	6.6%
DD other than MR	12.9%	4.8%
MR	10.1%	16.4%

Occupational therapy personnel are employed where there are populations at risk (i.e., premature births, adolescent parents, abused children), children with correctable impairments, and children with multiple/severe impairments that last throughout life. Programs for these populations include *prevention* through facilitation of the health aspects of development, *health maintenance* through the prevention of further dysfunction and the maintenance of competency, and *remediation* through the reduction of pathology-producing limitations in function (Banus et al., 1979).

The settings are varied from the home to short-term residential facilities (Clark & Allen, 1985). Specific places include but are not limited to the following:

Neonatal intensive care units

Public health departments

Well-baby clinics

Home health services/agencies

Physicians' offices and clinics

Community health centers

Health maintenance organizations

Pediatric units of general hospitals

Rehabilitation centers

Residential programs

Day training centers

Infant development programs

Public school systems

Private schools

Preschool programs

Private practice (individual or collaborative)

The Occupational Therapist as Member of the Interdisciplinary Team

The involvement of occupational therapists as team members varies from setting to setting and program to program. Inherent in team membership is the role definition for the occupational therapist, which is unique and also complementary to the knowledge and skills of the other team members. As a contributor to the master plan of habilitation for individual children/youth, the occupational therapist must be able to interpret assessment findings in the context of the total multidisciplinary evaluation for establishing long- and short-range goals.

To determine the unique role of the occupational therapist as a team member, it has been the responsibility of the occupational therapy profession to establish the perimeters and guidelines for occupational therapy personnel as in their *Uniform Terminology for Reporting Occupational Therapy Services* (American Occupational Therapy Association, 1979). Other guidelines are documented in the *Standards of Practice for Occupational Therapy Services* (1979–1980).

Ways of functioning by occupational therapists are dependent on the setting and the major objectives of services. In the health care-related program, the occupational therapist is a contributor to the individual program plan (IPP), and the objectives are health-related in focus. In the educational setting, the occupational therapist contributes to the individual educational plan (IEP) with education-related objectives. Other settings may have emotional/social primary objectives or prevocational/vocational goals.

Although the evaluation processes performed by occupational therapists are uniquely focused, the integrated plan of the interdisciplinary team should be holistic in the development of goals and objectives. Therefore, implementation of the plan in terms of specific occupational therapy objectives may be carried out by other team members, including parents, teachers, pediatric nurses, and other specialists who have frequent contact with the child/youth.

The lists of team members associated with specific settings vary according to the services. The most common associates of occupational therapists are physical therapists, speech and hearing therapists, nurses, and social workers. Other professional specialists include but are not limited to neurologists, orthopedists, pediatricians, neonatologists, prosthetists/orthotists, psychiatrists, psychologists, classroom teachers, special education/resource teachers, nutritionists and vocational rehabilitation counselors. Parents/guardians and the older child/youth capable of making informed decisions are a critical part of the team.

TRAINING OF OCCUPATIONAL THERAPISTS

According to *Occupational Therapy Manpower: A Plan for Progress* (1985), there are 60 colleges and universities that offer accredited entry-level preparation of occupational therapists. There are 57 community colleges, junior colleges, and technical institutes that offer approved educational programs for the occupational therapy assistant. Graduates of these programs are eligible to take the national certification examinations, and successful examinees are then designated as OTRs or COTAs. Twenty-seven states, the District of Columbia, and Puerto Rico require a license to practice in addition to certification. Some state boards of education require that occupational therapists meet their state certification requirements.

There are 23 universities offering postprofessional master's degree programs, of which two offer doctoral programs in occupational therapy. There are six programs in pediatrics and three in sensory-integration, which are areas directly related to services/research pertaining to children and youth.

The manpower report also indicates an increase in specialization with an increase in specialty certification among members of the American Occupational Therapy Association (AOTA) and the emergence of cross-discipline associations, i.e., sensory integration and neurodevelopmental treatment. There are two special interest sections within the AOTA—developmental disabilities and sensory integration—that are devoted to service, education, and research of dysfunction in children/youth.

UNMET NEEDS

Unmet needs of the young disabled and their families requiring professional occupational therapy services within a variety of settings are a problem of maldistribution of manpower and services. The supply of occupational therapy personnel is less than the demand nationwide, with a paucity in numbers of occupational therapists in southern states, which are increasing in population. There is a lack of services for populations in rural areas as well as in community-based facilities serving children and youth who are not placed in school system programs due to age or location. There is a greater need for respite programs for families that do not have extended family ties.

Societal problems have produced needs centered around incidence and prevalence of children born at risk. There is an increase of high-risk mothers under age sixteen and over age thirty-five. There is also a greater need for programs that offer early intervention and prevention.

There is a continuation of gaps in the eligibility for services, especially dyspraxic children who score high on achievement testing but rarely reach their full potential without intervention of occupational therapy services because sensory-integrated problems that result in specific learning disabilities. Another group of children having difficulty with eligibility for occupational therapy services is the group with severe/profound disabilities associated with oral–motor control and toilet training. In some school systems the interpretation of the law is such that priority for services or limited funding for services does not include all children in need.

There is a greater need for occupational therapists as well as other members of the interdisciplinary team to provide public and consumer education concerning the services and programs for disabled children/youth. This results in parents and guardians not being able to participate with informed consent in the habilitation process. Persons from low-income, educationally disadvantaged, poor-resource families are particularly vulnerable in their participation in the IPP and IEP.

SUMMARY

Occupational therapists and the profession of occupational therapy have a great involvement in the services for children and youth with disabilities. The focus of occupational therapy practice is the performance of life tasks in areas of self-maintenance, productivity (work), and leisure activities. The models of service, education, and research generated by occupational therapists are ever increasing for prevention of dysfunction and the development of function to improve the quality of life for children/youth and their families.

ACKNOWLEDGEMENTS

Shirley Holland Carr, MS, L/OTR, FAOTA; Elenora Hines, M. Ed., R.D.; selected members of the senior class 1986—Glendale A. Holmes, OTS; Hilary D. Lamar, OTS; Marcia V. Thomas, OTS; Gayle M. Williams, OTS—who served as editors for this chapter; and Mildred F. Moore, who prepared the manuscript.

REFERENCES

Ad Hoc Commission on Occupational Therapy Manpower. (1985). *Occupational therapy manpower: A plan for progress.* Rockville, MD: American Occupational Therapy Association.

American Occupational Therapy Association. (1979). *Uniform terminology for reporting occupational therapy services.* Rockville, MD: Author.

American Occupational Therapy Association. (1979–1980). *Occupational therapy standards of practice—physical disabilities, mental health, developmental disabilities, home health program, in the schools.* Rockville, MD: Author.

Ayers, A. J. (1972). *Sensory integration and learning disorders.* Los Angeles: Western Psychological Services.

Banus, B. S., Kent, C. A., Northon, Y. D., Sukiennicki, D. R., & Beckerr, M. L. (1979). *The developmental therapist* (2nd ed.). Thorofare, NJ: Charles B. Slack.

Clark, P. N., & Allen, A. S. (Eds.). (1985). *Occupational therapy for children.* St. Louis: C. V. Mosby.

Farber, S. D. (Ed.). (1982). *Neurorehabilitation of multisensory approach.* Philadelphia: W. B. Saunders.

Farber, S. D., & Williams, S. 1982. Neonatology. In S. D. Farber (Ed.), *Neurorehabilitation: A multisensory approach* (pp. 178–185). Philadelphia: W. B. Saunders.

Fiorentino, M.R. (1972). *Normal and abnormal development: The influences of primitive reflexes on motor development.* Springfield, IL: Charles C. Thomas.

Gilfoyle, E. M. (Ed.). (1979–1980). *Training: Occupational therapy educational management in schools (a competency-based educational program)* (Vol. 1–4). Rockville, MD: American Occupational Therapy Association.

Hopkins, H. L., & Smith, H. D. (Eds.). (1983). *Willard and Spackman's occupational therapy* (6th ed.). Philadelphia: J. B. Lippincott Company.

McKee, M., daCunha, K., Echols, L., Starr, C., Naskrent, D., & Urbanovsky, J. (Eds.). (1982–1983). *Occupational and physical therapy services. School based programs: An organizational manual.* Houston, TX: Psychological Services Division of Harris County Department of Education.

Moore, M. L. (1983). Movement: Therapeutic intervention. In *Programming for adolescents with cerebral palsy and related disabilities* (pp. 27–33). New York: United Cerebral Palsy Associations and Cathleen Lyle Murray Foundation.

Mosey, A. C. (1981). *Occupational therapy: Configuration of a profession.* New York: Raven Press.

Ramm, P. A. (1983). Pediatric occupational therapy. In H. L. Hopkins & H. D. Smith (Eds.), *Willard and Spackman's occupational therapy* (pp. 573–587). Philadelphia: J. B. Lippincott.

Reed, K. L. (1984). *Models of practice in occupational therapy.* Baltimore, Williams & Wilkins.

Reed, K. L., & Sanderson, S. R. (1983). *Concepts of occupational therapy* (2nd ed.). Baltimore: Williams & Wilkins.

Takata, N. (1969). The play history. *American Journal of Occupational Therapy, 23,* 314–318.

Chapter 14

THE ROLE OF PHYSICIANS WITH HANDICAPPED CHILDREN AND YOUTH

Clifford J. Sells

The role of physicians in the care of handicapped children and youth has changed dramatically during the past several decades and will undoubtedly continue to change as old medical problems are solved and new ones unfold. The problems brought to physicians 30 to 35 years ago and the diagnostic modalities and therapeutic agents available to them were far different from those of today. Yesterday's physicians caring for children spent most of their time managing infectious diseases and their sequelae. Uncomplicated bacterial infections of the ear, throat, and lungs frequently led to serious complications including chronic otitis media with spreading to the central nervous system, pharyngitis with subsequent rheumatic heart disease or acute glomerulonephritis, and pneumonia with its well-known associated pulmonary complications.

With the introduction of antibiotics in the early 1950s, the physician caring for children has been able to prevent many of the serious complications associated with bacterial infections. Today, although bacterial infections remain problematic, physicians caring for infants and children spend considerably less time than their earlier counterparts in treating and managing acute bacterial infectious diseases and their sequelae. Immunizations also have impacted dramatically on the practice of medicine. Effective vaccines have eliminated smallpox and have dramatically reduced the incidence of poliomyelitis, pertussis, rubeola, rubella, diphtheria, and tetanus. New vaccines promise to reduce further the incidence and sequelae of both bacteria-and virus-associated infections.

In addition to changes in the treatment of infectious diseases, other important changes have occurred that impact on the physician's time and practice. Whereas infant feeding used to occupy a significant amount of the physician's time, the introduction of excellent proprietary formulas and the increasing trend toward breast feeding have considerably reduced physician involvement in this area of patient care. Concomitant with the rapid and profound changes in medical practice, several important societal factors also have significant impact on the physician caring for children and youth. Decreasing family size, working mothers, child care concerns, the single-parent family, and altered life-styles have all influenced the types of problems presented to physicians who care for children. Central to these and other emerging societal changes is the concern for the individual and his present and future quality of life. Major controversy currently surrounds the quality-of-life issue. When, how much, and what services will be provided for individuals with identified or potential handicaps, particularly for infants who were born with various kinds of impairments, are but some of the questions being debated. Although medical issues are central to the problem, the decisions to be made are not merely medical and involve the ethical, moral, and legal arenas as well, as they are enmeshed in the basic fabric of society itself.

For years individuals with a variety of chronic handicapping conditions received no educational services and were either kept at home or placed in some type of institution. In recent years, largely because of concerned parents and various advocacy groups, educational services began to be developed. Two major events provided the stimulus for this movement: deinstitutionalization and the federal mandate that all handicapped children are entitled to an appropriate education in the least restrictive environment (PL 94-142, 1975, Education for All Handicapped Children Act). Removing children from institutions, placing them in the community, and providing an appropriate education for them has been and continues to be a major challenge not only for physicians but for educators and other health personnel. As a result, physicians caring for handicapped children now are being asked to provide a much broader array of services than in the past. What then should be the role of the physician in caring for handicapped children and youth?

GENERAL PRIMARY CARE

Today's children in the United States are cared for by various types of health professionals. Nevertheless, the vast majority of children receive their primary health care from either general pediatricians or family physicians. The primary care physician's role is, first and foremost, management. The concept of management is central to the care of the handicapped child as well as to the care of the nonhandicapped. Management involves doing all that is humanly and medically possible to improve the quality of life for the patient and his family.

The primary care physician's role is (a) to treat any medical condition that the child has or, if the problem is outside the primary care physician's area of expertise, to ensure that the child is referred to the appropriate specialist for treatment; (b) to provide ongoing health supervision for the child; and (c) to provide consultation and assistance to the family through interpretation, education, and counseling about the child's handicap and what can be done about it.

The child with a handicap often has other medical conditions that contribute to the severity of the impairment. Not infrequently, children with a chronic handicap receive less sophisticated basic health care because of their handicap. Providing the same type of care to the handicapped child as to his nonhandicapped peers often requires additional physician time and effort, for which the provider is often not reimbursed. The child with a handicap also may be less likely to be referred to a specialist because of the increased difficulty of providing the specialty care that may be indicated. Inadequate reimbursement for the additional time and effort required of the specialist is also problematic.

Physicians providing primary care for the child with a handicap often are uncomfortable caring for such children; thus, they may tend to do less for that child, with respect to diagnosis and, at times, to treatment, than they do for a nonhandicapped child. Primary care physicians often have had little training and experience in providing care for children with chronic handicapping conditions. They may be frustrated in trying to treat such patients. Physicians are trained to diagnose, treat, and cure medical problems. When a patient does not get well, and may even get worse during management, the physician's frustration is understandable. These feelings are usually readily apparent to the child's parents. Primary care physicians must be aware of their limitations. Yet they must also attempt to provide the most sophisticated care they can and to assume responsibility for ensuring that the care they cannot or do not provide is provided by another appropriate source.

Primary care physicians also should provide ongoing health supervision. Unfortunately, at times, even physicians who provide excellent, state-of-the-art health care supervision for normal children may provide less than ideal services for their handicapped patients. Handicapped children, no less than normal children, need immunizations, developmental screening, school-readiness evaluations, and help with behavioral management. Parents of handicapped children, possibly even more than parents of normal children, need help with anticipatory guidance, accident prevention, and feeding and nutrition concerns as well as with other developmental issues. Because of the myriad of services often required by the handicapped child, fragmentation is inevitable unless one individual assumes responsibility for coordinating the overall health care plan. Primary care physicians are uniquely positioned to orchestrate the handicapped child's care plan. Included in their responsibilities, in addition to ensuring that appropriate health care supervision and needed referrals are carried out, are interpretation, education, and counseling the family regarding the child's handicap and what can be done about it. Often the primary care physician also may be asked to interpret the results of medical subspecialist evaluations, explain nonmedical evaluation results, and help with implementation of the recommendations. Finally, the primary care physician, because he knows the child better than any other health care provider, is uniquely able to advocate for the child. Often major obstacles to treatment and program implementation can be overcome by the physician's expressed interest and input to the appropriate individual or agency.

ROLE OF THE PEDIATRICIAN

Most practicing pediatricians provide primary health care for their patients. Thus, the pediatrician's role in management of children with chronic handicapping conditions is to treat or refer for appropriate treatment any medical condition that arises, to provide general health supervision, and to support and guide the family through evaluation and counseling regarding the problem and what can be done abut it. In addition, as a specialist in child care, the pediatrician has specific expertise in normal child development as well as in the evaluation, diagnosis, and management of children with a vast array of medical disorders. Often the pediatrician is the first person the child's mother seeks help from when the child is not performing at age level in any of a number of areas. Parents often are the first to notice that their child has a problem, but unfortunately, some physicians dismiss or do not take seriously early parental concerns. Good pediatric practice mandates that infants and older children be regularly screened for certain metabolic disorders and medical conditions as well as for general development. When a possible problem is uncovered, a thorough comprehensive evaluation may be indicated and may include referral to the appropriate specialist for definitive diagnosis and treatment. A pediatrician is ideally suited to function as a case manager, orchestrating the child's overall care. He provides the parent with counseling and guidance regarding the problem, explains what the referral to the specialist will involve, interprets the subspecialty results to the family, helps to implement management plans, and, more important, discusses with the family what can be expected of the child in the future. Monitoring follow-along services and determining the need for appropriate reevaluations and/or additional subspecialty referrals are also key activities the pediatrician should provide.

In addition to the general responsibilities of the pediatrician in caring for his normal *and* handicapped patients, there are several responsibilities uniquely called for because of the child's handicap. Pediatricians are generally well-respected members of society and as such can very effectively advocate for more and improved services for handicapped children. As members of school boards, or by serving on the boards of a variety of agencies, the pediatrician can have significant influence on the development and improvement of services for the handicapped. A pediatrician also can be most helpful to parents of handicapped children by being knowledgeable about potential sources of support for the myriad services that the child or family may need. State-of-the-art services are of little value if the family cannot afford them or if parents are unaware of their availability.

A major service pediatricians should provide for their patients is counseling regarding unproved, untested, or questionable remedies. Parents of the handicapped are particularly vulnerable to newly touted "cures," and at any given time there are many controversial treatments purported by their proponents to be effective in the treatment of the handicapped. Pediatricians must be knowledgeable about these controversial "remedies" and must be able to discuss them objectively with parents, pointing out the merits, lack of merits, and possible harmful effects. Telling a parent that a particular treatment is worthless without an explanation or evidence supporting the statement may lead to parents' shopping for remedies and lack of confidence in the pediatrician. Parents are exposed to numerous medical articles in the lay press, and pediatricians also must be aware of these.

One of the pediatrician's most important roles in caring for the child with a chronically handicapping condition concerns proper diagnosis. Etiologic factors should be thoroughly investigated because most parents of handicapped children experience considerable guilt and spend vast amounts of time and effort searching for the cause(s) of their child's handicap. Because they lack accurate medical knowledge, parents often have considerable fear as well as guilt, and they may even misplace "blame." Medical shopping is not infrequent as parents seek diagnoses and treatments they are more comfortable with. Accurate medical information explained in understandable terms often can alleviate much of the parents' fear, guilt, and misplaced blame as well as prevent medical shopping.

A second reason for seeking a specific diagnosis is that it will assist in genetic counseling, should the parents want it. A specific diagnosis allows for a much more precise recurrent risk estimate than is possible without one. A specific diagnosis may in many instances prevent a similar problem in the future and, at times, permit implementation of a specific treatment. Finally, a specific diagnosis allows one to anticipate future complications as well as plan for whatever the child faces in the future.

In addition to providing a thorough diagnostic evaluation and treating the child's medical problems, a pediatrician should provide ongoing guidance and counseling for parents. "Why does my child have this problem?" and "What can I do about it?" are two of the questions most frequently asked of pediatricians. A pediatrician must deal with the family and the problem at the level on which it is presented. All parents exhibit some denial and guilt. A pediatrician must deal with this guilt in a straightforward, factual manner.

Often a thorough medical evaluation performed by the pediatrician will help parents to accept the problem; medical data from the evaluation will often clarify the etiology and thus alleviate the guilt parents feel regarding their role in causing the problem. How the pediatrician interprets to the parent the medical findings and what they mean to the child and his future is paramount in the management of the child. Will my child be independent as an adult? Is the disease progressive? What about children for my child? What resources are available to help me? Is there any hope? These are but a few of the delicate questions that often need to be answered. Information should be described in a factual manner. In counseling parents, the parent's own level of sophistication must be taken into consideration. Parents have "selected hearing" and may not carry away all that is intended. Thus, information may need to be repeated over time. The child's assets as well as his handicaps need to be addressed. Parents want to know what is right with their child as well as what is wrong with him. The pediatrician must share with parents easily comprehensible information regarding the diagnosis and treatment, being realistic rather than either overly pessimistic or overly optimistic. Pediatricians caring for handicapped children must remember that their management should be family-centered while focusing on the child's needs. A handicapped child does not exist in a vacuum. He is an integral part of the family who impacts and is impacted on by all of the family members. Chronic handicapping conditions are by definition long-term and as such require long-term care. Needs change over time and thus require the pediatrician to revaluate and update management strategies periodically.

Finally, health care is but one aspect of a handicapped child's overall needs. The pediatrician should help coordinate the resources necessary to address the child's physical, mental, emotional, educational, and social requirements over time. This requires the knowledge and the willingness to cooperate with and work with other disciplines as well as with various medical subspecialists on behalf of the handicapped child.

THE FAMILY

Handicapped children are part of a larger social unit—the family. Often the child's ultimate well-being to a large part depends on the family's adjustment to having a handicapped child. The physician can play a central role in helping the family cope with raising the child. Besides providing health care and health supervision and coordinating the many resources that may be necessary for the child, the physician must continually be aware of the interactive impact between the child and the family. Siblings frequently have difficulty adjusting and may need some assistance in coping with the presence of a handicapped brother or sister. Marriages are often strained. By helping parents recognize the problems the handicapped child presents for them and, more important, what can be done to lessen this burden, the physician can be of immense help to the family.

Helping to secure funding for needed medical and related services or helping parents secure baby sitting or other respite care may play a monumental role in improving the family's quality of life. Directing a family to an appropriate educational service and helping parents to get necessary medical services for their handicapped child offer additional assistance to the family. Central to helping the family deal with the handicapped child is directing efforts on activities that will improve the child rather than on accepting a child as is. There is an important distinction between a handicapped child and a child with a handicap: even children with severe handicaps have many more similarities to than differences from other children. Parents want to be reminded about what is right with their child, not just what is wrong. They also desire to be a part of the team caring for the child, not an "outsider." A recurrent theme of parents with a handicapped child in dealing with physicians is that they want to be treated as the physician would like to be treated. They want to be listened to and to actively participate in their child's management. They want to be recognized as having a child with a handicap, not as a "handicapped family." They also want normalcy for their normal children. As one parent stated so aptly when asked what she wanted for her handicapped child when he grew up, "I want my child to be happy and to be accepted by society for what he *can* rather than what he *can't* do."

THE SPECIALIST

Handicapped children may require an array of specialists in order to be provided the comprehensive services their disability dictates. These services generally are coordinated by the child's primary health care provider. Most medical schools and other large medical centers have available the type of services necessary for evaluation, diagnosis, and management of children with complex handicapping conditions. Nevertheless, children with various types of handicapping conditions do not always receive the types of services their impairment demands. Primary health care providers may be unaware of the services available to their patients or they may feel that referral to a specialist is unnecessary. Referral centers are often intimidating to parents, and there may be long waiting periods before they can be seen. Tertiary care services may be expensive, and reimbursement by third-party payers often may be inadequate. Some chronic handicapping conditions may not be reimbursed by third-party payers at all. In addition, specialty clinics may not be geographically accessible to families with handicapped children. In response to the latter, some medical centers have encouraged the development of community clinics staffed by hospital-based specialists. Coordination of such services creates some problems, but overall, community-based clinics may prove to be an efficient and effective way to provide specialty services in the families' own communities. Community clinics not only may provide appropriate care close to the child's home, but they also have the potential benefit of involving the child's primary care physician in the treatment/management. Thus, community clinics can help decrease the fragmentation often associated with the care of handicapped children by improving case management coordination.

Close cooperation between the child's primary care physician and the specialist is paramount if handicapped children are to receive optimal services. At the University of Washington a telephone consultation service—Medcon—is available for community physicians. Practicing physicians receive information from a battery of university consultants regarding patient-care matters. Many of these same physicians participate in a variety of continuing education and community clinic activities.

UNMET NEEDS

Despite the rather remarkable progress that has been made in the past decade, many children with chronic handicapping conditions continue to receive less and often far less than optimal care. According to the Task Force on Pediatric Education (1978), the care provided to children with chronic handicapping continues to be grossly inadequate. The Task Force noted that even though pediatricians are uniquely qualified to provide the care, too many pediatric residency programs underemphasize this aspect of pediatrics. Physicians and other health care professionals trained to provide care for children with chronic handicapping conditions remain in short supply in many parts of the country. Medical school curricula often place a lower priority on pediatrics than on adult medicine, and chronic disease in children may receive little emphasis. Training support has recently been drastically reduced, and quality training programs are far too few in number to meet current demands. Third-party reimbursement for pediatric services remains problematic, particularly for preventive services and for support of children with chronic handicapping conditions. Such services are frequently not covered by third-party payers; in addition, when services are covered, providers are only partially reimbursed. The Task Force on Pediatric Education noted the problem associated with the current fee-for-service reimbursement mechanism. They recommended that fair reimbursement mechanisms be developed for time spent, not for number of patients seen. Nonphysician health professionals caring for handicapped children are even less likely to have their services reimbursed by third-party payers. Thus, financing of comprehensive health care services for handicapped children remains a major problem.

In addition to the aforementioned issues of physician training and service reimbursement, geographic distribution of available services is also a major problem. The factors that affect the geographic distribution of physicians are multiple and include the site of medical and residency training, the location of the family and friends, the medical needs of the community, the personal life-style preference of the physician, and the income opportunity. The result is that the number of physicians available and the geographic distribution of physicians are equally important with respect to the provision of health care services for children.

Finally, one cannot stress too strongly the need for interdisciplinary cooperation and respect if handicapped children are to receive optimal care. Physicians cannot care for their patients properly without the help of numerous child-centered professionals. Physicians' educational colleagues must be informed about the medical needs of their students, particularly as they relate to the child's education. Teachers, on the other hand, are in a position to assist physicians in caring for their patients and have a unique opportunity to educate them regarding the educational aspects of their patients.

Providing comprehensive, quality health care services for children, particularly for children with chronic handicapping conditions, remains a challenge not only for physicians but for society in general. Medical technology has exceeded our ability and willingness to apply rationally the advances presented almost daily to physicians. With limited financial and manpower resources, it is most important that the well-being of children with handicapping conditions be given at least as high a priority by society as that of their normal peers.

References

The Task Force on Pediatric Education. (1978). *The future of pediatric education.* Evanston, IL: American Academy of Pediatrics.

Chapter 15

SERVICES FOR SPEECH AND COMMUNICATION DISORDERS

Betty Byers-Brown

A disorder of communication arises when a person cannot easily make himself understood through the language of his community or cannot fully understand that language when used by others. Because speech is the preferred medium for language exchange in our society, communication disorders will frequently manifest themselves in the form of disturbances of speech. Services for children with communication disorders must include specific remediation for speech problems but will be primarily directed to ensure that the person can use and understand the language that binds the community together.

Distinction must be made between those who use local or dialectal variants of a language and those who attempt to use the standard form but produce it defectively (Taylor, 1982). There also must be distinction made between people from other cultures who are capable of using the language of a new community but who have not yet mastered its code and those who grow up within the culture but cannot use its language adequately. Those who need to learn a new code may be helped by teachers; those who fail to master their own will require the help of those professionals who specialize in speech, language, and hearing pathology and in remediation.

Disorders of communication may be caused by hearing loss, anatomical or structural defects of the organs of speech and hearing, neurological impairment, emotional disturbance, or severe environmental deprivation. In many cases the communication disorder is a secondary handicap associated with primary motor or cognitive impairment. However, as the child develops, the emphasis may change. Lencione (1966) has pointed out that in persons with cerebral palsy the associated language disabilities may prove a greater handicap to learning and to social intercourse than does the restriction on mobility.

In other cases the communication disorder constitutes the primary handicap. The child shows no gross neurological disability, hearing loss, psychiatric impairment or cognitive deficit. Nevertheless, he is slow to develop speech, and that speech is disordered (Ingram, 1976).

PROFESSIONALS CONCERNED WITH COMMUNICATION DISORDERS

The complex nature of communication problems means that many different professionals are involved in their management. These include pediatricians, neurologists, otolaryngologists, orthodontists, plastic surgeons, audiologists, psychologists, psychiatrists, speech-language pathologists, classroom teachers, and learning consultants. Some professions carry more responsibility than others for creating and maintaining services for the communicatively handicapped. The profession that has communication disorders as its central concern is that of speech-language pathology. This title was adopted in 1979 in the attempt to clarify the professional role. It superseded the term speech therapy, which is still retained in the United Kingdom for want of a better alternative (Byers-Brown, 1981). In other countries the professional is variously known as language-speech pathologist (Canada), speech pathologist (Australia), and logopedist (several European countries).

The difficulty in determining a title arises from the wide range of disorders that constitute communication impairment and the very varied nature of the diagnostic and remedial tasks.

SPEECH-LANGUAGE PATHOLOGY

The science and practice of speech-language pathology is not generated by one theory as to the nature of communication. It is nourished by research from many disciplines, including acoustics, neurophysiology, and linguistics, and its application is influenced by both medical and educational practice (Flower, 1985). The field is rapidly expanding because there has been considerable growth in all of the subjects with which it is associated. It is now no longer possible for a practitioner to keep abreast of developments across the whole field (Travis, 1971). The work of the whole profession embraces every aspect of communication disorder: perceptual and productive language problems, vocal disorders, stuttering, and articulatory disabilities. Because hearing loss is highly correlated with most of these, the speech-language pathologist also must be able to identify hearing problems and work with the hearing-impaired. However, the main responsibility for assessing the nature and extent of any hearing loss and advising on management lies with the audiologist. These two professional groups, speech-language pathology and audiology, together constitute the majority of those enrolled in the professional association predominatly associated with communication disorders in the United States, the American Speech-Language-Hearing Association (ASHA). ASHA is responsible for determining the standards for professional entry and for maintaining the code of ethical practice.

TRAINING

To qualify as a speech-language pathologist the candidate must follow a program of general education, specialized academic requirements, and practical clinical training. Students who terminate their studies at the bachelor's level are not entitled to use the term speech-language pathologist. They may be employed as speech correctionists in some institutions if they have taken the requisite course work at an accredited university. The standard of entry into the profession of speech-language pathology is that of the master's degree obtained at an institution accredited by ASHA. The doctorate has not been required for clinical practice, but its role is now under active consideration (Feldman, 1984; Punch & Fein, 1984).

REGULATION OF PRACTICE

The public may be protected from unqualified practitioners through the procedures of the state licensing board and those of ASHA. The latter requires candidates who have completed their academic requirements to undertake a year of supervised clinical practice. After the completion of this clinical fellowship year they may be awarded a Certificate of Clinical Competence in Audiology (CCC/A) or Speech-Language Pathology (CCC/Sp). Foreign-trained applicants may submit their qualifications to ASHA. Recognition may be granted to those whose standards are equivalent to those operating in the United States. However, all candidates are required to pass the national examination, which is part of the certification procedure. State licensure is now in effect in 37 states. Speech and hearing professionals serve on the licensing boards and are thus able to coordinate state and professional demands.

Speech-language pathologists working in the school systems must have a certificate issued by the state department of education.

THE NATURE OF THE SERVICES

The clinical work carried out by speech-language pathologists may be classified under three headings: prevention or prophylaxis, assessment and monitoring, therapeutic intervention.

Prevention

Screening programs are an essential component of prevention. They are carried out through the public schools, which since the passage of the Education for All Handicapped Children Act (PL 94-142) have extended their responsibilities to preschool children. Speech-language pathologists and audiologists are active in promoting early communication screening for infants and young children by primary care personnel. Among the measures that will encourage this tendency has been a grant awarded by the Robert Wood Johnson Foundation to five medical education institutions for the specific purpose of training primary health clinicians in the early identification and management of communication disorders. These institutions are housed in the universities of Colorado, Iowa, and South Florida, the University of Medicine and Dentistry of New Jersey-Rutgers Medical School, and Vanderbilt University.

The screening of high-risk populations for hearing impairment is now widespread. Provision and criteria are under regular review by state and professional bodies (American Academy of Pediatrics, 1982; Gerkin, 1984).

Professionals are recognizing their responsibility to inform the public of the need for early identification of communication handicaps. Outreach procedures include the distribution of posters and brochures to guide parents, open houses at speech and hearing clinics, television and radio interviews, and articles written for local papers. The telephone numbers of ASHA and local speech and hearing associations are given maximum publicity.

Assessment and Monitoring

Assessment and monitoring procedures go into operation once a potential problem has been identified. Normal young children vary in their rate of speech acquisition (Morley, 1972), so regular monitoring is the best way to determine whether the child is having real difficulty or is simply taking a slower route. Unfortunately, it is not always possible to provide this monitoring without direct cost to the parents if the child shows no medical pathology. When a child is classified as handicapped or medically at risk, he may be monitored by the speech–language pathologist as a member of the high-risk follow-up team. Children also may be seen by the speech–language pathologist alone.

A number of tools for the assessment of communication skills is available for preschool and school-age children. However, the number available for the very young is more restricted (Lewis & Byers-Brown, 1985).

Therapeutic Intervention

Therapeutic intervention may be undertaken at any age, through infancy to adolescence. In infants with severe neurological dysfunction, intervention may take the form of promoting the primary functions of sucking, chewing, and swallowing. Not only are these essential for life but they pave the way for secondary function, or the adaptation of the vocal–respiratory tract for speech.

Early intervention programs may promote communication skills in the handicapped by improving the quality of the parent-child interaction. Speech-language pathologists work as members of the early intervention teams, sharing their expertise and benefiting from the expertise of others.

Multidisciplinary teaching programs are particularly applicable to children with pervasive language disorders. These programs cover the development of both cognitive and linguistic skills and are carried out within a number of institutions.

Other types of intervention are carried out by the speech–language pathologist in order to effect a specific change in language use, articulation or voice production, or fluency control. Here the speech-language pathologist may work alone or in conjunction with a physician or teacher.

The teams in which the speech-language pathologist participates to serve the communicatively handicapped will vary in composition with the type of child served. If the disorder from which the child suffers is a pervasive one, as is common in early language problems, the team is likely to be large. If the problem is restricted to one element of the communication process—for example, the malproduction of a group of consonants associated with tongue thrust—the speech-language pathologist may work on his own or in association with the orthodontist. Listed below are some of the teams within which the speech–language pathologist may be included.

High-risk follow-up—neonatologist, pediatrician, nurse practitioner, physical therapist, occupational therapist, audiologist, psychologist, speech-language pathologist.

Cleft palate—plastic surgeon, orthodontist, otolaryngologist, audiologist, speech-language pathologist.

Child study team—school physician, psychologist, learning consultant, social worker, classroom teacher, speech-language pathologist.

Rehabilitation—pediatrician, physical therapist, occupational therapist, speech-language pathologist.

Language class—teacher, psychologist, learning consultant, speech–language pathologist.

Stuttering treatment program—speech-language pathologist.

These teams are not comprehensive but illustrative of the professionals
involved in different types of treatment and management programs. Parents
are members of all preschool teams, but the amount of emphasis placed on
their role will vary with the program.

In accordance with the ruling of PL 94-142 that handicapped children
must be placed in the least restricted environment, children will be mainstreamed, or integrated into the normal classroom, wherever possible. The
teacher and the speech-language pathologist will work together to promote
the children's language skills, and the latter may work as consultant or resi-
dent staff member according to need. Many speech-language pathologists
now also see their role as helping to create a school environment conducive
to language learning.

Augmentative communication, or the use of mechanical aids and non-
verbal language systems, is one of the major developments in the field of
communication management (Holland, 1984) and is enabling very handicapped pupils to participate in group activities as well as developing individual language skills.

WORK SITES

The last 20 years has seen a considerable change in the work setting of
speech-language pathologists. Prior to that time they were mainly employed
in school settings or university speech and hearing clinics, with a few employed in community agencies. Now many more are providing services
through hospitals and private practice. The increase in private practice has
been a highly conspicuous feature of the profession's growth (Feldman, 1984).
Work settings include neonatal follow-up clinics, early intervention programs, preschool language programs, public school systems, community
speech and hearing centers, hospital speech and hearing departments, private schools, private practice, and university speech and hearing centers.

UNMET NEEDS

The services offered to those handicapped by communication disorders
are expanding to meet the needs of a population that is only now being sys-
tematically identified. There is a danger that failure to coordinate these
services could reduce their efficiency. This is particularly important when the
child's problems stem from central nervous system deficit. There is likely to

be a number of behavioral and linguistic manifestations of these deficits, which might appear to be unrelated unless the nature of the condition is thoroughly understood. It is important that professional patterns of referral do not themselves reinforce division. In their *Survey of Professionals Who Assess Young Children for Communicative Disorders,* Lewis and Byers-Brown (1985) found that there was a two-track referral structure. Physicians apeared to refer to otolaryngologists and audiologists, whereas parents referred their children to speech-language pathologists and psychologists. So long as the two-track structure is permeable and allows for cross-referral there is no cause for concern. If it operates too rigidly, a child may recieve only part of the assessment he needs. Thus, a child with recurrent otitis media might have his hearing assessed and improved, but the language disorder consequent on his impaired hearing might remain undetected.

The most conspicuous need is therefore for full cooperation between professionals and agencies working in this complex field. This would be greatly assisted by more joint interdisciplinary programs of continuing education.

It is also desirable that the general public take more responsibility for helping those with communication handicaps. The extent to which any handicap becomes a disability depends on the attributes of the individual and the attitudes of society. Of all handicaps, communication is the one most dependent on society's action. Society is itself a product of communication. It creates and maintains the system that allows it to operate. It is therefore society's business to see that the system does not exclude its members. It is the professional's business to ensure that the nature of any communication handicap is fully understood.

REFERENCES

American Academy of Pediatrics. (1982). Joint committee on infant hearing: Position statement. *Pediatrics, 70,* 496–497.

Byers-Brown, B. (1981). *Speech therapy: Principles and practice.* Edinburgh: Churchill-Livingstone Edinburgh.

Feldman, A. S. (1984). In support of the professional doctorate. *ASHA, 26,* 28.

Flower, R. M. (1985). Presidential address. *ASHA, 1,* 21–25.

Gerkin, K. P. (1984). The high risk register for deafness. *ASHA, 26,* 17–23.

Holland, A. (1984). *Language disorders in children.* San Diego: College Hill

Ingram, T. T. S. (1976). Speech disorders in childhood. In Lenneberg & Lenneberg (Eds.), *Foundations of language development.* New York: Academic Press.

Lencione, R. M. (1966). Speech and language problems in cerebral palsy. In W. Cruikshank (Ed.), *Cerebral palsy* (2nd Ed.). Syracuse: University Press.

Lewis M. & Byers-Brown, B. (1985). *Survey of professionals who assess young children for communication disorders.* New Brunswick, NJ: UMDNJ-Rutgers Medical School, Institute for the Study of Child Development.

Morley, M. E. (1972). *The development and disorders of speech in childhood* (3rd Ed.). Edinburgh: Churchill-Livingstone.

Punch, J. L., & Fein, D. J. (1984). Profile of educational programs in speech-language pathology and audiology. *ASHA, 26,* 43–48.

Taylor, O. L. (1982). Language differences. In Shames & Wiig (Eds.), *Human communication disorders.* Columbus, OH: Charles E. Merrill.

Travis, L. E. (1971). Preface to L. W. Travis, (Ed.), *Handbook of speech pathology and audiology.* New York: Appleton-Century-Crofts.

Chapter 16

NURSING SERVICES

Kathryn K. Peppe

An important aspect of the care of handicapped children in the community is the provision of nursing services. Nurses in varying levels of professional preparation work with handicapped children in newborn intensive care units, nurseries, inpatient and outpatient units of hospitals, local health departments, schools, residential facilities, clinics, and private physicians' offices. Few nurses serve only handicapped children; rather, the child who has a handicap and his family are most likely to be just a small segment of the total patient population of the nurse. The amount and kind of service that nurses can offer to handicapped children and their families depend on their own education, experience, and position within the employing agencies. Although the majority of nurses have only a basic education in nursing, a small number of nurses have chosen to specialize in pediatric nursing and care of the handicapped child through graduate education. These clinical nurse specialists serve as consultants to other nurses as well as direct care givers in any of the settings mentioned above.

Nursing services in care of handicapped children and their families can be broadly classified into the areas of prevention, case finding, treatment, continuity of care, and research. Although these functions normally overlap, they will be treated as distinct entities for the purposes of this chapter.

PREVENTION

In recent years, activities to prevent handicaps in children have received increasing attention from health care planners and providers. Nurses are making a significant contribution in this regard through their participation in preventive health programs. They promote health maintenance activities such as routine well-child care and physical examinations, developmental screenings, and immunizations. They encourage good health practices such as giving nutrition education to an expectant mother. They offer health supervision of families by guiding them in the need for early prenatal care or genetic counseling, or in seeking appropriate medical attention for illness. Health supervision also encompasses giving parents anticipatory guidance about safety measures to prevent childhood accidents. The nurse helps parents to understand normal growth and development and to adapt this information to stimulate the child's development. The prevention of secondary problems for the child and his family when a diagnosis of a chronic disability is made may require more specialized nursing services. The need for these services may begin with the birth of the affected child or the confirmation of a diagnosis and extend over the lifetime of the family members. Nurse specialists understand the grieving process and are in a position to assist the family to cope with their own feelings. In this way the nurse helps to prevent the disorganization of the family.

CASE FINDING

Wherever nurses work with children and families, they should know what constitutes normal growth and development and be able to recognize deviations. Knowledge of developmental screening tools such as the Denver Developmental Screening Test or the Nursing Child Assessment Tools are critical to the early detection of delays in development. These tools permit the nurse to screen the child and can serve as the basis for referral to community resources able to provide comprehensive evaluation and diagnosis. Nurses are alert to child development regardless of the setting in which the child is seen. Although the functions of the nurse may vary depending upon the employing agency, collecting developmental and health histories may be a routine activity that yields valuable information for the family and all members of the health care team.

TREATMENT

Once the child is diagnosed, a variety of services are put into action to promote optimal development. Nursing services are frequently required for both the child and the family to achieve this goal. Specific recommendations may demand that the nurse counsel the family, interpret the medical treatment, teach child-care or self-care skills, encourage the family to carry out the recommended treatment modalities from a number of disciplines, offer guidance concerning discipline and behavior problems, suggest toys and play activities to promote motor development and socialization, or any number of other nursing care activities. Normally, the nurse prepares a nursing care plan to set mutual goals with the family. In this plan the nurse identifies the problem areas needing attention and prioritizes interventions. The nurse may deliver services to the handicapped child in his home, during clinic or office visits, or during hospital stays. In many large clinics the nurse specialist on the team refers the child back to the public health nurse who then implements the recommended plan of care. The public health nurse frequently knows the family and may be of help during times of crises affecting the child or can assist in management of day-to-day problems in the home. Through ongoing contacts with the handicapped child and his family, the nurse observes and reports on situations that may necessitate a change in the treatment plan.

CONTINUITY OF CARE

Nurses assure continuity of care for handicapped children by other community resources. They stimulate frank discussions and information sharing among professionals to minimize confusion and maximize the benefit to the child and family. According to the American Nurses' Association (1975), continuity of care can be attained by identifying and linking health care providers, having each provider contribute to the care plan, and reaching mutually set goals through planning, coordinating, communicating, referral, and follow-up services. For the handicapped child who is hospitalized, planning needs to occur prior to admission so that the child and family are prepared. Planning also needs to occur prior to the discharge of the child. Discharge planning is designed to help the family make a smooth transition from the hospital to home and may require that referrals be made to agencies that can provide needed care. Once a referral has been made and the child has been discharged, follow-up is needed to assure that the services being given remain appropriate. With the recent advent of the diagnostic-related group as the foundation for reimbursement under the Medicaid program, lengths of hospital stay are being shortened. Early discharge of handicapped children necessitates that nurses advocate for adequate discharge planning, including assessment of the physical, psychosocial, and environmental factors concerned in the child's care in the home (DeRienzo, 1985). The immediate goal is to assure that services are "continuous and uninterrupted . . . to meet both actual and anticipated patient needs" (Povse & Keenan, 1981, p. 668).

RESEARCH

Although the need to conduct research is not often thought of as part of the nurse's role in care of the handicapped child and his family, it is nevertheless critical to nursing services. Research is directed toward questions whose answers are not immediately known. It can be evaluative and look back to assess what has already been done, or it can be aimed at discovering new facts. Research also can be descriptive or explanatory in nature. Nurses have a responsibility to conduct research to advance knowledge and improve the practice of nursing. However, little attention has been paid by nurse researchers to questions about the care of handicapped children. Nursing research can help the nurse who teaches clean catheterization techniques to a child with spina bifida to know which of the techniques are the most effective in promoting independence in bladder control. Nurses who work with handicapped children have a wealth of experience and data available to them that can readily form the basis for many research studies. These studies either can be carried out in concert with other researchers or can be designed to be studied alone (*Proceedings and recommendations,* 1979, pp. 63–65).

There are three major settings in which nurses provide care to handicapped children in the community. These settings include public health agencies delivering care in clinics, patient homes, or other locales outside of the hospital; public and private schools in which children with handicaps are mainstreamed or in schools specially designed to serve the handicapped child; and rehabilitation centers, long-term care facilities, or other residential settings. The rest of this chapter describes the role of nurses working in these various environments.

PUBLIC HEALTH NURSES

Although most health care professionals are aware of the common activities of public health nurses, such as home visitation, conducting immunization clinics, coordination of services and referrals, the potential capabilities of the public health nurse may not be so fully recognized. Public health nursing is a field of specialization that exists within both the practice of professional nursing and the broad area of public health practice. It utilizes the philosophy, content, and methods of public health as well as professional nursing. Public health nurses are responsible for providing nursing services on a family-centered basis for individuals and groups at home, work, schools, public health centers, and clinics. Public health nursing interweaves its services with those of other health care workers, such as physicians, nutritionists, and social workers, and participates in the planning and implementation of community health programs. Assisting and supporting individuals and families to meet their multifaceted needs as a result of having a handicapped child in the community can be considered an integral function of the public health nurse.

The role of the public health nurse includes the general nursing functions of prevention, case finding, treatment, and continuity of care and also includes case management and health promotion as treatment services. The specific activities of public health nurses in each general functional area are diverse. Activities that contribute to prevention of handicapping conditions in children may include providing instruction regarding infant feeding and care of the newborn or encouraging routine preventive medical care. In the area of case finding, the nurse may perform developmental screenings and observe the child's attainment of developmental milestones, whether these are physical (such as height and weight), or psychosocial (such as the ability to socialize and play with peers). With the advent of early hospital discharge, many health problems of the newborn or young child are not recognized until a public health nurse makes an assessment. Case management is a major treatment service and requires that the nurse select appropriate community resources and services for potential or identified health problems, such as genetic disease evaluation or mental health counseling. The nurse refers the client and family to agencies providing needed services and also serves as the focal point for coordination of all of the community-based services that the family receives. The nurse assures that channels of communication are maintained between the client and all agencies and professionals. This is accomplished by providing agencies with appropriate reports such as dietary records or a description of the family's coping skills, interaction patterns, and home environment. The nurse also would seek detailed instructions for a handicapped child's home care from other professionals. This activity may occur, for example, when a child receives hyperalimentation or the complex respiratory care necessary for treatment of cystic fibrosis. The nurse's activities include providing individuals and families with the information needed to assist them to maintain a healthy state of being through health education and counseling. Typically, the public health nurse becomes a trusted home visitor to whom the family of a handicapped child turns for advice, support, and guidance.

SCHOOL HEALTH NURSES

School health nursing is a specialized field within pediatric and community health nursing practice. School health services to handicapped children may be given either by school nurses employed by the educational agency for this sole purpose or by public health nurses a part of the broad range of services that they offer in a community. Provision of school nursing services is highly variable nationally. Some school districts do not provide school health service programs and thus do not employ nurses. Other school districts may assign one nurse to anywhere from 1,200 to 6,000 students (American Nurses' Association, 1980). With such wide disparity across the country, it is difficult to describe school nursing services for handicapped students in any but the ideal situation. Obviously, the extent of services actually given by a school nurse to handicapped students directly depends on the overall case load.

The passage of the Education for All Handicapped Children Act of 1975 (PL 94-142) enhanced the role of the school nurse with handicapped children. The act required that "related" services be provided to evaluate, develop, and implement the educational plan for each handicapped student. It also required the early identification and assessment of students eligible under the act (American Nurses' Association, 1980). Nursing provides an integral service helpful in carrying out the mandatory provisions of this federal law.

The school nurse works in concert with the children, parents, teachers, school administrators, and other members of the school health team to achieve the highest possible level of care for handicapped students. Within this context the school nurse is responsible for obtaining information about the health status of every handicapped student, including a comprehensive health and developmental history as well as a health assessment and physical examination. The nurse can provide the appropriate health information for the development of the individual education plan. The school nurse also may be called on to provide special health services or procedures at school while the child is present. Examples of such services include catheterization of a child with spina bifida, administration of medications to a child with epilepsy, nutrition education of a child with diabetes, and care of a child who requires the support of a ventilator. These services are provided in addition to the customary duties of maintenance of school health records, immunization status checks, screenings, preventive health education, first aid, and safety programs that are required for all students in a comprehensive program. Leadership and direction of the school health program comes from nurses who are educationally prepared and experienced to provide comprehensive programs reflective of the needs of handicapped students and their families.

REHABILITATION NURSES

The scope of nursing practice is broad, and, not surprisingly, nurses have a broad knowledge and skill base on which to build their philosophy of care. Rehabilitation principles are woven into the philosophy of nurses regardless of their area of specialization. These principles help the nurse to internalize the values of concern for the client as an individual with specific needs and as part of a family and to translate these values into practice in a variety of health settings.

By definition, rehabilitation is considered tertiary care. However, it is actually a component of each part of the health care delivery system. Therefore, a handicapped child's rehabilitation potential must be considered wherever he enters the health care system. For example, a primary intervention might dictate the handicapped child's education to prevent a complication from developing. A secondary intervention occurs when the handicapped child receives treatment but is also evaluated for potential complications. Tertiary interventions occur when the handicapped child receives specific treatments designed to make the most of his functional abilities (Fanslow, 1979). From these examples, it can be seen that rehabilitation principles are applicable to nursing care of handicapped children.

There are two types of rehabilitation nurses: the nurse generalist who specializes in rehabilitation and the rehabilitation clinical nurse specialist. The former is a nurse functioning in a rehabilitation setting but lacking advanced preparation other than on-the-job training, experience, and continuing education. The rehabilitation clinical nurse specialist has an advanced degree in rehabilitation nursing (Fanslow, 1979). It is rare to find a rehabilitation nurse who is also a specialist in pediatrics. Therefore, the handicapped child may have his rehabilitation nursing care needs met by pediatric nurses who incorporate the principles into their practice or, more rarely, rehabilitation nurses may incorporate the developmental model into their practice. Nurses specialized in pediatric rehabilitation may be employed in a wide variety of settings, including hospitals, rehabilitation centers, long-term care facilities, community agencies, and other residential settings.

The roles of nurses working in rehabilitation settings with handicapped children include providing preventive health education to the child and his family. Thus, a child with a chronic respiratory disorder might be taught to recognize early signs of infection and to take appropriate actions such as increasing fluid intake to help reduce the viscosity of secretions. The rehabilitation nurse also provides direct care to the child and family. The impact of the disability needs to be explored and plans made to facilitate transition from the rehabilitation facility to the community and home. The rehabilitation nurse also may serve as an expert consultant to whom other nurses in the community turn for information and direction in the care of a specific handicapped child. For example, the rehabilitation nurse can provide the community health nurse with specific instruction on the care and use of adaptive equipment. Nurses specialized in the rehabilitation of handicapped children are helpful to all members of the health care team.

SUMMARY

Nurses of differing educational preparation make a significant contribution to the prevention, case finding, treatment, continuity of care, and research needs of handicapped children and their families. Although nurses work in a variety of settings, it is frequently public health nurses, school nurses, and rehabilitation nurses who are intimately involved in provision of care to these children. When the diagnosis of a handicapping condition is made, the nurse assists the families with management of day-to-day problems as well as with guidance in the often complex medical treatment program. Using a family-centered approach to delivery of their services, nurses can coordinate the treatment programs offered by numerous agencies. Nursing is a key member of the health care team serving the handicapped child and his family.

REFERENCES

American Nurses' Association, (1975). *Continuity of care and discharge planning programs in institutions and community agencies.* Kansas City, MO: Author.

American Nurses' Association. (1980). *School nurses working with handicapped children.* Kansas City, MO: Author.

DeRienzo, B. (1985). Discharge planning. *Rehabilitation Nursing, 10,* 34–36.

Fanslow, C. A. (1979). The rehabilitation clinical nurse specialist. In R. Murray & J. C. Kijek (Eds.), *Current perspectives in rehabilitation nursing* (Vol. 1, pp. 21–26). St. Louis, MO: C. V. Mosby.

Povse, S. M., & Kennan, M. E. (1981). Discharge planning for the transition from a health care facility to the community. In N. Martin, et al. (Eds.), *Comprehensive rehabilitation nursing* (pp. 668–686). New York: McGraw-Hill.

Proceedings and recommendations. First national conference on nursing in CCS-SSIDC programs. (1979). Dayton, OH: Wright State University.

Chapter 17

EARLY INTERVENTION PROGRAMS FOR HANDICAPPED PRESCHOOL CHILDREN

E. J. Bailey
Diane Bricker

Currently, educational programs and related services are available through-out the nation for handicapped preschool children and their families. A historical review of federal mandates and regulations suggests a progressive trend in the development of social policy for the education of young handicapped children

In 1968 the U.S. Congress passed the Handicapped Children's Early Education Assistance Act (PL90-583), which has supported a nationwide network of model demonstration programs designed to serve handicapped children. Although the provision of educational programs for non-school-age children is not mandated, the Education for All Handicapped Children Act (PL94-142) has been a most influential piece of legislation for handicapped preschool children (Bricker, 1986). Interpretation and implementation of PL 94-142 has varied; however, the law appears to be clear in mandating educational rights for handicapped children, such as the right to nondiscriminatory evaluation, placement in the least restrictive educational setting, and parental participation (Gallagher, 1984). The recent passage of the Education of the Handicapped Act Amendments of 1983 (PL 98-199) specifically addresses young handicapped children. This revision and extension of PL 94-142 provides two mandates that are particularly pertinent to handicapped infants and preschool children and their families. First, the preschool incentive grants program has been amended to include children from birth to three years. In programs for handicapped children the definition now explicitly "includes children from birth through eight years of age" and makes clear that state plans must include "all handicapped children from birth through five years of age" (Section 623, PL 98-199). Second, the crucial role that parents have in the education of their handicapped children is emphasized by specifying a variety of roles for parental participation (e.g., that the majority of board members for private non-profit programs be parents of handicapped children).

Although critics argue that the implementation of federal policy at state and local levels is often compromised by lack of necessary resources, public opinion, and interpretation of non-specific mandates (Noel, Burke, & Valdivieso, 1958), federal policy has influenced major changes within states to ensure the availability of appropriate services for young handicapped children and their families. According to a survey completed by O'Connell (1983), eight states mandate special education services to all handicapped children from birth to five years of age; 12 states mandate special education services to all handicapped children from three to five years of age. Four states mandate services at birth, and seven states mandate services at three years of age for certain subgroups of handicapped children (e.g., hearing-impaired, visually impaired).

Despite variations in the interpretation and implementation of federal policy at state and local levels, a network of early intervention programs for handicapped infants and preschool children exists and the number of programs is increasing (Bricker, 1986). The purpose of this chapter is to describe the consistencies and variations in early intervention approaches. Following are a series of questions concerning the who, why, and what of early intervention programs that will provide the framework in which to describe contemporary early intervention efforts.

1. Who receives early intervention services?
2. What are the goals of early intervention programs?
3. What service delivery models are available?
4. How are personnel trained and deployed in early intervention programs?
5. What is the curricular content of early intervention programs?
6. What instructional approaches and strategies are used in early intervention programs?
7. How are parents/families involved in early intervention programs?
8. How is program effectiveness evaluated?

EARLY INTERVENTION PROGRAMS

Who Receives Early Intervention Services?

In general, early intervention programs serve children from birth through five years of age, ranging from those identified as at risk for developmental delays or problems to profoundly impaired; in some cases, nonhandicapped children who serve as normal models may participate in early intervention programs (Bricker & Sheehan, 1981). Some programs are designed to serve groups of children who have been diagnosed as having a variety of handicapping conditions and etiologies such as Down syndrome, general development delay, motoric impairments, and sensory impairments (Bricker & Sheehan, 1981). Other programs may be designed to serve children with specific etiologies such as Down syndrome children (Clunies-Ross, 1979; Hayden & Haring, *1977*) or disabilities such as cerebral palsy (Haynes, 1976).

In addition, the backgrounds of the enrolled children vary. Demographic characteristics of families involved in early intervention programs can be as diverse as the population characteristics of handicapped children. Families included in programs often have widely disparate cultural, socioeconomic, and educational backgrounds.

What Are the Goals of Early Intervention Programs?

In part, the goals of programs reflect the potential benefits of early intervention. A direct benefit of early intervention refers to positive changes in the child and family members. For example, early intervention can enhance the behavioral repertoire of the child and assist the family to maintain the child in the least restrictive educational setting and in the home.

Many programs suggest that early intervention produces indirect benefits for society as well as positive outcomes for the child and family. Early intervention assists parents in maintaining their child at home versus institutionalization; maintaining disabled children in their homes and in the mainstream of regular education produces significant savings to the community (Bricker, Bailey, & Bruder, 1984; Garland, Swanson, Stone, & Woodruff, 1981). The more disabled the child, the more costly the program; therefore, early habilitative efforts that lead to the placement of the child in a less restrictive environment potentially save finite educational resources.

What Service Delivery Models Are Available?

There are three major early intervention service delivery models: home-based, center-based, and home-center-based combination (Filler, 1983). Programs for infants often deliver services in the home (Hanson & Schwartz, 1978). The target in the home-based approach is often the parent or care giver who is helped to acquire effective intervention skills to use with the child. The center-based model requires that the infant or child be brought to an educational setting on a regular basis. The focal target in center-based models is usually the child; however, many center-based programs stress parental involvement (Hayden & Dmitriev, 1975) and may even provide structured training for the parent (Bricker, Seibert, & Casuso, 1980).

Some programs have adopted a combined home–center model. There are programs that stress training simultaneously in the classroom and in the home (Bricker & Sheehan, 1981) and others that serve the child initially in the home and transfer the child to a center setting after a certain age or when the child develops targeted skills (Kysela, Hillyard, McDonald, & Taylor, 1981).

How are Personnel Trained and Deployed in Early Intervention Programs?

Many early intervention programs are operated by staff members (e.g., teachers, administrators) who have had minimal formal training in the area of early childhood/special education. In addition, state standards and regulations for certifying teachers of preschool handicapped children vary. Currently, 18 states have established certification standards, 12 states are developing standards, and 21 states report no specific standards (O'Connell, 1983).

The lack of formal training and certification can lead to two unfortunate outcomes: (a) personnel poorly prepared concerning content and strategies required to work effectively with preschool-age handicapped populations and (b) personnel prepared to work with school-age children inappropriately assigned to programs that serve preschool handicapped populations. The uniqueness of handicapped infants and young children and the recent focus on the importance of involving the family in intervention programs requires that early intervention personnel receive specialized training in order to maximize the effectiveness of early intervention efforts.

Overall, personnel working in early intervention programs can be divided into two categories: direct service and support service. Direct service personnel are those individuals who interact with the child/family in a regular and consistent manner (e.g., interventionists, aides, parents, or others). Early interventionists and other direct service personnel have numerous responsibilities and assume a variety of roles, such as child developmental specialist, behavior manager, parent trainer, and program evaluator.

Support personnel are specialists who have been trained in a specific discipline such as physical or occupational therapy. In addition, bus drivers, administrative personnel, and others who provide services that are necessary for the operation of a program also fall into the category of support personnel.

What Is the Curricular Content of Early Intervention Programs?

Although programs operate using a variety of orientations, two theoretical perspectives have influenced the major curricular efforts for handicapped infants and young children. These perspectives are (a) developmental and (b) functional.

The developmental approach is based on the assumption that development is hierarchical and sequential; developmental progress is viewed as the integration and reorganization of earlier acquired behavioral schemes in a generally consistent sequential order. Age-related developmental milestones, such as those identified by Arnold Gesell (Gesell & Amatruda, 1962) often comprise the curricular content for this approach.

A frequently used developmental approach is based on the work of Piaget (1970) in which curricula for handicapped infants and young children center on sensorimotor and pre-operational skills. Personnel using a Piagetian perspective focus training efforts on the acquisition of developmental processes, such as object permanence and means–ends, through the accommodation and assimilation of progressively more complex skills.

The functional model is based on the premise that developmental progress is the acquisition of skills that will immediately or in the future improve a child's ability to interact with the environment and become self-sufficient and independent. The content of such a curriculum is often task-analytical in nature and contains skills that are or will be "functional" for the child.

What Instructional Approaches and Strategies Are Used in Early Intervention Programs?

Because handicapped infants and young children tend to have deficits in many critical areas of functioning, there is often a need to assist children to gain cognitive, communication, social, self-help, and motor skills. Therefore, the majority of programs offer a comprehensive menu of educational targets. Instructional strategies used by programs to present curricular content rely on some form of environmental engineering (i.e., arrangement of antecedent events to elicit and reinforce the occurrences of targeted behaviors). However, the rigor and rigidity with which behavioral technology is used varies considerably across programs. Programs that use a "teacher directed" approach tend to initiate training by focusing on specific targets, using highly controlled presentation formats (e.g., specific cues/stimuli, expected performance responses, and predetermined consequences). As children show progress in the acquisition of target responses, instructional presentations shift to encourage generalization of responses to other conditions (e.g., settings, individuals). Programs that are more "child directed" tend to use a more flexible application of behavioral principles. From the onset, children are encouraged to use targeted responses in a variety of settings, and once the responses are functional, artificial contingencies are eliminated.

Other programs use instructional approaches that specify goals and objectives for children by allowing, in part, the environmental events and the seemingly apparent interests of the children to guide the implementation of specific instructional strategies. For example, a training goal might be to assist a child in using agent-action-object phrases, rather than drilling a number of predetermined phrases; the interventionist might use opportunities that arise during the day that target the activity (e.g., use of a book chosen by the child to teach agent-action-object sequences).

Some programs focus on reinforcement of desired responses using some form of tangible or verbal feedback. Often this feedback is in the form of verbal comments such as "good boy," "that's right," "you did that well," and so on. In programs where children have more freedom to determine the activities in which the training exercises will be imbedded, reinforcement is often inherent in the activity (Mahoney & Weller, 1980). For example, pouring juice into a cup provides practice in wrist rotation and self-help skills, and getting to drink the juice may be reward enough to continue to practice the behavior.

How Are Parents/Families Involved in Early Intervention Programs?

Parents of young handicapped children have increasingly become active participants in their children's educational programs. First, federal legislation (e.g., PL 94-142, PL 98-199) mandates the inclusion of parents in program efforts such as individualized education program (IEP) development and the provision of training to assist parents in becoming more effective when dealing with professionals. Second, parents can provide valuable educational information (e.g., instructional strategies) concerning their children and can accurately assess their children's developmental status (Gradel, Thompson, & Sheehan, 1981). Finally, the professional community has become aware that involving all family members (e.g., siblings, grandparents) in intervention efforts can provide benefits to the family (e.g., coping strategies for siblings, support to parents) as well as enhance the developmental outcome of the handicapped children.

Families participating in early intervention programs represent a wide range of backgrounds (e.g., education, socioeconomic status) and usually have a variety of different educational and support needs. For these reasons, family involvement is usually highly individualized based on individual family needs. The types of family programs and services offered by early intervention programs can range from providing the family respite time to involving the family directly in the delivery of services (e.g., assisting in a classroom, working with other parents) to providing training to assist parents to become effective change agents with their children (Bricker & Casuso, 1979). Often programs offer social service assistance and counseling as well as educational information and skill training.

How Is Program Effectiveness Evaluated?

Evaluation of early intervention programs generally has been focused on measuring child change (Bricker, Bailey, & Bruder, 1984). A few programs have measured training impact on parents, and even fewer have collected information on other relevant variables such as changes in attitude, cost factors, or longitudinal effects (Ramey, MacPhee, & Yeates, 1983).

Although child change is a consistent outcome variable used to index program effectiveness, methodologies used to measure child change differ considerably across programs. A variety of evaluation designs and analytical procedures (e.g., statistical tests, frequencies, and percents) are used, and the dependent measures range from standardized test scores to the number of training objectives completed during the intervention period. In addition, many programs use several varied measures (e.g., test scores, parent impressions) to index child change, whereas others use only one measure.

A few programs use either a nonequivalent contrast group design or a one-group post-test–only design (Brassell & Dunst, 1978; Moore, Fredericks & Baldwin, 1981); however, the majority of programs use a one-group pre- and post-test comparison design. Typically, some type of measure (e.g., standardized test) is administered prior to the intervention period and readministered following the intervention period; the time interval between the two measures (e.g., six-month pre-test–post test interval) varies for different programs. Frequently, the resulting data are aggregated across subjects, and the difference between performance on the pre- and post-test measure is compared to examine the nature or degree of child change (e.g., performance gains).

SUMMARY

The purpose of this chapter was to provide some general information about the nature of early intervention programs. A review of programs reveals considerable variability in the way intervention for handicapped infants and young children is conceived, implemented, and evaluated. Although staffing patterns, family involvement, curricular content, instructional strategies, and evaluation systems differ among many dimensions, some consistencies do exist among programs. For example, most programs appear to operate from a rationale that argues positive change can be made in the target children and families, which in turn may produce other indirect positive outcomes.

Advances in the early intervention field will evolve from the need to improve the quality of current intervention practices. There is a general trend in education toward cost-effective accountability; the move for programs to become more accountable should lead to improvements in the areas of assessment, curricula, and instructional technologies. There is a growing trend in early intervention toward greater parent and family involvement; this trend will continue to develop (Walker, Slentz, & Bricker, 1985). In recognition of the need for specialized training to work adequately with handicapped infants and preschoolers, there will continue to be an increase in the number of early childhood/special education training programs offered by universities and colleges and an increase in the number of states offering preschool teacher certification (Cohen, Semmes, & Guralnick, 1979). A final future emphasis will be on research designed to determine what intervention approaches produce the more significant outcomes, what program elements contribute substantially to child/family growth, and the comparative cost outcomes of specific intervention procedures.

REFERENCES

Brassell, W., & Dunst, C. (1978). Fostering the object construct: Large scale intervention with handicapped infants. *American Journal of Mental Deficiency, 82,* 507–510.

Bricker, D. (1986). *Early education of at-risk and handicapped infants, toddlers, and preschool children.* Chicago, IL: Scott, Foresman & Co.

Bricker, D., Bailey, E., & Bruder, M. (1984). The efficacy of early intervention and the handicapped infant: A wise or wasted resource? *Advances in Behavioral Pediatrics, 5,* 373–423.

Bricker, D., & Casuso, V. (1979). Family involvement: A critical component of early intervention. *Exceptional Children, 46,* 108–116.

Bricker, D., Seibert, J., & Casuso, V. (1980). Early intervention. In J. Hogg & P. Mittler (Eds.), *Advances in mental handicap research.* London: Wiley & Sons.

Bricker, D., & Sheehan, R. (1981). Effectiveness of an early intervention program as indexed by child change. *Journal of the Division for Early Childhood, 4,* 11–27.

Clunies-Ross, G. (1979). Accelerating the development of Down's syndrome infants and young children. *The Journal of Special Education, 13,* 169–177.

Cohen, S., Semmes, M., & Guralnick, M. (1979). Public Law 94-142 and the education of preschool handicapped children. *Exceptional Children, 45,* 279–285.

Filler, J. (1983). Service models for handicapped infants. In G. Garwood & R. Fewell (Eds.), *Educating handicapped infants* (pp. 369–386). Rockville, MD: Aspen.

Gallagher, J. (1984). Policy analysis and program implementation/PL 94-142. *Topics in Early Childhood Special Education, 4*(1), 43–53.

Garland, C., Swanson, J., Stone, N., & Woodruff, G. (1981). *Early intervention for children with special needs and their families (Series Paper No. 11). Seattle, WA: WESTAR.*

Gessell, A., & Amatruda, C. S. (1962). *Developmental diagnosis.* New York: Paul B. Hoeber.

Gradel, K., Thompson, M., & Sheehan, R. (1981). Parent and professional agreement in early childhood assessment. *Topics in Early Childhood Special Education, 1*(2), 31–39.

Hanson, M., & Schwarz, R. (1978). Results of a longitudinal intervention program for Down's syndrome infants and their families. *Education and training of the Mentally Retarded, 13,* 403–407.

Hayden, A., & Dmitriev, V. (1975). The multidisciplinary preschool program for Down's syndrome children and the University of Washington model preschool center. In B. Friedlander, G. Sterritt, & G. Kirk (Eds.), *Exceptional infant* (Vol. 3, pp. 193–221). New York: Brunner/Mazel.

Hayden, A., & Haring, N. (1977). The acceleration and maintenance of developmental gains in Down's syndrome school age children. In P. Mittler (Ed.), *Research to practice in mental retardation. Volume I: Care and intervention* (pp. 129–141). Baltimore, MD: University Park Press.

Haynes, U. (1976). The national collaborative infant project. In T. Tjossem (Ed.), *Intervention strategies for high risk infants and young children* (pp. 509–534). Baltimore, MD: University Park Press.

Kysela, G., Hillyard, A., McDonald, L., & Taylor, J. (1981). Early intervention, design and evaluation. In R. Schiefelbusch & D. Bricker (Eds.), *Early language: Acquisition and intervention* (pp. 341–388). Baltimore, MD: University Park Press.

Mahoney, G., & Weller, E. (1980). An ecological approach to language intervention. In D. Bricker (Ed.), *A resource book on language intervention with children* (pp. 17–32). San Francisco: Jossey-Bass.

Moore, M., Fredericks, H., & Baldwin, V. (1981). The long-range effects of early childhood education on a trainable mentally retarded population. *Journal of the Division for Early Childhood, 4,* 93–110.

Noel, M., Burke, P., & Valdivieso, C. (1985). Educational policy for the severely mentally retarded. In D. Bricker & J. Filler (Eds.), *The severely mentally retarded: Research to practice* (pp. 12–35). Reston, VA: The Council for Exceptional Children.

O'Connell, J. (1983). Education of handicapped preschoolers: A national survey of services and personnel requirements. *Exceptional Children, 49*(6), 538–543.

Piaget, J. (1970). Piaget's theory. In P. Mussen (Ed.), *Carmichael's manual of child psychology* (Vol. 1, pp. 703–732). New York: Wiley & Sons.

Ramey, C., MacPhee, D., & Yeates, KI. (1983). Preventing developmental retardation: A general systems model. In L. Bond & J. Joffe (Eds.), *Facilitating infant and early childhood development* (pp. 343–401). Hanover, NH: University Press of New England.

Walker, B., Slentz, K., & Bricker, D. (1985). Parent involvement in early intervention. In *Rehabilitation Research Review*. Washington, DC: Catholic Universal Rehabilitation Information Center.

Chapter 18

SPECIAL EDUCATION

Eleanor Whiteside Lynch

Special education encompasses a wide range of programs and services designed to help exceptional students learn. Although special educators work with gifted and handicapped students in programs for children from infancy through young adulthood, this chapter focuses on the role of special education for handicapped students from age three through twenty-one.

DIFFERENCES BETWEEN REGULAR EDUCATION AND SPECIAL EDUCATION

Regular educators and special educators share a similar goal, to help students acquire the skills and knowledge to become informed, productive citizens; but they differ in what they teach, how it is taught, and where it is taught. Public Law 94-142 (U.S. Office of Education, 1977) defines special education as "specially designed instruction, at no extra cost to the parent, to meet the unique needs of a handicapped child, including classroom instruction, introduction in physical education, home instruction, and instruction in hospitals and institutions" (p. 42480). In addition to the legislation that defines and regulates the delivery of special education services (PL 94-142, PL 98-199, and Section 504 of the Rehabilitation Act of 1973, discussed in Chapter 6), five primary differences separate special education from regular education: curriculum, focus on the individual learner, instructional process and procedures, emphasis on evaluation of student progress, and extent of parental involvement.

Curriculum refers to content, or what is taught. Although curricula vary from district to district and state to state, there is a generally agreed-on set of skills that are taught at each grade level. The curriculum in special education programs usually deviates in breadth, depth, and/or content from the regular academic curriculum. For example, students with mild handicaps that interfere with learning may be taught basic arithmetic skills such as counting, adding, subtracting, multiplying, and dividing, but they may not be introduced to higher-level math such as algebra or geometry. This alteration limits the breadth and content of the curriculum. The depth of the curriculum, or how much is taught, also might be limited. Although students may learn to count and use numbers for basic computations, they may not be taught that there are Arabic and Roman numerals, ordinal, cardinal, prime, and root numbers, or that there are systems of numbers that are not designed around a base of 10. The curriculum for students whose handicaps are more severe differs dramatically in content. Students may be taught to use coins in vending machines or make simple purchases at a fast-food restaurant, but they would not be taught formal arithmetic. This type of curriculum, which focuses on teaching life skills that the student can use now and in the future, is referred to as a functional curriculum (Guess et al., 1978) and is being used increasingly in programs for students with moderate and severe mental retardation.

A second difference between regular and special education is the focus on the individual student. PL 94-142 mandates that each student receiving special education services have an individualized education program (IEP). Following assessment of the student's current level of performance by a multidisciplinary team, the IEP team determines the goals and objectives that are to be the focus of instruction. The IEP clearly specifies the instructional objectives for the year. Just as no two students are alike, no two IEPs are exactly alike. Thus, each student in special education receives instruction that has been tailored to his needs.

The instructional process and procedures also differ in special education. Students who are receiving special education services are those who, by definition, need a specially designed educational program. Often they have not been successful in school because of their inability to attend, to work in a large group, or to learn at the same rate as their nonhandicapped peers. In order for them to achieve, the instructional process must be modified. Some need only to be taught at a slower pace with more opportunities to practice; others need to have material sequenced into small steps; still others may require very systematic teaching that includes direct instruction and immediate reinforcement of correct responses (Lewis & Doorlag, 1983).

Although all teachers measure student progress, special educators are especially concerned with the student's rate of learning and skill acquisition. When a student has learning problems, there is no time to waste on methods that do not work. Daily or weekly measurement of the student's progress can alert the teacher to needed changes in the program or provide documentation that skills have been mastered (Bagnato & Neisworth, 1981; McLoughlin & Lewis, 1986).

Finally, the degree of parent involvement in special education is higher than in regular education. PL 94-142 requires that parents be included in the assessment process and in the decision-making of the IEP team (Turnbull, Turnbull, & Wheat, 1982). Consequently, parents' priorities for their child's education are included in the instructional program. Some families may ask teachers to include behavior management goals so that they can take their son or daughter on family outings without fear of disruption. Others may want teachers to concentrate on basic academic skills to increase their child's opportunities for higher education; still others may want help teaching their son or daughter how to eat, bathe, or toilet independently.

THE PURPOSE OF SPECIAL EDUCATION

Although the overall goal or purpose of special education is to help students become more informed, productive, responsible individuals, that goal is interpreted differently for various groups of students. For those with mild handicaps, the purpose may be to improve their academic skills so that they can succeed in the regular education curriculum. For students with more severe handicaps, the goal may be to teach life skills that enable students to live as independently as possible. Thus, "education" is used in its broadest context, referring to traditional, academic experiences as well as instruction in toilet training, dressing, or communicating.

Using the word *education* to apply to instruction in such basics skills has at times sparked controversy. Some authors use the word *habilitation* to describe programs for students with more severe handicaps (Bernstein, Ziarnik, Rudrud, & Czajkowski, 1981); others use *education* and *habilitation* interchangeably (Fink, 1982). Regardless of the term one uses, education is a process that helps students acquire new behaviors or utilize existing behaviors in ways that enable them to function more effectively in their total environment (Roos, cited in Burton & Hirshoren, 1979). This definition also describes special education.

PERSONNEL PREPARATION IN SPECIAL EDUCATION

Each state has its own requirements for teacher certification or credentialing in special education, and teacher training programs to meet these requirements are offered at colleges and universities throughout the country. Although training in some states can be completed in an undergraduate program, an increasing number require post-baccalaureate or graduate work.

In some states special education teachers must first be trained in regular education; in others, certification to teach in a regular classroom is not required. Many university training programs have organized course work around the competencies that teachers need in order to be successful. Often, those competencies include skill development in areas such as assessing students, planning and delivering instruction, managing behavior, and interacting with parents and other professionals. In addition to developing skills that are generic to all special education programs, university students may specialize in a particular level or category of special education. Some may train to work with mildly handicapped students; others may focus their preparation on students with more severe handicaps. Or special educators may be trained to work in particular categorical areas such as mental retardation, learning disabilities, behavior disorders, or physical or sensory handicaps.

THE SPECIAL EDUCATION PROCESS

The provision of PL 94-142 that has received the most attention in the popular press is that of mainstreaming. The word *mainstreaming* was coined to describe the requirement that handicapped students be educated in the least restrictive environment, i.e., the setting which, for that student, is the least isolated and segregated with the greatest number of opportunities for normal interactions with nonhandicapped peers. Unfortunately, this concept has often been misunderstood (Meyen, 1982). As Cartwright, Cartwright, and Ward (1981) have pointed out, mainstreaming does not mean that all handicapped children will be put into regular classrooms. It does, however, mean that those who can succeed in regular classrooms with help will be placed there.

Recently, the term *integration* has been used to describe the process of moving programs for more severely handicapped students out of institutions and special schools onto regular school campuses. It is also used to describe the movement of more mildly handicapped students out of special classes and into regular classrooms. According to U.S. Department of Education (1984) figures, fewer than 7 percent of the students enrolled in special education programs are educated in segregated schools for handicapped individuals or in institutional settings; and of the more than 93 percent who attend regular schools, nearly two-thirds are educated in regular classrooms with their nonhandicapped peers. These students usually get extra help from a special education resource room teacher. This integration has provided opportunities for handicapped and nonhandicapped students to learn, work, and play together in ways that were not possible just a few years ago. It also has brought regular and special educators together to examine ways to teach all children more effectively.

Because of the emphasis that PL 94-142 placed on the setting for special education programs, some of the other issues of special education programming were temporarily obscured. In discussing policy issues as they relate to students with mental retardation, Forness and Kavale (1984) state, *"Where we teach may not be as important as what and how we teach the mentally retarded."* It is likely that special educators will begin to place renewed emphasis on curricular content and the instructional process.

The IEP mandated by PL 94-142 is an essential aspect of special education. IEP development is a process that includes assessment of the student, program planning, placement, program implementation, and program monitoring. Throughout the process, parents' and students' rights are protected. Parents have access to all school records about their child, and records must be maintained and stored according to strict rules of confidentiality. If at any point in the process parents and school personnel cannot agree on the program or placement, the parents have the right to challenge the school through a due process hearing.

The first step in the process of IEP development is assessment of the student. By law the student must be assessed by a multidisciplinary team; the assessment instruments must be unbiased, reliable, and valid for the purpose for which they are being used; and the tests must be administered in the language normally used by the student. No single test can be used as the basis for decision-making; and the assessment must be comprehensive, examining all aspects of the student's handicap (McLoughlin & Lewis, 1986).

Following the assessment, the IEP meeting is convened. The meeting must include a school system representative who is charged with supervising the proceedings, the student's teacher or teachers, one or both parents, the student when appropriate, and a member of the assessment team or someone familiar with the assessment procedure and findings. It is the team's responsibility to develop the written IEP document that will serve as the plan of the instruction. PL 94-142 mandates that an IEP contain the following: (a) the student's present levels of educational performance; (b) a statement of annual goals and short-term objectives; (c) specification of the special education and related services (e.g., transportation, physical therapy, counseling, etc.) that are to be provided, along with a statement about the student's extent of participation in regular education programs; (d) the date that the services are expected to begin and the probable duration of the services; and (e) objective criteria for determining on an annual basis whether or not the short-term objectives have been met (U.S. Department of Education, 1977). Each student's IEP is reviewed at least yearly to evaluate progress, determine whether services should be continued, and determine what (if any) modifications are needed. Although the IEP is not a formal contract between the school and the family, it serves as an agreement about what is to be taught, the setting in which it is to be taught, the additional services that will be provided, and how progress will be evaluated.

THEORETICAL APPROACHES TO SPECIAL EDUCATION

Special education has been influenced by many theories over the years. Those that have withstood empirical tests of effectiveness have been retained and incorporated; those that have not have been discarded. Although each categorical area of special education has its own history, some generalizations about underlying theory can be made. In many areas, early approaches relied on theories of perceptual development or psychological processing (Lewis, in press). Because it was believed that basic perceptual and psychological processing skills were prerequisite to more complex academic skills, teachers worked to improve students' skills in these areas. Training in eye tracking, balance, and laterality, as well as verbal and visual memory, were included in the students' educational program. However, studies of these approaches demonstrated that neither perceptual-motor training (Kavale & Glass, 1982) nor training in psycholinguistic processes (discrete elements of language) (Larsen, Parker, & Hammill, 1982) are related to improving academic skills. Thus, these approaches to special education have fallen into disfavor (Kavale & Glass, 1982).

A theoretical approach that has proved to be effective in educating handicapped students is that of behaviorism. The principles of applied behavioral analysis include a clear delineation of what is to be taught, task analysis of each skill, and instruction that makes use of reinforcement, fading, chaining, and other behavioral principles. This methodology, built on behavioral theory, has been effective with students of all ages with all handicapping conditions regardless of the extent of their disability and is an important part of many special education programs (Bernstein et al., 1981).

Another approach that is currently being incorporated into special education classrooms has its basis in the research on teacher effectiveness, teacher behaviors that seem to increase student learning (Rieth, Polsgrove, & Semmel, 1981). In this approach teachers demonstrate skills to be learned, maintain high expectations for student performance, provide frequent, supervised practice with corrective feedback, and keep students actively engaged in learning (Lewis, in press). Although the research on the effectiveness of direct instruction in special education classrooms is just beginning to be reported, preliminary findings suggest that it may be appropriate for some special education students (Lewis, 1983).

As researchers from a variety of disciplines learn more about the teaching-learning, new theories will be tested in special education classrooms. As the past has demonstrated, those that improve student performance will be adopted.

TRENDS IN SPECIAL EDUCATION

Several trends that have influenced special education programs and services in the 1980s will continue to shape the field in the next decade. Early intervention, parent/professional partnerships, new methods of instruction, transition planning based on collaboration across agencies and disciplines, preparation for adulthood, and normalization have all contributed to the improvement of special education programs. Increasingly, handicapped infants, preschoolers, and their families are served by health, social service, and/ or educational agencies. It has been documented that early educational intervention can significantly improve the child's functioning and reduce the need for later special education services (DeWeerd, 1981; Schweinhart & Weikart, 1980). These programs also increase parental knowledge about their rights and those of their handicapped child, resulting in more effective advocacy for quality services.

The parent/professional partnership that was supported in the provisions of PL 94-142 has evolved into a movement of its own. Many parents have become exceedingly successful advocates and are taking roles of importance in the service delivery system. Their continued participation, advocacy, and monitoring will enhance the range and quality of special education programs.

Renewed emphasis on curriculum and methods of instruction for students in special education programs also will affect special education. In programs for students with more severe handicaps, community-based instruction is again receiving attention. Instead of teaching life skills in the classroom, teachers work with their students where the behavior is expected to occur. For example, students would learn how to use the city bus system by riding buses and receiving instruction in the "real" world instead of practicing in the classroom. Technology also has influenced curriculum and instruction. Handicapped students have begun to gain skills in the use of technology; and technology, especially the microchip, has enabled students with physical and sensory handicaps to learn more easily. The current research on teacher effectiveness and the direct instruction movement are additional examples of new trends in instruction.

Though most often associated with the movement from school to the world of work, transition planning includes all changes from one program or service to the next. For example, handicapped infants move from an infant program to a preschool program. Adolescents and young adults move from school into higher education, vocational training, or the work place. A major trend in special education is work with parents, professionals, and other agencies to assure that the handicapped student and his family are adequately prepared for the transition (Will, 1984). Early intervention programs must prepare infants and their parents for the new demands of preschool programs, just as high school programs must prepare students for employment or continued education.

Programs for handicapped students often have been far less demanding than those for their nonhandicapped peers. Because it was assumed that many of the students would not continue their education or function independently as adults, students were not prepared for adulthood and maturity. More recently, it has become clear that most handicapped students can continue their education or hold jobs and participate quite fully in the mainstream of adult life. Thus, special education programs are changing their emphasis to include the academic and/or life skills that students will need when they leave school.

Finally, normalization, or the provision of programs and services that are as near to the cultural norm as possible, has dramatically influenced all programs and services for students with handicaps (Wolfensberger, 1972). The affirmation that handicapped individuals have the same rights as their nonhandicapped peers and the development of programs and services that support those rights will continue to influence special education.

UNMET NEEDS

Despite the gains made in special education programs and services since the enactment of PL 94-142, some needs are still unmet. Only 38 states mandate early-intervention services for any portion of the population below age six; and in those, the services are generally for those children from three through five (U.S. Department of Education, 1984). These services need to be extended to all young handicapped children and their families.

Providing appropriate special education services for students from diverse cultural backgrounds continues to be a need (Cegelka, in press). Although the numbers of non-English-speaking, handicapped students is increasing, methods and materials for these students have not kept pace.

Training that prepares special education students to continue their education or enter the job market is another area of need. Special education programs are not successful when students do not have the skills to make the transition into the world of work.

Finally, ongoing, systematic evaluation of special education programs and services continues to be a need. Only through careful study of current practice and outcomes can programs be improved.

SUMMARY

Special education is a discipline that is concerned with providing instruction to both gifted and handicapped students. Educational services for handicapped students are mandated and regulated by PL 94-142, the Education for All Handicapped Children Act. This act, which guarantees a free and appropriate education in the least restrictive environment for all handicapped students, has been extremely beneficial in improving programs and services in both regular and special education throughout the United States.

REFERENCES

Bagnato, S. J., & Neisworth, J. T. (1981). *Linking developmental assessment and curricula.* Rockville, MD: Aspen Systems.

Bernstein, G. S., Ziarnik, J. P., Rudrud, E. H., & Czajkowski, L. A. (1981). *Behavioral habilitation through proactive programming.* Baltimore: Paul H. Brookes.

Burton, T. A., & Hirshoren, A. (1979). Some further thoughts and clarifications on the education of severely and profoundly retarded children. *Exceptional Children, 45,* 618–625.

Cartwright, G. P., Cartwright, C. A., & Ward, M. J. (1981). *Educating special learners.* Belmont, CA: Wadsworth Publishing.

Cegelka, P. (in press). Multicultural considerations in special education. In E. W. Lynch & R. B. Lewis (Eds.), *Introduction to exceptionality.* Glenview, IL: Scott, Foresman & Co.

DeWeerd, J. (1981). Early education services for children with handicaps— Where have we been, where are we now, and where are we going? *Journal of the Division of Early Childhood, 2,* 15–24.

Fink, W. (1982). Education and habilitation of the moderately and severely mentally retarded. In P. Cegelka & H. Prehm (Eds.), *Mental retardation—From categories to people.* Columbus, OH: Charles E. Merrill.

Forness, S. R., & Kavale, K. A. (1984). Education of the mentally retarded: A note on policy. *Exceptional Children, 19,* 239–245.

Guess, D., Horner, R. D., Utley, B., Holvoet, J., Maxon, D., Tucker, D., & Warren, S. (1978). A functional curriculum-sequencing model for teaching the severely handicapped. *AAESPH Review, 3,* 202–215.

Kavale, K. A., & Glass, G. V. (1982). The efficacy of special education interventions and practices: A compendium of meta-analysis findings. *Focus on Exceptional Children, 15* (4), 1–14.

Larsen, S. C., Parker, R. M., & Hammill, D. D. (1982). Effectiveness of psycholinguistic training: A response to Kavale. *Exceptional Children, 49,* 60–66.

Lewis, R. B. (1983). Learning disabilities and reading: Instructional recommendations from current research. *Exceptional Children, 50,* 230–240.

Lewis, R. B. (in press). Learning disabilities. In E. W. Lynch & R. B. Lewis (Eds.), *Introduction to exceptionality.* Glenview, IL: Scott, Foresman & Co.

Lewis, R. B., & Doorlag, D. H. (1983). *Teaching special students in the mainstream.* Columbus, OH: Charles E. Merrill.

McLoughlin, J. A., & Lewis, R. B. (1986). *Assessing special students* (2nd ed.). Columbus, OH: Charles E. Merrill.

Meyen, E. L. (1982). An overview. In E. L. Meyen & D. H. Lehr (Eds.), *Exceptional children in today's schools: An alternative resource book*. Denver: Love Publishing.

Rieth, H. J., Polsgrove, L., & Semmel, M. I. (1981). Instructional variables that make a difference: Attention to task and beyond. *Exceptional Education Quarterly, 2*(3), 61–71.

Schweinhart, L., & Weikart, D. (1980). *Young children grow up: The effects of the Perry preschool program on youths through age 15*. Ypsilanti, MI: High/Scope Educational Research Foundation.

Turnbull, H. R., Turnbull, A. P., & Wheat, M. J. (1982). Assumptions about parental participation: A legislative history. *Exceptional Education Quarterly, 3*(2), 1–8.

U.S. Department of Education. (1984). Executive summary—Sixth annual report to Congress on the implementation of Public Law 94-142: The Education for All Handicapped Children Act. *Exceptional Children, 51*, 199–202.

U.S. Office of Education. (1977). Implementation of part B of the Education for the Handicapped Act. *Federal Register, 42*, 42474–42518.

Will, M. C. (1984). Let us pause and reflect—But not too long. *Exceptional Children, 51*, 11–16.

Wolfsberger, W. (1972). *The principle of normalization in human services*. Toronto: National Institute on Mental Retardation.

Chapter 19

SEXUALITY AND THE DEVELOPMENTALLY DISABLED

Marilyn J. Krajicek

The sexual developmental issues encountered by children and youths with handicapping conditions are similar to those facing the general population. However, special problems—including the nature of the handicap, environmental restrictions, and the lack of opportunity for social interactions—pose barriers that may prevent persons who are developmentally disabled from developing self-confidence and the social skills that are so necessary for appropriate psychosexual adjustment in society.

Parents and care givers, who are expected by society to help their children reach responsible sexual adulthood, are often unprepared to counsel their special-needs child. They are frequently uncomfortable with discussing sensitive personal issues with their young adult and are unsure both how to approach the topic and what to teach. Therefore, parents and caretakers often look to health professionals for expert help.

Unfortunately, too few professionals are adquately prepared for this role. Like parents and caretakers, professionals often are uncomfortable discussing human sexuality. In addition, few professionals have adequate preparation in this area. This chapter will address major issues of which the professional should be aware, and will suggest resources to aid the professional.

A Helpful Professional Orientation

Professionals who would be effective in counseling children and youths with handicapping conditions and their families/caretakers about sexuality must first be comfortable with their own sexuality. It is important that the professional be honest and straightforward, demonstrate an open attitude, be comfortable using both technical terminology and slang words (which may be all that the young person knows), and be able to simplify complex ideas when necessary (Kempton, 1974). In addition, the professional needs to understand handicapping conditions and their implications for human sexuality.

Assessment and Teaching

The professional should first meet with the young person's parents/caretakers to learn their expectations from the professional. Developing rapport with the parents/caretakers, gaining insights into their concerns, and finding out how they perceive the young person's needs are important first steps in the assessment process.

Next the professional will want to assess the young person's level of understanding of human sexuality. Yet such assessment may not be simple if the young person is severely mentally retarded, lacks communication skills, or is hearing-impaired. Fortunately, materials are available to help with assessment. In some cases, a sign interpreter may be needed during the assessment.

To be effective during both assessment and teaching, the professional must present information that interests the young person and is at his level of understanding. In addition. the professional must be creative, imaginative, and flexible in working with the individual who has a handicapping condition (Kempton, 1974). Assessment and teaching often go hand-in-hand, with the professional providing the child or young adult with accurate words for body parts and functions during the assessment process. Sometimes the professional will want to provide more formalized teaching, either one to one or in groups. If teaching is to be provided in groups, it is important that the individuals involved be at a similar functional level.

Socialization

As was mentioned previously, children and youths who are developmentally disabled face a number of barriers to their development as sexual adults. A major problem for many of these young people is a lack of self-esteem, of feeling "OK" about themselves. Unfortunately, there are few social programs designed to develop their social skills, including self-esteem.

Therefore, the professional should help the client to develop the self-esteem that is essential for all successful interpersonal interactions, whether psycho-social or sexual (Blum & Blum 1981).

Activities that encourage self-esteem may be conducted individually or in groups. Role modeling, slides and movies, pictures, flannel boards, be-havior modification techniques, and so on may be useful. Emphasis should be on helping the young person who is developmentally disabled to learn to be intimate in ways that can be but are not necessarily sexual. For example, the young person can be helped to share feelings, express concerns, be sen-sitive, feel close, touch and hold, and kiss and snuggle (Gunn & Poore, 1984).

MARRIAGE AND THE FUTURE

The professional may be asked to counsel a young adult who has a handicapping condition and who is considering marriage. Such a situation requires assessment of many factors. These include assessment of the young couple's self-help skills, skills in managing money, ability to work, ability to be responsible for living arrangements, and appropriate problem-solving skills. It also requires indentification of the couple's support systems (such as families) and helpful community resources.

When a young couple in which one partner is developmentally disabled considers marriage, the issue of child-bearing needs to be discussed. The professional can assess whether the couple have adequate parenting skills or can benefit from parenting classes. Can they cope with the stresses of mar-riage life and realistically care for a child? If not, the couple should be coun-seled as to appropriate birth control measures.

CONTRACEPTION

A major concern as the young person approaches maturity or marriage is contraception. Decisions about contraception must be made by the indi-vidual, often with the help and guidance of the professional and parents or caretakers.

The professional probably should begin by determining the parents' or caretakers' perceptions. Developing a good working relationship with these significant others is essential, for their assistance may be necessary to ensure that come contraceptive measures are successful (Chamberlain, et al., 1984).

One role of the professional regarding contraception involves teaching the importance of sexual responsibility. Another involves assessing the per-son's need for the control of fertility (Chamberlain, et al., 1984).

A third role involves providing the individual with information so that he can determine which type of contraception is most appropriate. Certain kinds of birth control may be contraindicated for various handicapping conditions. For example, a person with cerebral palsy may have difficulty applying a mechanical or chemical contraceptive; an oral contraceptive may be ruled out for a person with a seizure disorder; or a severely mentally retarded young woman may be unable to successfully take "the pill" (National Clearing House for Family Planning, 1980).

STERILIZATION

The issue of sterilization is one that is controversial and emotionally "loaded," yet is is one for which the professional must be prepared.

Because the laws of each state regarding sterilization differ, the professional will have to become informed about local requirements. New Jersey has developed due process standards to protect the mentally retarded under certain circumstances (Passer, et al., 1984), and approximately 20 states have laws permitting the review of requests for sterilization. However, many states have eliminated the eugenic sterilization statutes but have not passed new legislation permitting sterilization under certain conditions.

In Colorado, for sterilization to occur, the consent of the individual, the parent or legal guardian, a psychologist or psychiatrist, and one other professional must be obtained. (These latter professionals must have interviewed the client.) If there is a question about the person's mental capacity to give voluntary informed consent, Colorado law provides for a hearing procedure; court approval must be obtained before sterilization of a minor.

The point is not that the health professional should attempt to become a legal expert. Instead, the professional should learn the general provisions of the state's laws and should know where to refer parents/caretakers who are considering sterilization for their young person.

SEXUALLY TRANSMITTED DISEASE

Persons who are developmentally disabled are as prone as members of the general population to contract a sexually transmitted disease (STD). As a result, individuals who are developmentally disabled must be taught to protect against these diseases. The professional should have a basic understanding of the signs and symptoms of these diseases and how they are transmitted.

STD refers to infections caused by micro-organisms that are transmitted by intimate contact (usually genital, sometimes oral). The most frequent STDs include gonorrhea and syphilis, which can be asymptomatic (Rosenfeld & Litman, 1984).

Gonorrhea can cause pelvic inflammation in women; it is often associated with right-lower-quadrant pain, elevated temperature, problems in walking, and a possible vaginal discharge and burning sensation. In men there may be puslike discharge and burning on urination, or there may be no symptoms at all (Harger & Britton, 1984).

Syphilis is marked by a chancre (lesion) that appears more often in men than in women. This chancre can heal even without treatment, but a secondary stage will follow. If untreated, a third or latent phase develops; the disease has no signs or symptoms in this phase but can result in a fatal condition (such as organic brain syndrome) (Harger & Britton, 1984).

Herpes simplex virus I is another common STD. This infection most often appears as sores or blisters on the lips, eyes, nose, and/or genitals. It can be spread by using another's glass, towel, and so on. Any kind of sexual play involving the genitals during the infected stage can spread the virus (Gunn & Poore, 1984).

Chlamydia is primarily transmitted during intercourse and can cause pelvic inflammatory disease. It also can be transmitted to an infant during birth.

Clients can be taught that the use of condoms on a regular basis will prevent the spread of STD (Harger & Britton, 1984).

MASTURBATION

Masturbation is normal in both handicapped and non-disabled people and can relieve stress, boredom, and depression. However, in some individuals who have a handicapping condition, it becomes a compulsive behavior that warrants assessment and evaluation. The issue becomes more concerning when masturbation is carried out in public; then it can be a very real barrier to socialization (Kempton, 1974).

If masturbation is occurring in public, the professional should determine whether the developmentally disabled young person has been taught what is and is not socially acceptable behavior. If it appears obsessive, the professional should determine whether excessive masturbation may be caused by infection or genital irritation. Explanation, teaching, and/or behavior modification may be needed to ensure that masturbation does not become a barrier that results in isolation of the person with a developmental disability.

SEXUAL ABUSE AND EXPLOITATION

Unfortunately, children and youths who are developmentally disabled are as likely to be sexually abused or exploited as so-called normal youngsters. This vulnerability reaches into adulthood in many cases. Persons who are severely handicapped may not know they have been exploited and may not know how to seek help if they are victimized. Therefore, one role of the professional is to be alert at all times to any signs or symptoms of sexual abuse, assault, or exploitation. Any suspicion of sexual abuse must be reported to social service agencies.

THE PROFESSIONAL'S ONGOING ROLE

It is essential that the professional be prepared to be involved with a young developmentally disabled child and his family/caretakers over time. As the youth approaches adolescence, questions about sexuality inevitably arise. The professional may be asked to assess the youngster's level of understanding and provide training regarding socialization and human sexuality. As the youth matures, the professional may be asked for help with questions of marriage, child-bearing, contraception, and/or sterilization.

The professional must consider how he will be involved with the young person who is developmentally disabled and his family/caretaker over time. The special trusting relationship that will develop over the years can greatly help the individual, can ease the stresses on the family or caretakers to a considerable extent, and will be especially rewarding to the professional.

REFERENCES

Blum, G., & Blum, B. (1981). *Feeling good about yourself*. Mill Valley, CA: Feeling Good Associates.
Chamberlain, A., Rauh, J., Passer, A., McGrath, M., & Burket, R. (1984). Issues in fertility control for mentally retarded female adolescents: I. Sexual activity, sexual abuse and contraception. *Pediatrics, 73,* 445–450.
Gunn, T., & Poore M. (1984). *The herpes handbook* (5th ed.). Portland, OR: The Venereal Disease Action Council.
Harger, D., & Britton, T. (1984). *Chlamydia and NGU*. Portland, OR: The Venereal Disease Action Council.
Kempton, W. (1974). *A teacher's guide to sex education for persons with disabilities that hinder learning*. Belmont, CA: Wadsworth Publishing.
National Clearing House for Family Planning. (1980). *Information Services Bulletin* (#20852, No. 14). Rockville, MD: National Clearing House for Family Planning.
Passer, A., Rauh, J., Chamberlain, A., McGrath, M., & Burket, R. (1984). Issues in fertility control for mentally retarded female adolescents: II. Parental attitudes towards sterilization. *Pediatrics, 73,* 451–454.
Rosenfeld, W., & Litman, N. (1984). Sexually transmitted diseases. In S. Shelov, H. Mezey, & C. Edelmann (Eds.), *Primary care pediatrics* (pp. 549–550). Norwalk, CT: Appleton Century-Crofts.

Chapter 20

CARE OF HANDICAPPED CHILDREN AND YOUTH AWAY FROM THEIR OWN HOMES

David E. Loberg

In the life of a family, few events are so devastating, especially for young parents, as the discovery at the birth of a child, or soon after, that their new-born son or daughter has one or more severe handicaps (Blacher, 1984; Waisbren, 1980). A second related event with comparable significance and added tragedy for the young family is the moment of reluctant recognition that the severely handicapped child cannot be maintained indefinitely, for a variety of possible reasons, in the family home and that their young disabled child will require placement in some form of residential setting outside of the family. Although parents will subsequently be thrust into the process of making periodic changes in the living arrangements for their child with handicaps as they continue to arise in later years, the family may never be so distressed over the special problems associated with meeting the needs of this child as they are during the difficult period just prior to and during the first few weeks after the child's initial out-of-home placement.

The burden of having a child with a severe handicap is not only the bit-ter sense of disappointment and the dashed hopes of the parent for the ful-fillment of the potential of the child, it is also the recognition that the severely handicapped child will be required to live out most of his life in an unfa-miliar, stranger-staffed service facility that is most likely outside of the usual experience of the family, their relatives and neighbors, and the community. An added burden is the fear, often validated, that the child will be the life-long object of the curious stares and the stereotyping treatment that is commonly encountered by severely handicapped individuals, especially if they are associated as residents or clients with mental health or mental retardation service facilities. The separation of parents and their handicapped children that is the significant outcome of out-of-home placement is made all the more stressful by the sense of helplessness of parents in being unable to prevent the anticipated suffering, real and imagined, of their least capable child that is feared, even when mistaken, to be a common element of any out-of-home placement.

It is often pointed out that, in the past, families were commonly advised by pediatricians and family physicians, psychologists, social workers, and teachers that their severely handicapped child should be "put away" in an appropriate setting and that the family must "try to forget" that the handicapped member had "ever been born." At the time that such advice was typically given, large, overcrowded state institutions were frequently the only residential placement alternative available for consideration by parents of severely handicapped children. These publicly operated residential facilities were often castle-like, forbidding structures that were located in remote rural areas. They were the heritage of the eugenics movement of earlier generations of professionals during which the recognized leaders of the field argued confidently that the social problem of subnormal intellectual functioning and the related problems of "degeneracy," "criminality," and "pauperism" would be ultimately eliminated by a policy of firmly limiting any opportunity for social interaction and any consequent reproductive relationships between individuals with mental deficiency and others of normal intelligence (Brown, 1898/1976; Goddard, 1908/1976; Kerlin & Greene, 1884/1976; Powell, 1886/1976; Rogers, 1890/1976).

It was not until the middle of this century that the choices available to families whose severely handicapped children required out-of-home placement began to change. The post–World War II period brought about global changes in social attitudes and behavior in the areas of family life, education, social services, employment, civil rights, health services, and many others. The increasing use of a variety of newly developing media by business for marketing products and later by organized interest groups for influencing public opinion also began to stimulate associations with charitable purposes to influence public opinion and, ultimately, legislation. The role of the consumer of products and services began to emerge as a dominant force, not only in the marketplace but also in the areas of health, education, and social services. Greatly expanded opportunities for higher education became available through the G.I. Bill, and the post-war "baby boom" encouraged college students to seek careers in education and human services. It was in this context that parents, with the assistance of professionals in social services, were stimulated to organize, first, local associations and, later, state and national associations that focused on the special problems and needs of handicapped children and their families. The National Association for Retarded

Children was founded in 1950, and United Cerebral Palsy was founded in 1951 (Lippman & Loberg, 1985).

In the 1960s, President John F. Kennedy was a major stimulus for the start of the present era in the provision of services to severely handicapped children and adults. In 1961 he appointed the President's Panel on Mental Retardation, which in 1963 issued its landmark report entitled "A Proposed Program of National Action to Combat Mental Retardation." In that same year he gave a Special Message to Congress in which he called national attention to mental illness and mental retardation as occurring more frequently, affecting more people, requiring more prolonged treatment, causing more suffering by families, and costing both the public and families more than any other condition, and he called for a "bold new approach" (*Public Papers of the Presidents*, 1964, p. 126). It marked the point when new federal legislation in support of the systematic mental disabilities planning by states began to be passed by the Congress, and the choices confronted by parents whose children, because of their handicapping conditions, needed special education and residential placement began to change.

The work of Goffman (1961), Blatt and Kaplan (1966), Wolfensberger (1972), and others precipitated the movement of "de-institutionalization," a major and continuing critical assessment of the role and value of all large institutions in the provision of services to groups of individuals regardless of the particularity or intensity of their needs. The broad consensus has now been fairly well established that institutional placement should be regarded only as the "last resort" for anyone needing to be placed out-of-home for whatever reason and that the special needs of children dictate that their placement in large institutions be avoided if at all possible.

There is still a lack of consensus as to the defining criteria of institutions in terms of appropriate size. The definition of an institution may vary from, for example, the Federal Regulations for Intermediate Care Facilities for the Mentally Retarded, which uses a minimum of *four* residents to a facility with a bed capacity that exceeds "3 times the average number in a family household within the geographic area," as used in U.S. Senate Bill 873, Chaffee, Rhode Island, 1985. The fire and life safety codes adopted by many states use 15 residents or fewer as the capacity below which boardinghouse fire and life safety standards versus institutional fire and life safety standards may normally be applied. More recently, the *characteristics* of residents of facilities in terms of their ability to respond to alarms and be self-preserving in an emergency are increasingly being employed, along with numbers of residents to gauge appropriate levels of fire protection (MacEachron, & Janicki, 1983). Also, state laws governing the enactment of zoning ordinances that preempt local government from imposing zoning restrictions or special use permits on family-size residential facilities vary from state to state but are normally limited to facilities that range in maximum size from four to six or eight residents.

There were other factors that led to an increasing emphasis on the avoidance of large institutions for children. The community mental health movement, aided by the success of dramatic advances in psychotropic medications, began to expand and demonstrate that many individuals who had been treated as inpatients in psychiatric facilities also could be treated effectively in outpatient clinics, with the added benefit of avoiding the disruption, cost, and discontinuity in lives that almost always accompanies long-term, out-of-family placement. Further, the success of child guidance clinics in the years following World War II fostered an optimism that resulted in increasing efforts to treat children, even those with problems of relatively severe emotional disturbance, while they continued to reside at home with their families. This approach began to extend to the services provided to children whose handicapping conditions were increasingly complex and ultimately came to include children with the problems of mental retardation and other severe handicaps.

One of the major trends that contributes to the increased numbers of choices available to parents seeking out-of-home placement for their handicapped child has been the recent expansion in number and variety of community residential facilities for individuals with increasingly wide ranges of needs, ages, and disabilities. More than one-half (8,065) of the total number of facilities responding to a survey for a national census of mental retardation residential facilities in 1982 reported that they had opened services for mentally retarded residents since January 1, 1977. Ninety-six percent of those facilities were smaller residences with a median size of four residents (Bruininks et al., 1983).

One of the more recent developments that has helped to reduce the number and the proportion of handicapped children who are at risk of out-of-home placement is the increased availability of family support services: respite care, parent training, parent counseling, referral services, special transportation services—virtually any supportive help that will make it possible for families to defer the out-of-home placement of their handicapped child. In a few states, cash payments are being made directly to families to provide assistance with the excess costs of caring for a severely handicapped child in the family home. This "family support approach" contains the added advantage of achieving significant savings of tax dollars by avoiding or deferring the high costs of out-of-home placement in exchange for the relatively small costs required for the provision of family support services.

The optimism concerning the possibility of meeting the needs of severely handicapped children within the family home has been increasingly accompanied by the view that when out-of-home placement cannot be avoided or deferred, a foster home is the most appropriate first alternative to be considered. If a foster home placement is not feasible for whatever reason, case managers are encouraged to refer families seeking out-of-home placement for their son or daughter to a conveniently located group home in the nearby community. The theme is to make every effort to ensure that the family is encouraged to seek a small, home-like, family-scale living arrangement for the child with severe handicaps.

There is a working assumption by many first-line professionals that, in spite of the promises held out by the de-institutionalization movement, in spite of the availability of family support services, and in spite of the dramatically increased numbers and variety of family-size, community-based residences, there is a residual group of the most severely handicapped children that will require the services of relatively large, 24-hour congregate care facilities. Although the pervasiveness of this view may be challenged, the fact is that the proportion of handicapped children who fit this description is constantly *decreasing*. Today young children whose needs require a large residential setting are a relatively small number—only those children with multi-handicapping conditions, i.e., severe physical disabilities, sensory handicaps, or behavior disorders combined with, for example, the problems of severe or profound mental retardation. Additionally, it is recognized that a negligible number of handicapped children, although they may not have multiple severe handicaps, may be from family situations with special factors unrelated to the child's needs that require that their services be provided in larger residential settings.

In the mid-1980s, the choices that are presented to families for the out-of-home placement of their severely handicapped children are significantly greater than the choices that were available in the 1960s. In nearly every state the adoption of a state policy of seeking to reduce reliance on larger publicly operated institutions and to foster the development of community-based services has stimulated private agencies and individuals to establish residential facilities: nursing homes, group homes, supervised apartments, private residential schools—a veritable *continuum* of living arrangements. These facilities are licensed, regulated, and funded usually by the state agencies that are responsible for operating the public institutions that serve individuals with severe handicaps. In some states these same agencies have the responsibilities for case management and referrals as well; however, that is a changing pattern, with the functions of diagnostic evaluation, assessment of needs, and referral for services to the appropriate agencies in the continuum of services being increasingly the responsibility of case management agencies, sometimes called "service brokers," that are *not* directly affiliated with the provision of residential services.

One of the legislative landmarks that is well recognized as the direct result of parent and professional advocacy and successful litigation was the passage in 1975 of Public Law 94-142, the Education for All Handicapped Children Act. This act had the effect of requiring the states to offer *all* handicapped school-age children, regardless of the severity of their disability, a free, appropriate (individualized), publicly funded education. The outcome, a rapid expansion on a nation-wide scale of the availability of special education services, is making it possible for many parents to maintain their handicapped child satisfactorily in their homes for an indefinite period, even up to young adulthood. This development is considered one of the major factors, along with the declining overall birthrate, that accounts for the greatly reduced percentage, as shown by Table 20-1, of children being served in public residential facilities in the 1980s compared to the 1960s (Bruininks et al., 1983; Scheerenberger, 1976).

The significance of these data becomes clearer when viewed in the context of the changes shown in Table 20–2 of the population of all ages of residents of public residential facilities of the United States over the past 20 years (Lakin, 1979; Rotegard, Bruininks, & Krantz, 1984; Scheerenberger, 1982).

It is widely recognized that these trends for public residential facilities are broad, strong, and expected to continue for the indefinite future. Although comparable data are not readily available for private facilities, studies have reflected similar patterns in the services for children in private residential facilities as well. A 1982 survey of each of the states to determine the national scope of group home programs found that of the residents identified by age in the sample ($N = 54,158$ residents), 7,954 or 14.7 percent were less than eighteen years of age, and most of these children or adolescents (62.6 percent) resided in homes of fewer than 15 residents (Janicki, Mayeda, & Epple, 1983). A related finding of the 1982 National Census of Residential Facilities (Bruininks et al., 1983) is that proportionately more children are served by private residential facilities than by public residential facilities.

There are issues that continue to dominate the dialogue concerning the out-of-home placement of severely handicapped children and youth. States vary greatly in their progress thus far in reducing their reliance on large state-operated residential facilities. Families express reservations about the stability, reliability, and quality of residential facilities that are smaller, decentralized, less frequently monitored, and operated as businesses, whether for profit or as non-profit agencies. Residential service providers frequently point out that state governments have not re-directed sufficient resources from state-operated facilities that are declining in population to community-based programs to be able to provide for the stability, reliability, and assurance of quality that families seek. State officials point out that although the population of state institutions is declining, the residents who remain and who are now being admitted constitute a single concentration of the most medically involved, behaviorally difficult, or multiply handicapped residents within a state. Although the legal system has been comparatively active in the area of rights for people with handicaps, the needs of young individuals with severe handicaps who come to the attention of the courts as a danger to self or others are not yet being adequately addressed in the development of new community-based residential programs. Also, the needs of young individuals with the so-called dual diagnosis of mental retardation accompanied by severe emotional disturbance are not yet being met in existing small community residential facilities.

It is widely acknowledged that the current emphasis on community-based

Table 20-1. Percentage by Three Age Groups of Residents of U.S. Public Residential Mental Retardation Facilities from 1964 to 1982

Chronological Age	Year			
	1964[a]	1973–74[a]	1975–76[a]	1982[b]
0–2	1.5	0.3	0.3	0.4[c]
3–21	49.2	42.3	36.3	21.4[d]
22+	49.3	57.4	63.4	78.2

[a]From Scheerenberger, 1976.
[b]From Bruininks et al., 1983.
[c]Birth through four.
[d]Five through twenty-one.

Table 20-2. The Changes in Population of Residents of All Ages in Public Residential Facilities in the United States from 1960 through 1982

1960	1965	1970–71[a]	1975–76[a]	1980–81[a]	1982[a]
163,730[b]	187,305[b]	189,546[c]	153,584[c]	125,799[c]	117,160[d]

[a]Average daily population for year as shown.
[b]From Lakin, 1979.
[c]From Scheerenberger, 1982.
[d]From Rotegard et al., 1984.

care for children has not yet addressed the needs of young children and youth with severe handicaps who have chronic medical problems. The choice is still too often among (a) nursing homes that are oriented to the care of adults; (b) state hospitals that, by state policy, are seeking to deflect clients of all ages to less expensive, less restrictive, and more normal living arrangements; or (c) group homes that have minimal medical services. The California Department of Developmental Services conducted a state-wide study of small community facilities serving medically fragile persons with developmental disabilities and found that approximately 800 people in 200 facilities were receiving inadequate nursing care and developmental services (California Department of Developmental Services, 1981). The California legislature addressed this problem with legislation sponsored by the California Department of Developmental Services that created a new health facility category for medically fragile persons with developmental disabilities, particularly infants and children (Senate Bill 851 by Senator W. Craven, 1985).

These new facilities are designed to care for four to six residents and provide on-site nursing care, supportive, developmental, and administrative services on a 24-hour basis with an ultimate potential benefit to 2,400 residents across the state. California is also the recipient of a U.S. Department of Health and Human Services grant that is being used to develop and pilot standards for small community-based facilities for medically fragile children for use by other states as well. In this connection the state of New York is similarly engaged in a project that is designed to meet the special needs of medically fragile young children in community-based living arrangements (Arthur Webb, personal communication). Larger private residential schools for children with severe handicaps also report anecdotally that an increasing proportion of their referrals are children with chronic medical conditions whose needs require 24-hour access to nursing care services along with more traditional educational or developmental services.

The period of rapid development of varied programs and services for children and youth with severe handicaps may be drawing to a close. The overall continuing decline in the birth rate is the most significant factor affecting the incidence of children with handicapping conditions and there are indications that the present trends in the child-bearing patterns of the middle class will continue. The postponement of first births by inevitably more mature mothers does concern some professionals that older mothers are more likely to bear infants who will be born at risk. However, the relatively recently increased availability and use of prenatal diagnosis and intrauterine intervention or termination of pregnancy already can be observed in the ethnic and socioeconomic composition of samples drawn from the case loads of state mental retardation and developmental disabilities agencies. The extent to which biomedical measures will be adopted by other ethnic and socioeconomic groups, especially in the present political climate, is an open question.

Although epidemiological studies appear to indicate that the overall *prevalence* of developmental disabilities is increasing (Lubin & Kiely, 1985), it is still possible to conclude that other evidence of the decreased *incidence* of certain birth defects will eventually result in a further reduction in the numbers of young disabled children who will need out-of-home placement in the future. There is some concern that welcome improvements in obstetric care, with resulting decreases in the incidence of infant mortality, may be accompanied by an increased prevalence of severely handicapped children who in the past might not have survived childbirth. It seems clear that the continuing extension of the life span and resulting increases in the numbers of adults with developmental disabilities will work to give children with the need for residential services a less dominant influence than adults in the planning and development of residential resources for severely handicapped individuals for the indefinite future. In this context, the continued expansion of the availability of family support services for families with severely handicapped children is a trend that deserves the strong support and encouragement of professionals, government officials, friends, and especially the families of severely handicapped children.

REFERENCES

Blacher, J. (1984). Sequential stages of parental adjustment to the birth of a child with handicaps: Fact or artifact? *Mental Retardation, 22,* 55–68.

Blatt, B., & Kaplan, F. (1966). *Christmas in purgatory: A photographic essay on mental retardation.* Boston: Allyn & Bacon.

Brown, G. A. (1976). President's address. *Journal of Psycho-Asthenics, 3*(1), 7. In W. Sloan & H. A. Stevens (Eds.), *A century of concern: A history of the American Association on Mental Deficiency 1876–1976* (p. 42). Washington, DC: American Association on Mental Deficiency. (Original work published 1898).

Bruininks, R. H., Hauber, F. A., Hill, B. K., Lakin, K. C., McGuire, S. P., Rotegard, L. L., Scheerenberger, R. C., & White, C. C. (1983),. *1982 national census of residential facilities: Summary report* (Brief No. 21). Minneapolis: University of Minnesota, Center for Residential and Community Services.

California Department of Developmental Services. (1981). *A study of community residential facilities serving medically fragile clients with developmental disabilities.* Sacramento, CA: Author.

Goddard, H. H. (1976). Impressions of European institutions and special classes. *Journal of Psycho-Asthenics, 13*(1, 2, 3, 4), 21. In W. Sloan & H. A. Stevens (Eds.), *A century of concern: A history of the American Association on Mental Deficiency 1876–1976* (p. 70). Washington, DC: American Association on Mental Deficiency. (Original work published 1908).

Goffman, E. (1961). *Asylums: Essays on the social situation of mental patients and other inmates.* Chicago: Aldine.

Janicki, M. P., Mayeda, T., & Epple, W. A. (1983). Availability of group homes for persons with mental retardation in the United States. *Mental Retardation, 21,* 45–51.

Kerlin, I. N., & Greene, H. M. (1976). The obligation of society to its defective members: Report of the standing committee to the eleventh national conference of charities and reforms. In W. Sloan & H. A. Stevens (Eds.), *A century of concern: A history of the American Asssociation on Mental Deficiency 1876–1976* (p. 2). Washington, DC: American Association on Mental Deficiency. (Original work published 1884).

Lakin, K. C. (1979). *Demographic studies of residential facilities for the mentally retarded: An historical review of methodologies and findings.* Minneapolis: University of Minnesota, Department of Psychoeducaltional Studies.

Lippman, L., & Loberg, D. E. (1985). An overview of developmental disabilities. In M. P. Janicki & H. M. Wisniewski (Eds.), *Aging and develop-*

mental disabilities: Issues and approaches (pp. 41–58). Baltimore: Paul H. Brookes.

Lubin, R. A., & Kiely, M. (1985). Epidemiology of aging in developmental disabilities. In M. P. Janicki & H. M. Wisniewski (Eds.), *Aging and developmental disabilities: Issues and approaches* (pp. 95–113). Baltimore: Paul H. Brookes.

MacEachron, A. E., & Janicki, M. P. (1983). Self-preservation ability and residential fire emergencies. *American Journal of Mental Deficiency, 88* 157–163.

Powell, F. M. (1976). President's address. *Proceedings of the association of medical officers of american institutions for idiotic and feeble minded persons, 10,* 388. In W. Sloan & H. A. Stevens (Eds.), *A century of concern: A history of the American association on mental deficiency 1876–1976* (pp. 12–13). Washington, DC: American Association on Mental Deficiency. (Original work published 1886).

Public papers of the presidents. John F. Kennedy, 1963. (1964). Washington, DC: U.S. Government Printing Office.

Rogers, A. C. (1976). President's address. *Proceedings of the association of medical officers of American institutions for idiotic and feeble minded persons, 14,* 31. In W. Sloan & H. A. Stevens (Eds.), *A century of concern: A history of the american association on mental deficiency 1876–1976* (p. 19). Washington, DC: American Association on Mental Deficiency. (Original work published 1890).

Rotegard, L. L., Bruininks, R. H., & Krantz, G. C. (1984). State operated residential facilities for people with mental retardation. *Mental Retardation, 69*–74.

Scheerenberger, R. C. (1976). *Public residential services for the mentally retarded.* Madison, WI: National Association of Superintendents of Public Residential Facilities for the Mentally Retarded.

Scheerenberger, R. C. (1982). Public residential services, 1981: Status and trends. *Mental Retardation, 20,* 210–215.

Waisbren, S. E. (1980). Parents' reactions after the birth of a developmentally disabled child. *American Journal of Mental Deficiency, 84,* 345–351.

Wolfensberger, W. (1972). *The principle of normalization in human services.* Toronto: National Institute on Mental Retardation.

Chapter 21

RESPITE CARE

Ludmilla Suntzeff Gafford

Respite care is the provision of appropriate services on a short-term basis in a variety of settings to individuals unable to care for themselves because of the absence, illness, emergency, or need for periodic relief of persons normally providing care (Lakin, Greenberg, Schmitz, & Hill, 1984). In early 1970s respite care emerged because of the normalization movement and the concept that persons who are handicapped are entitled to live in the least restrictive environment. Professionals began to recognize that unremitting care of handicapped persons at times brought about unwarranted placement in a residential facility due to disintegration of some families experiencing this stress.

Chronic problems such as managing hyperactivity in a non-verbal child or lifting a spastic teenager out of a wheelchair are often physically exhausting. Developmentally delayed children by definition have a longer period of dependency than normal children (Wikler, 1983).

Actually the concept of respite care had been practiced with non-handicapped children for thousands of years in most countries when the family became a viable social unit. In the United States the role of relatives in providing child care, or baby sitting, has been recognized as an important contribution to family mental health. By this means the parents obtained relief from constant demands of child care, assistance during illness or emergencies, and an opportunity to engage in recreational pursuits or attend to family business. More recently, as our society became more mobile, with families

239

moving away from their relatives, many parents began to rely on their friends or to hire teenagers as baby sitters. Some couples exchanged care for each other's children to obtain some time to themselves. Thus, intermittent relief for parents form child care is an accepted norm in our society.

What happens to these natural support systems for the parents of children and youth who are handicapped? Families of retarded children have decreased access to these resources (Wikler & Hanusa, 1980). Often the relatives are geographically unavailable. Even when they are available, some may be depressed themselves because of their grief over the birth of a child who is handicapped. Grandparents worry about the impact of their grandchild's condition on their own sons' and daughters' mental health. Hence, the relatives may be limited in their ability to assist with child care. Those who have adjusted to the reality of the child's handicap may be well able to provide respite care to a child who is only mildly retarded or handicapped but may not know how to look after a child who is substantially handicapped or has serious health problems.

Despite these problems, relatives are still the first source of respite care. When this support system is deficient, the pressures on the family are intensified, and need for respite care becomes more acute (Lakin et al., 1984; Parham, 1983). Friends and neighbors may be willing but are usually lacking in specific skills. In a study of 339 families, Upshur 1982a) reported that respite or evening care, when available, was mot often provided in their own home by other family members, relatives, neighbors, or family with no special training in working with handicapped individuals.

Significantly handicapped children and youth have only limited access to the usual sitter and day-care services in the community. The individuals providing such child care lack familiarity with the skills needed and perhaps react to the stigma associated with a child who is mentally retarded, developmentally delayed, or handicapped (Wikler & Hanusa, 1980).

TARGET POPULATION

As evident from research, the severity of the child's handicap, the extent of related health or behavioral problems, and the drain on the family's physical and emotional health are the chief reasons for the family seeking respite care. Other reasons are unexpected illnesses, emergencies, absence of the primary caretaker, and vacations (Upshur, 1982a, 1982b). The nature of the handicapping condition seldom affects the need for respite care though it may influence where it is sought and its availability. According to several studies in different parts of the country, children and youth who are profoundly handicapped, those with severe medical problems, those exhibiting serious emotional/behavioral problems and self-destructive tendencies are often excluded from respite care available to others who are handicapped. Autistic children are also frequently excluded (Apolloni & Treist, 1983; Joyce,

Singer, & Isralowitz, 1983; Upshur, 1982a). Major users of respite care were those whose children were identified as mentally retarded, the next largest groups being those with cerebral palsy and multiple handicaps (Appollini & Treist, 1983; Joyce et al., 1983; Upshur, 1982a). No information on programmed respite care for emotionally disturbed children and youth was found in literature review nor in interviews with the local mental health facilities, who expressed belief that there may be need for such service (University of Tennessee, Department of Child Psychiatry, Center for Health Sciences, 1985).

There is little information about sociocultural influence on the use of programmed respite care services. However, in a study of 330 families of mentally and physically handicapped children and youth in Lake County, Illinois, nonwhite, currently unmarried, and mothers with less than high school education were significantly more likely to use family and friends as respite providers. In contrast, higher-income, white, and more highly educated mothers were more likely to use professional respite providers (Suelzle & Kennan, 1981).

IMPACT OF RESPITE CARE ON FAMILIES

Professionals working with the handicapped population have begun to examine, through research methodology as well as through documented clinical impressions, the impact of specific interventions on grief process and stress experienced by their families. The effect of one of these interventions—respite care—has recently been studied.

Wikler's research (Wikler & Hanusa, 1980) measures the effect of in-home respite care on families. Though very limited in scope (ten families), this study documents by means of three assessment instruments that respite care does significantly reduce stress experienced by the families of handicapped family members. College students trained in behavioral techniques were respite care providers for ten weeks, offering a maximum of six hours time per week to families to which they were assigned. There were nine moderately retarded children and one severely retarded child, all with major behavior problems. Their additional handicaps were diverse, including cerebral palsy, autism, microcephaly, and hearing impairment. Significant reduction of stress in all families was shown by all measures used.

According to the Holyroid scale, there were decreases in negative attitudes toward the handicapped persons and decreases in the reported difficult personality characteristics. This was indicative of persons with developmental delay becoming more acceptable within the family. Improvement in social support and activities for persons with developmental delay also was noted. The qualitative assessments of observed familial stress estimated by respite care providers indicated a decrease from baseline of 4.0 (6 = extreme stress) to an average of 1.8 during the final visit. On Wikler's Life

Changes Questionnaire 100 percent of changes were positive, though the extend of reported change varied from 58 to 14 percent. The parents frequently did not know how to make use of leisure time and needed some suggestions. Automatic provision of respite care was found to be more helpful than respite care on demand. Continuity and positive nature of the relationship with the respite care provider were factors in stress reduction.

Research conducted by Joyce et al. (1983) provides further empirical evidence that respite care helps to improve family relations, increases social activities by family members, and alleviates the family's physical and emotional stress. In-home respite care was furnished by trained respite providers to the families of disabled/chronically ill children and adults living in a metropolitan area. After respite care, most parents (53 percent) related better to their handicapped family members. The majority (68 percent) felt that respite care relieved family stress and enabled non-handicapped family members to spend more time with each other (52 percent). Consequently, more social activities were possible (76 percent). The emotional strain of caring for their handicapped child was significantly relieved (95 percent), as was the physical strain (67 percent). The impact of the program was perceived as helpful by most families (86 percent), and the majority (95 percent) considered that in-home respite care can help parents avoid residential care for their handicapped sons and/or daughters. Although respite care was helpful to most families of handicapped children and youth, it was critically needed for families whose children were recently disabled.

RESPITE CARE STRUCTURE

Parents possess a wide spectrum of desires, needs and capabilities, and no assumptions or judgments concerning their capacity or interest should be made until the staffs of agencies have fully explored these areas with family members. Many times the staff disagrees about the parents' ability to become viable partners on the health care team and about the amount of information that should be shared with them. To achieve better collaboration between the parents and the professionals, several specific techniques are helpful: (a) encourage a system of record keeping and health maintenance by parents; (b) facilitate orientation to the role of each involved discipline; (c) acquaint the parents with community resources and ways of securing services; (d) foster communication with team providing service through role playing, encouraging questions, and providing an advocate, if necessary, to assist in communication; and (e) nurture advocacy skills. Successful home care depends on a strong alliance between the professional and the family. Both parents and siblings, if possible, should be involved. Communication between parents and professionals is essential, and it must be constructive and ongoing. Each family's circumstances are unique, and the planning process must be individual, flexible, and constantly evolving. No model, regardless of how effective it has been for someone, can be applied without individualization to each and every family (Golden, 1984).

Until the 1980s, respite care for handicapped children and youth was largely available through state institutions or community group programs, with a few beds set aside for this purpose. Many families used this as a "trial" placement, to be followed later by long-term placement. With the impetus of de-institutionalization and normalization, many respite care beds in state residential facilities were terminated (Parham, Hart, Newton, & Terraciano, 1983; Upshur, 1982b). Some parents began to "trade off" with each other in providing respite care for their handicapped child and to seek in-home services. The passage of Public Law 95-602, the Rehabilitation, Comprehensive Services, and Developmental Disability Amendments of 1978, with emphasis on life-span rehabilitation services for independent/semi-independent living, gave impetus to the development of a comprehensive approach to respite care in early 1980s (Parham et al., 1983).

A range of respite services is recommended in order to meet the diverse needs and preferences of the handicapped children and youth and their families. For optimal coverage, respite services in any community should contain the following options: community in-home approach, which offers respite providers, homemaker services, home health aide services, and companion services; community out-of-home approach, which offers respite care in the providers' own home, placement in group homes, group treatment facilities, and pediatric nursing homes; and out-of-community approach, which provides short-term placement in a public or private residential facility for children and youth with complex medical, psychiatric, or behavioral problems whose care requires expertise beyond that of other respite care facilities.

States differ in provision of respite care. Sometimes respite services are administered by the departments of developmental disabilities or their equivalent, with contracts to community agencies for provision of services (Apolloni & Triest, 1983).

CASE MANAGEMENT

A case manager is a designated person or an organization that assists the families with locating, coordinating, and monitoring the use of biomedical and psychosocial services needed by handicapped individuals and their family. Most families consider this to be a valuable service because they often are not familiar with the complex array of community resources. Case management includes an assessment of the handicapped individual's condition (Lakin et al., 1984) and the family situation, as well as knowledge of resources for respite care. Frequently, social workers function as case managers because they have generic training and understanding of community resources. Optimally, an MSW degree is desirable, but social workers with a BSW degree can perform this task if consultation is available. Nurses, especially those with training and/or experience in public health, also provide this service. Professionals in other related disciplines can function in this capacity if they have training in case management.

IN-HOME RESPITE CARE

Respite care most frequently requested and preferred by the families is in-home respite care. This has been documented in many studies, such as Hagan (1980), Upshur (1982a, 1982b), Apolloni and Triest (1983), and Smith (1984). Many families still rely on informal in-home respite care by relatives, friends, or neighbors when the children' handicapping condition does not present significant medical or behavioral problems. However, even those families tend to use this informal system sparingly, possibly lacking confidence in ability of such caretakers to handle potential problems or because they feel over-protective or guilty about leaving their handicapped child or youth while attending to their own needs. Informal arrangements between families who take turn in providing respite care for each other's handicapped children have had a measure of success (Smith, 1984).

Respite Care Providers

In-home respite care by trained respite providers is a fast-expanding service as information about such programs is disseminated. In some communities respite care is an additional function in existing agencies; in other places respite placement agencies are organized under private or public auspices. Respite providers are intensively trained in behavior management, specialized aspects of health care, infant stimulation, safety practices, and other relevant aspects of care of handicapped children and youth. Many respite providers are already technically or professionally employed in health care or special education settings or may be college students with these as career interests. As respite providers they usually have the option of part-time employment. Housewives and retired persons sometimes become respite providers. In-service training may be developed by their host agencies or by agencies already working with handicapped children and youth. Care is provided in the home of the handicapped person when the caretaker family member needs some relief, is attending to an emergency, or is absent or incapacitated. Continuity of the same respite provider is of great importance because they usually develop a positive relationship with the handicapped child or youth and his family. This reduces the parent's concern about their child's care (Wikler & Hanusa, 1980). Since trained respite providers have diverse personal and technical skills and have undergone intensive training, they constitute a manpower pool that can match the widely varying health needs and behavioral problems of this target population. The time frame for respite care is flexible, differing with the needs of the clients and ranging from a few hours to several weeks' duration. In research done by Wikler (Wikler & Hanusa, 1980) it was found that automatic provision of respite care on a regular basis is more useful to families than respite care on demand because initially some families may not know how to make use of available leisure time and may need some suggestions.

Homemakers

Another means of in-home respite care is provision of homemakers trained to work with handicapped children and youth. This service is available in most urban and rural communities through state departments of human services and sometimes through United Way-funded agencies. In addition to general housekeeping, the homemakers may offer training to families of those handicapped children and youth whose care requires expertise beyond that of other respite care facilities.

Home Health Aides

When requested by an agency or a client, Home Health Aide Services extend their coverage to include handicapped children and youths in their community. According to the regulatory definition, this involves performing "simple procedures such as the extension of therapy services, personal care, ambulation exercises, household services essential to health care at home, assistance with medications that are ordinarily self-administered, reporting changes in the patients' condition and needs and completing appropriate records" (Lakin et al., 1984). Personnel are professionally qualified registered nurses, MSW social workers, and other relevant disciplines. Some of these services also may be provided by such organizations as Visiting Nurses' Association and public health nurses in health departments. The respite feature of these services is the provision of health care or specific services to handicapped individuals in their home, so saving their primary caretakers the extra burden of transporting a non-ambulatory or difficult-to-manage handicapped individual to a health care facility.

Companion Services

In implementation of these services, volunteers or paid sitters/companions provide recreational opportunities for handicapped children and youth and assist them with developing specific skills or areas of interest. This may involve recreational experience at home or elsewhere, such as taking the handicapped persons to a ball game, a movie, a special Olympics event, or a party. Programs similar to Big Brothers, Big Sisters, or Foster Grandparents may be placed in this category (Parham et al., 1983). In addition to the socializing aspects of these programs, they offer temporary relief from child care for the primary caretakers.

OUT-OF-HOME RESPITE CARE

Many families still rely on informal out-of-home respite care provided by relatives, friends, or neighbors during the handicapped children's and youth's visits to their homes. Usually these opportunities exist for children who do not have a serious medical or behavioral problem. There are informal arrangements between families for providing respite care to each other's handicapped children. The extend-a-family system arranged by respite placement agencies matches a handicapped child's needs to those of a child in another family. This is an economical approach that enables the children to make new friends and have normalizing "out in the world" experiences, living, sleeping, eating, and playing with others (Smith, 1984).

Respite Care Provider

Some respite providers are certified to offer respite in their own home. Certification includes inspection of the home for safety and sanitary conditions by the coordinator of respite care. Exploratory interviews with members of the respite providers' families are held because they become temporarily a part of the psychosocial environment for the handicapped person, and consequently their reactions and attitudes toward the child's condition become matters of considerable importance. Services offered by respite providers are similar to those offered in the home of the handicapped youth. For children who are mildly or moderately retarded, this out-of-home experience has some normalizing aspects by making it possible for them to adjust to a different but accepting social environment and strengthening their capacity to cope with change. For their families it provides an opportunity to engage in some social activities, such as vacations, without having to consider the special needs of the handicapped member of their family.

Weekend Respite Camps

Such camps provide recreational experience with physical activities, games, and special Olympics for those able to participate, as well as simple crafts. The families gain relief from the constant care of their handicapped children and a chance to engage in social activities without feelings of guilt. In Memphis, MARC operates these weekend respite camps eight times a year. Only respite providers with a minimum of 1 year of satisfactory performance qualify for this assignment (MARC, 1985).

Respite Foster Homes

In most communities this service is provided by public or private agencies specializing in foster home placement, with some foster homes specializing in the care of handicapped children. In recruitment of foster parents their emotional response to handicapped children and their knowledge about such conditions are some of the factors considered (Coyne, 1983). Foster parents are usually given special training for working with this target population. Such training may include the following aspects: identification of foster parents' common concerns and problems about their foster children who may be mentally retarded, physically handicapped, and/or emotionally disturbed; reactions of foster parents to their foster child's handicaps; coping with their behavior problems; talking to their foster child about his condition; the role of foster parents; and collaboration with the agency in planning for the future (Park, 1983).

Temporary Group Home Placement

Group homes that are live-in facilities for persons enrolled in community training programs or employed during the day may have a few beds set aside for overnight respite care. Some may even have all or most beds available during vacations or holidays. The staff is already trained to work with handicapped children.

For handicapped children and youth with emotional/abehavioral problems respite care may be offered during vacations and holidays in some residential treatment facilities. There is already trained staff available for this purpose, and the facilities are adapted to such use (Upshur, 1982a).

Pediatric Nursing Homes/Hospitals

These primarily serve as long-term nursing care facilities or acute hospitals buy also may provide overnight or daytime respite for handicapped children and youth with significant medical needs, which make other kinds of placement difficult (Upshur, 1982a). Such facilities meet an urgent need because many handicapped persons with significant medical problems are often difficult to place. Most facilities do not offer respite care for handicapped children with significant medical problems. Facilities that do provide this service tend to give insufficient consideration to the stress experienced by the families.

OUT-OF-COMMUNITY RESIDENTIAL RESPITE CARE

For a few families the final solution to seeking respite care may still be a residential facility. Some have a few beds set aside for providing overnight care to older children and youths when there is no medical or psychosocial alternative. Most prefer to serve only their former inpatients (Upshur, 1982a). Such facilities have a built-in advantage in skilled staff and appropriate technology for treatment of medically fragile children.

SOURCES OF FUNDING

Many families pay for the services received, usually on a sliding scale or through special grants or funds that respite placement agencies secure to make up for difference in costs (Upshur, 1982a). Partial or total reimbursement through some health insurance companies or third-party payment through Champus, Supplemental Security Income, or other sources may be available. Some agencies have the cost of respite services as a line item in their budgets.

The funding conduit model allows families to select their own care giver for daytime or overnight services in their own home or that of the care giver. The respite placement agency merely reimburses the family (within agreed-on limits) for costs incurred in obtaining respite care. There is more potential for problems and a poorer quality of service because this is a contractual arrangement between the respite provider and the family, with no supervision provided (Upshur, 1982a).

A new concept that is rapidly changing the funding for some programs for the handicapped and bringing about more ready access to respite care is contained in Section 2176 of the Omnibus Budget Reconciliation Act of 1981 (PL 97-35). This statute grants the Secretary of Health and Human Services the authority to waive existing Medicaid (Title XIX) statutory requirements to permit states to finance non-institutional, long-term care services for Medicaid-eligible individuals. The waiver legislation and regulations allow states maximum flexibility in designing their home- and community-based programs within general restrictions controlling their size and cost. The participating states are free to establish programs for specific target populations. In addition, the states have the option to establish higher income and resource standards of Medicaid eligibility and may choose not to "deem" the parents' income to be available to the children and so omit it from eligibility considerations. Section 2176 specifies seven basic services that the states may offer under the waiver program: (a) case management, (b) homemaker services, (c) home health aide services, (d) personal care services, (e) adult day health services, (f) habilitation services, and (g) respite care. As of February 15, 1983, 16 states have elected to participate in the Medicaid waiver program (Lakin et al., 1984).

Congregational respite care to persons who are handicapped has emerged in the 1980s as an interfaith ecumenical movement. In some communities Christian and Jewish denominations collaborate in providing in-home and out-of-home respite care. The volunteer respite providers are members of participating congregations. They receive intensive training in respite care by qualified professionals. Referrals are non-denominational; *no fee is charged*. Congregational respite care supplements but does not compete with the existing services. The purpose is to provide services to families of handicapped persons and to enrich personal and spiritual growth of the volunteers by serving those in need and learning how to interact with persons who are handicapped. (Garberich, Kidd, Sherrill, & Gaventa, 1985) A manual containing guidelines for congregational respite care is provided by the National Council of Churches (Murphy, 1985).

CONCLUSION

An increasing number of mentally retarded/physically handicapped children and youth are living at home as a result of de-institutionalization. Some of their families need periodic, short-term relief from unremitting child care to prevent "burnout," as well as time for handling family emergencies and engaging in activities unsuitable for a handicapped family member. Respite care is a rapidly developing service for meeting those needs. National Medicaid waiver legislation of 1981 opened the way for funding diverse respite care programs for the handicapped population and made it financially feasible for most families living in participating states to utilize such programs.

Scarcity of respite care for emotionally disturbed children and youth is an unmet need.

REFERENCES

Apolloni, A. H., & Triest, G. (1983). Respite services in California: Status and recommendations for improvement. *Mental Retardation, 21*(6), 240–243.

Coyne, A. (1983). Techniques for recruiting foster homes for mentally retarded children. In L. Wikler & M. Keenan (Eds.), *Developmental disabilities no longer a private tragedy* (p. 196). Washington, DC: American Association on Mental Deficiency.

Garberich, R. T., Kidd, I. J., Sherrill, J., & Gaventa, B. (May 1985). *Respite care: Tapping the natural resources in the religious community.* Paper presented at the annual meeting of the American Association on Mental Deficiency, Philadelphia, PA.

Golden, D. (1984). Encouraging early family involvement. In *Home care for children with serious handicapping conditions* (pp. 41–43). Houston, TX: Association for the Care of Children's Health.

Hagan, J. (1980). *Report on respite care services in Indiana.* South Bend, IN: Northern Indiana Health Systems Agency.

Joyce, K., Singer, M., & Isralowitz, R. (1983). Impact of respite care on parents' perceptions of quality of life. *Mental Retardation, 21*(4), 153–156.

Lakin, K., Greenberg, J. N., Schmitz, M. P., & Hill, B. K. (1984). A comparison of Medicaid waiver applications for populations that are mentally retarded and elderly disabled. *Mental Retardation, 22*(4), 182–192.

MARC (Memphis [Tennessee] Association for Retarded Citizens). (May 1985). Interview by author.

Murphy, J. K. (1985). *Sharing care: The Christian ministry of respite care.* New York: National Council of Churches.

Parham, J. H., Hart, T., Newton, P., & Terraciano, T. L. (1983). Complementary concepts: Independent living and in-home respite care. *Journal of Rehabilitation, 1,* 70–74.

Park, D. N. (1983). A workshop for foster mothers of special children. In L. Wikler & M. Keenan (Eds.), *Developmental disabilities no longer a private tragedy* (pp. 166–171). Washington, DC: American Association on Mental Deficiency.

Porter Leath Children's Center, Memphis, TN. (May 1985). Interview by author.

Smith, P. M. (1984). Approaches to respite care. In *Home care for children with serious handicapping conditions* (pp. 52–53). Houston, TX: Association for the Care of Children's Health.

Suelzle, M., & Keenan, V. (1981). Changes in family support networks over the life cycle of mentally retarded persons. *American Journal of Mental Deficiency, 86*(3), 270.

University of Tennessee (Memphis), Department of Child Psychiatry, Center for Health Sciences. (May 1985). Interview by author.

Upshur, C. C. (1982a). Respite care for mentally retarded and other disabled populations: Programs, models and family needs. *Mental Retardation, 20*(1), 2–6.

Upshur, C. C. (1982b). An evaluation of home-based respite care. *Mental Retardation, 20*(2), 58–62.

Wikler, L. (1983). Chronic stresses of families of mentally retarded children. In L. Wikler & M. Keenen (Eds.), *Developmental disabilities no longer a private tragedy* (pp. 102–114). Washington, DC: American Association on Mental Deficiency.

Wikler, L., & Hanusa, D. (May 1980). *The impact of respite care on stress in families of developmentally disabled.* Paper presented at American Association of Mental Deficiency Annual Meeting, San Francisco, CA.

Chapter 22

TRANSPORTATION

Leonard F. Bender
Melinda K. Conway-Callahan

Significance of the Problem

The structure of our society imposes a stringent demand for personal mobility if one is not to be isolated socially and vocationally. When a person's mobility is limited, many of life's goals are unattainable. For the disabled child or adolescent, the parent or guardian is the primary person responsible for transit. However, that transportation is often limited to school or a very few scheduled activities. Transportation to social and informal leisure activities is likely to be nil. As the impaired child becomes an adult, the problems are intensified. Those with disability generally find it difficult or impossible to obtain essential transportation because taxis or other types of private services are very expensive or non-existent. In addition to the expense of purchasing transportation services, the isolation of the disabled is compounded by their problems with access to public and private transportation systems. According to Bookis (1983), a main factor in the social isolation of the handicapped in the United Kingdom is lack of mobility; the problem is worldwide.

More than one million physically disabled persons who live within a short walk of transit service cannot use it. Those who suffer the most severe problems are 409,000 wheelchair users, whose handicap poses exceptional problems for bus and subway operators attempting to serve them. Some wheelchair users who lack access to cars are too poor to pay taxi or ambulance fares have very few opportunities to visit friends, shop, go to the doctor's office, or pursue leisure activities. An additional four million handicapped persons live near transit but find it difficult to use (Congressional Budget Office, 1979).

In a comprehensive survey of the needs of the severely disabled, 60 percent of the individuals interviewed indicated that their need for transportation was not being met (Revis & Betty 1978).

The primary problem that inhibits transportation for the disabled is low income that does not allow for the purchase of equipment to facilitate travel. Transportation services are either unavailable, inconvenient, or available at the wrong time and the wrong place. Incidents have been reported where lift-equipped buses pass by disabled individuals because the drivers do not know how to operate the lifts. The disabled who are located in rural areas often are isolated from any type of transportation other than personal vehicles. Finally, there are many design problems that reduce accessibility both of vehicles and fixed facilities such as terminals and stations.

With the transportation limitations and restraints placed on disabled persons total community integration becomes difficult and in many instances impossible. In order for disabled individuals to claim their rightful place in the school system, work environment, and community, changes within our public transportation system are essential.

NEEDS

The specific problems handicapped persons face vary, depending on health, income, age, access to car, availability of family and friends, and location of residence.

Decreased mobility for the disabled typically means fewer trips and limited choices as to where they can go, especially if public transit routes are largely oriented toward work locations. To a considerable extent, the nature of these trips is determined by the character of the system available to the disabled. Most special transportation systems tend to provide for only limited trip purposes because they are designed that way. Some special systems provide access to social services or school *only* and cannot provide services for recreation trips, visiting, socializing or shopping. Similarly, public transit systems do not provide a wide network of ubiquitous service and may impose limitations by their fixed-route and fixed schedule characteristics (Revis & Betty 1978).

What is needed includes availability of handicapped driver evaluation and training programs, barrier-free public and private transportation systems, increased flexibility of public transportation routes, and improved provision and coordination of community agency transportation efforts. These needs are emphasized in *Conference Report: Critical Needs of the Child With Long Term Orthopedic Impairment* (American Academy of Orthopaedic Surgeons, 1985).

Requirements

In 1973, national policy was established that expressly forbids discrimination against the handicapped in federally funded programs. Specifically, Section 504 of the Vocational Rehabilitation Act of 1973 stated that "no otherwise qualified handicapped individual can be denied the benefits of or excluded from participating in, any program or activity receiving federal assistance." In addition, the Rehabilitation Act defines a handicapped person as "any person who has a physical or mental impairment which substantially limits one or more of such person's major life activities, has a record of such impairments, or is regarded as having such an impairment" (Congressional Budget Office, 1979).

The current proposed rule to enforce the accessiblity of mass transit for handicapped individuals will require providers to meet six service area criteria (U.S. Department of Transportation, 1983):

1. Availability throughout the same general service area as transit service for the general public.

2. Availability on the same days and during the same hours as service for the general public.

3. Fare for a handicapped person comparable to the fare for a member of the general public.

4. Prohibition of the establishment of special restrictions or priorities based on the trip purposes of the handicapped person.

5. Limitation of waiting period to a "reasonable time."

6. Prohibition of waiting lists for the provision to eligible users.

Each local transit authority is to develop "special efforts" to ensure accessible transportation if they receive federal funding. For some cities this means purchasing new buses with wheelchair lifts and/or modifications. Some cities opted for a "door to door" system that provides services to handicapped individuals through call-in reservations. However, these services may have long waiting lists, limited hours and restricted travel destinations. The new proposed rules will require transit authorities to meet more adequately the needs of the handicapped in their communities.

Provision of Transportation

Handicapped persons currently have four general types of transportation available to them in cities (Congressional Budget Office 1979): (a) private motor vehicles, (b) public transportation, (c) transportation provided by social service and voluntary health organizations, and (d) commercial services for handicapped persons. A study of the number of trips taken by handicapped and nonhandicapped persons in each mode of transportation was performed in 1977; the results are shown in Table 22-1 (U.S. Department of Transportation, 1978; 1979).

Private Automobiles

Handicapped persons typically own fewer vehicles and are less likely to drive than non-handicapped persons, thus indicating that the handicapped are often forced to schedule their trips to accommodate those who drive them.

In recent years rehabilitation centers have begun to provide driver evaluation and training programs for the handicapped. This service not only trains the handicapped to drive but prescribes adaptive equipment appropriate to the needs of each client. Equipment requirements range from simple adaptations such as steering knobs to compensate for the partial loss of use of an upper extremity to a complete system of adaptive aids such as a wheelchair lift, sensitized accelerators, braking and steering mechanisms to compensate for partial or total loss of use involving all four extremities.

Traditionally, government agencies such as the Rehabilitation Services Administration have assisted in the funding for training and adaptation for purchase. Costs do, however, affect the feasibility of independent driving. The adaptation of a van for a person with quadriplegia requires major modification and can approach a cost of $30,000.

Public Transportation

A few cities have buses with wheelchair lifts on their main transit lines, and some cities provide door-to-door service similar to a taxi service. The door-to-door service generally requires advance reservations and usually has very limited hours. The Metro system in Washington, DC, and the BART system in San Francisco are two subway systems that are fully accessible to the handicapped and will serve as examples for future mass transit projects; they have elevators to station platforms from ground level, auditory signals for the blind, visual signals for the deaf and flush entry for wheelchairs.

Transportation Provided by Social Organizations

Many cities through the United States have special projects operated by public or private non-profit agencies, such as Easter Seal Societies and Muscular Dystrophy Associations that provide transportation for the handicapped. However, they have two major shortcomings. First, many of them

Table 22-1. Proportion of Total Daily Trips Taken with Each Mode of Transportation by Handicapped and Non-Handicapped Persons, 1977

Transportation	Nonhandi-capped[a] (%)	All Handi-capped[b] (%)	Handicapped With No Car Usually Available (%)	With Car Usually Available (%)
Car	78	72	26	85
As driver	62	38	2	66
As passenger	16	34	24	19
Bus	9	9	33	5
Subway	3	2	8	1
Taxi	1	3	7	2
Specialized service	—	1	1	1
Walking	5	7	23	3
Other	4	6	3	4

[a]Persons aged 16 years or more living within a half-mile of a transit stop.
[b]Persons aged 5 years or more living in urban areas.
SOURCE: Compiled by Congressional Budget Office from U.S. Department of Transportation, 1978, 1979.

carry passengers only to specific destinations, and second, most social agencies offer transportation only to their own clients. Many agencies are attempting to coordinate transportation service, which would reduce costs and allow for greater service opportunities.

Commercial Service for Handicapped Persons

Individuals living in urban areas often utilize taxi service for their transportation needs. In addition, private companies offer van and limousine services, using vehicles equipped with lifts that are operated by drivers who provide specialized services by physically assisting the handicapped traveler. The fares tend to be very high, often as much as $45 per trip, (U.S. Department of Transportation, 1978; 1979) making this service unrealistic for most handicapped individuals.

Other commercial services such as airlines and trains are now beginning to provide services for the handicapped. Airplanes have been designed with wider aisles, and airports have increasing numbers of barrier-free ramps and airplane loading facilities. Some trains have special accommodations for wheelchair users, and large stations usually have elevators and level entry to trains.

UNMET NEEDS

The barriers in overcoming the transportation needs for the handicapped are indeed great and are not new. However, there are also societal barriers that need to be overcome before the handicapped can fully integrate within the community. By limiting handicapped individuals' ability to function independently within our society, we impact significantly on the quality of their lives. A group of physical impaired people proposes to define disability "as the disadvantage of restrictions of activity caused by contemporary social organization." (Finkelstein 1980) To the extent that barriers to attainable and practical mobility exist we need to continue and to renew efforts to reduce and remove them.

REFERENCES

American Academy of Orthopaedic Surgeons. (1985). *Conference report: Critical needs of the child with long term orthopaedic impairment*. Chicago: Author.

Bookis, J. (1983). *Beyond the schoolgate: A study of disabled young people aged 13–19*. London: Royal Association for Disability and Rehabilitation.

Congressional Budget Office. (1979). *Urban transportation for handicapped persons: Alternative federal approaches*. Washington, DC: Author.

Finkelstein, V. (1980). *Attitudes and disabled people: Issues for discussion*. New York: World Rehabilitation Fund.

Revis, J. & Betty, D. (1978). Transportation and disability: An overview of problems and prospects. *Rehabilitation Literature, 39*, 170.

U.S. Department of Transportation. (1978). *Technical report of the national survey of transportation of handicapped people*. Washington, DC: Author.

——. (1979). *Top-line presentation of transportation of handicapped people who do not have a car available and who do not use public transit*. Unpublished draft tabulations.

——. (1983). *The Department of Transportation's regulation implementing Section 504 of the Rehabilitation Act of 1973 in the urban mass transit program*. Washington, DC: Author.

Chapter 23

THE TEAM

Allan C. Oglesby

The "team," as it applies to community services for disabled children and their families, implies interdisciplinary collaboration and cooperation by professionals who assist the child and family to identify and achieve their goals.

It has long been recognized that disabling conditions in children cannot be approached successfully by any single discipline. The complexity of interacting factors in the internal and external environment of the child and the family require multidisciplinary involvement if optimal outcomes are to be achieved. Client and family expectations and clearly articulated goals are essential at the onset. These goals must be the basis for any professional relationship with the child and family in delivering direct services, planning, consultation, and family support.

The comprehensive and often non-technical nature of tasks required to achieve goals for the disabled person includes a large number of tasks that cannot be accomplished effectively by one person. Many models of teams have been described. They vary from the highly specialized surgical team, whose task is very specific and time-limited, to the consulting team in case management that is concerned with the ongoing and ever changing needs of a child and the family. All disciplines in health, welfare, and education may be members of the team as specific goals are defined. Although all persons require the collaborative and cooperative interaction of professionals in some aspects of their lives, the disabled, because of special needs, interact with more disciplines than the non-disabled throughout their life spans. The composition of a team is defined by the tasks to be accomplished and the purpose of the professional effort in accomplishing those tasks.

A group of professionals working with a child and the family will represent a number of different disciplines, but they may have no interaction related to their efforts. The lack of or limited interaction among disciplines means a more limited perspective for each discipline and less effectiveness in meeting the needs of the disabled person. This is seen in the multidisciplinary approach without the team effort.

Using the definition that a team is a group of individuals who must work together collaboratively and interdependently to accomplish a task, we imply interdisciplinary functioning of the team.

The team must have the client as its primary focus. This implies the inclusion of the family and other significant persons who influence the client's life. The client's needs and goals are the purpose for the existence of a team. Team functioning must transcend ethnic, cultural, socioeconomic, religious, political and geographic influences in defining and accomplishing tasks.

For effective interdisciplinary functioning, understanding and communication are essential to cooperative work in identifying client goals and what is needed to accomplish those goals. The goals may be related to procedures, priority setting, treatments, implementation strategies, planning, equipment and materials, education, ethical decisions and continuing evaluation of outcomes as goals are achieved and change. There is a shared responsibility with the client and the family.

Teams do not automatically function effectively. There is a continuing need for development of each member. Team development has been studied extensively and involves the application of principles of certain applied behavioral sciences and management concepts that increase team efficiency. This requires the collaborative development of skills and rules governing the team work in accomplishing tasks. The skills and rules include setting team goals, defining and clarifying roles, decision making, setting priorities, effective communication, team leadership, and conflict management. If the team is to function interdependently to assure comprehensive and coordinated services, each member must give great importance to the interactional process of the team.

LEADERSHIP

Leadership implies a hierarchical model. In functional interdisciplinary teams the leadership may be the responsibility of any member of the team based on the task to be accomplished.

Nominal leadership may occur at the organizational phase of an interdisciplinary team. If there is trust and openness among the members, other leadership may emerge and roles may change. Studies have demonstrated that democratic leadership in a group results in more creativity and collaboration. Autocratic leadership is not compatible with effective team functioning.

When the leadership role does not facilitate effective problem solving, the functional interdisciplinary team will resolve the conflict to the satisfaction of team members by clarifying the role in order to successfully complete the team tasks. Attention to the dynamics and team goals are an essential responsibility of each team member.

ROLE

Each individual member brings unique facets to the team. The special skills of the discipline that one represents help define the role that is played as a team member. There is also the team role that is not defined by discipline, such as leader, facilitator, negotiation, and so on. Each team member also brings his own philosophy, beliefs, biases, and personality.

Interdisciplinary team functioning is based on respect for each team member. It is not necessary to acquire another discipline's skills and knowledge, but it is essential that each member learn enough about each discipline to understand that discipline's perspectives. Many problems that impede interdisciplinary functioning are related to perspective and territorial misunderstanding. Role clarification both for the discipline and the expected functioning on the team is basic to effective functioning in problem solving if tasks are to be successfully accomplished.

An increased knowledge by team members of the training, methods of professional practice, diagnostic and treatment modalities, licensing requirements, and terminology unique to that discipline all improve the ability to collaborate in a positive manner. Areas of disciplinary interface and overlap must be clarified to prevent conflict and dissonance as the team approaches its tasks.

COMMUNICATION

Interdisciplinary team development and functioning is dependent on the effective use of communication. Verbal, non-verbal, and listening skills are essential for all team members.

Communication is much more than specific content messages. It is the basis for sharing technical information, expressing ideas and opinions, and showing feelings about team action, especially approval and disapproval. It is facilitated by feedback, which regulates the team functioning. There is unique disciplinary terminology that must be defined and understood and that must be avoided with the client and family if not clearly understood.

Nonverbal communication is often used, but communication should be verbal in feedback to facilitate the team process. Agreement, disapproval, pleasure, and anger must be expressed verbally in order to sustain the team collaboration in problem solving.

If client and family goals are to be expressed so that team goals and tasks can be identified, each team member must develop listening skills. It is as important to receive messages from others in interpersonal interaction as to express oneself verbally or nonverbally.

DECISION MAKING

Decision making and setting priorities by the team are the outcome of team collaboration. Knowledge and skills in processes that enhance team consensus in accomplishing tasks can be developed. The child and/or the family or primary caretaker must be involved in this process before any decision is made regarding their goals. Differences or conflicts will occur at all levels of team functioning, and the members must understand and practice effective methods of conflict resolutions.

An issue that frequently must be considered by the team is whether the client and family will be members of the team. This issue should always be considered and agreement reached regarding their participation and role in the team functioning. Whatever the relationship may be with the disabled person, the team is responsible for selecting the most appropriate member to communicate and interpret decisions.

Evaluation of team functioning is a responsibility of the team and of each member. There should be agreed-on methods for the team to review its process regularly. Each individual member should review his own performance on the various components necessary for successful functioning, and the team should evaluate itself in order to identify factors causing conflict and obstructing progress. As these factors are addressed, team development progresses, resulting in the effective accomplishment of the team's tasks.

Interdisciplinary teams working with disabled children and their families may vary considerably in composition, the tasks they undertake, and the site in which they function. However, with client and family goals clearly as the purpose of the team and with concern for process, the team will continue to develop the ability to function collaboratively to reach the optimal outcome in achieving client goals.

Chapter 24

EVALUATION OF STATE AND COMMUNITY PROGRAMS SERVING CHILDREN AND YOUTH WITH CHRONIC CONDITIONS

Henry T. Ireys
Phyllis R. Magrab

As this book illustrates, a broad array of health, education, and social service programs are available to meet the needs of children and youth with chronic conditions. Efforts to evaluate the effects of these programs, however, lag behind their considerable ingenuity and achievement in providing care. Many factors may account for this relative neglect, including a lack of appropriate methodology or expertise, an absence of funds to support evaluation efforts, or political forces that discourage careful assessment of a particular program. An evaluation project also requires a great deal of time for planning, for implementing, and for disseminating results—time that may be elusive in the press of delivering care.

The primary aim of this chapter is to provide a general overview of evaluation strategies pertinent to programs serving children and youth with diverse chronic conditions. Throughout the chapter, we use examples of specific evaluation projects to illustrate general concepts and problems. Our chapter is much influenced by major evaluation studies conducted in various domains (for example, Anderson & Ball, 1983; Attkisson, Hargreaves, Horowitz, & Sorensen, 1978; Price & Smith, 1985; Starfield, 1974; Struening & Guttentog, 1975).

We define evaluation as the systematic ordering of evidence, a perspective borrowed from Anderson and Ball (1983, p. 12). The key word here is *systematic*. Almost every program will be judged informally and haphazardly by the public, by legislators, and by other administrators—all of whom have little access to the kind and amount of information required for an informed appraisal. Unless there is a specific reason not to conduct an evaluation, most programs are far better served by a systematic ordering of evidence (i.e., a well-planned evaluation) than by haphazard and fallible judgments.

PRAGMATICS OF EVALUATION

To many program administrators, evaluation may be a frightening prospect. Without experience in evaluation efforts, administrators may believe that the results of an evaluation will be used to discredit the program, to show only the program's weaknesses. Such concerns are important because most evaluations do in fact have social and political consequences; some of these consequences may indeed be injurious to the program (Cambell & Kimmel, 1985). Yet these possible consequences, rather than forestalling an evaluation effort, underscore the necessity for carefully developing an evaluation plan. This plan should take into account both the environment in which an evaluation will occur and the context in which the results of the evaluation will be announced. In developing such a plan, several factors are wisely considered.

First, many experts stress the importance of starting small and of evaluating carefully selected aspects of an overall program. Administrators may believe that a particular program truly makes a difference in the lives of the children it serves. They may be right, but the difference is likely to be relatively small. The best evaluation typically illuminates modest effects (Anderson & Ball, 1983; Haggerty, 1978; Rogers, Blendon, & Hearn, 1981).

Second, administrators must anticipate the possibility of negative findings from an evaluation. If an evaluation uncovers evidence about areas of relative weakness, it should also discover means of addressing these areas. A well-planned evaluation effort can collect information sufficient to identify both problems and potential solutions.

Finally, evaluation is value-laden. Determining what is a worthy objective for a program, identifying the specific means for conducting an evaluation, even believing that evaluation is necessary, all of these invite decisions that often rest on convictions and beliefs held strongly by program administrators. These beliefs frequently find expression in the criteria by which a program's resources are allocated. For example: Is it better for a state health care program for handicapped children to support all needed services for a few seriously ill children or some needed services for many moderately ill children? Definite answers are elusive for these types of questions. Yet the underlying issues can play a major role in shaping an evaluation and its conclusions. Recognition of the values that play upon a particular program may result in an improved understanding of obstacles to and consequences of the program's evaluation (Suchman, 1976).

GOALS, METHODS, AND MEASURES

The evaluative approach best suited for a particular situation will depend on such factors as the experience of the program director, the speed with which an evaluation must be completed, available financial and technical supports, the immediate political context, and, most importantly, the overall goal of the evaluation. Clear specification of the intentions of an evaluation is crucial to the success of the project. Evaluative efforts may serve many goals, but the following three are common: (a) assisting in the development of a new program or initiative, with continuing feedback to refine the program (often termed formative evaluations); (b) helping in decisions about how or whether an existing program should change (often termed summative evaluations); or (c) obtaining evidence to justify a program's continuing existence.

Depending in part on the goal of the evaluation, an appropriate methodolgy will be needed. Scrutiny of published evaluations of programs serving children and youth with various chronic conditions reveals a wide range of methodologies: a pediatric home care program serving children with serious, ongoing physical illnesses was evaluated with a randomized, controlled clinical trial (Stein & Jessop, 1984); the efforts of local school districts to provide related services to children in special education under the provisions of PL 94-142 (The Education for All Handicapped Children Act of 1975) have been evaluated using a comparative case-study method (Boston Children's Hospital, 1984); a similar approach was used to examine selected state Crippled Children's Service programs (Ireys, 1980); survey methods were used to evaluate the Supplemental Security Income/Disabled Children's Program (SSI/DCP) (Pratt & Bachman, 1979); a comprehensive account of a program's philosophy and functional components formed the basis for an evaluation of new community residential programs for emotionally disturbed children (Hobbs, 1982). These efforts represent only some of the varying purposes and approaches to evaluation in this field. Many other examples are available (for example, Haggerty, 1978; Pless, 1978, Starfield, 1974; Wallace, Siffert, Tobis, Losty, & Elledge, 1956).

In addition to examining programs as a whole, evaluation studies also may focus on any of three different aspects of a given program. One aspect concerns the necessary elements for a program to exist: the required resources, staff, and expertise. Evaluation of these elements (input evaluation) leads to conclusions concerning the adequacy of a program's foundation. The second aspect, often referred to as process evaluation involves the monitoring and appraisal of the activities that enable a program to achieve its goals. From this type of evaluation emerges evidence regarding strengths and weaknesses in a program's current functioning. In most instances, input and process evaluations are formative in nature, directed at specifying ways of improving a program. The third aspect of a program concerns its effect or

264   HANDICAPPED CHILDREN AND YOUTH

outcome. Outcome evaluations typically focus on the changes that a program has effected or the products that it has produced.

Table 24-1 is a way of conceptualizing the varying approaches to program evaluation; it lists evaluation methods that range from those that meet standards of a scientific enterprise (the first four items) to those commonly used by many programs with limited resources (the last five items). Experimental studies using appropriate control groups tend to provide the strongest evidence from a scientific vantage point (for example, Stein & Jessop, 1984), but such studies often have limited generality and typically require a long time to complete. Correlational and quasi-experimental studies may be somewhat less methodologically rigorous in comparison to studies that use true control groups, but in many instances these approaches may be the most feasible (see Cook & Campbell, 1979). For example, consider a state program for home visits by public health nurses to mothers of high-risk infants. Rather than being based on experimental and control groups (i.e., randomly assigning families to receive a visit and comparing those families with families who do not receive a visit), an evaluation of such a program might have to rely on approximate comparison groups (for example, families before the program began or families in a similar program elsewhere) or on correlational approaches (for example, correlating the number of home visits with measures of subsequent use of health services). The fourth approach is illustrated in the work of Pless (1978) and his colleagues (Haggerty, Roghman, & Pless, 1975), who used a wide variety of sample survey and epidemiological studies to examine patterns of health behaviors and of health service utilization within a single community.

The last five items in Table 24-1 rest on more informal but potentially no less powerful methods of collecting data. Many program administrators employ variations of the discrepancy evaluation, in which a program's current functioning is compared to an explicit standard that defines a program's expected performance (Yavorsky, 1984). A final report using this approach would identify where a program is achieving its goals and where it is failing to live up to expected standards. An example of the last three methods are combined in a series of reports by a collaborative study of five special education programs (Boston Children's Hospital, 1984). In these reports, intensive case studies of selected schools were used to illustrate successful special education programs. Personnel and client assessments, informal testimonies, expert judgments, and careful examination of available program data provided the basis for the evaluation.

From our perspective, there is no one correct method for evaluation. Different situations demand different approaches; in many instances several approaches together will yield the strongest evidence (Webb, cited in Anderson & Ball, 1983, p. 50).

In most evaluations of programs serving children and youth with chronic handicapping conditions, there is a need to define appropriate measures.

Table 24-1. Evaluation Methods

Experimental studies or randomized controlled clinical trials
Correlational studies
Quasi-experimental studies
Sample surveys or epidemiological studies
Discrepancy evaluations: the ideal vs. the present
Personnel or client assessment
Systematic expert judgment
Clinical or case study
Informal testimony

Adapted from Anderson & Ball, 1983.

Attkisson and colleagues (1978) suggest a series of general criteria from which specific measures can be derived:

> Improvement in client's status
>
> Reduction in incidence and prevalence of problems addressed
>
> Awareness of services among citizenry
>
> Acceptability of services to clients
>
> Level of service availability and continuity achieved over time
>
> Adequacy of service volume relative to need
>
> Appropriateness of clients served relative to high-risk groups or mandated target populations
>
> Linkage of clients to other necessary and appropriate services
>
> Cost–effort–outcome–effectiveness comparisons for different target groups
>
> Financial viability of component services and organizations

A somewhat overlapping approach is illustrated in Table 24-2. The general categories in this table and the specific items within them are directly relevant to state Crippled Children's Service programs but can be applied to other programs as well (Magrab & Ireys, 1985).

In specifying measures, it is also helpful to distinguish between categorical measures and generic measures (Jessop & Stein, 1983). Categorical outcomes relate to specific conditions or subpopulations and usually lack generalizability. For example, over the last several years the Association for Maternal and Child Health and Crippled Children's Programs has mounted a major effort to improve methods of collecting program outcome infor-

Table 24-2. Possible Outcome Measures for State Child Health Programs

Measures of program impact on health status, daily function, or family life
   Health status measures
   Impact on family
   Functional indices
Measures of program function or performance
   Penetration of target population
   Scope of services provided
   Extent of coverage of diagnostic conditions
Measures of service usage
   Clinic visits
   Physician or provider "encounters"
   Hospital days
Measures of cost
   Clinic visit costs per patient with a given diagnosis
   Hospital costs by diagnosis
   Average costs
Measures of the population served or targeted
   Number of children previously lacking a primary care physician
   Number of low-income families previously lacking a social worker
   Number of families requiring home care visits
Measures of relationships with other health care programs
   Families served who have no other coverage
   Services provided for which there would be no other source of support
   Quantity and quality of interagency collaborative agreements
Measures of leadership and advocacy
   Publication of standards
   Number of site visits to clinics or hospitals
   Presence on relevant policymaking boards
Measures of community involvement
   Who participates on program's advisory board
   Knowledge of programs within the community
   Contact with schools
Measures of historical continuity
   Trends in number served or penetration rates
   Trends in diagnosis covered
   Trends in relative state-federal contributions

mation related to the Maternal and Child Health Block Grant. As a part of this effort, specific, categorical health-status indicators or health outcomes for defined groups have been identified (Van Dyck & Nangle, 1983). For example, for children with cleft palate, outcome indicators include the number of children with a complete plan for total palate correction as well as the number of children with no hearing loss; for cystic fibrosis, outcome indicators include the number of children in the appropriate school grade and the number of school absences; for seizure disorders, indicators include the number of children with therapeutic drug levels as well as the number of children seizure-free for one year; and for prenatal care, measures include the neonatal mortality rate and the low birthweight rate. These measures are part of a data set that combines both process and outcome information.

    Generic outcomes are more cross-cutting and may have broader implications for services and care. In terms of conceptualizing program outcomes, there is an increasing trend to examine more generic outcomes, such as the impact of an illness on family functioning or on the child's school attendance. An excellent example of a generic outcome approach is contained in the studies conducted by Stein and Jessop (1984). These investigators mounted a comprehensive assessment of an ongoing service delivery program entitled Pediatric Home Care (PHC). PHC is designed for children with a variety of chronic illnesses and conditions; it includes a team composed of pediatricians, social workers, and nurse practitioners who work closely with the family, the school, and subspecialty physicians. The evaluation took the form of a controlled clinical trial; it was based on a randomized pretest–posttest design in which 219 children were followed over a period of several years. Half of the children were assigned to the PHC program; the other half received standard care. Noncategorical or generic outcome measures included assessment of the child's functional status and psychological adjustment, the impact of illness on the family, the mother's psychological adjustment, family satisfaction with care, the unmet health needs of the family, levels of self-care knowledge, and service utilization. Using these outcomes, the investigators were able to identify important psychological and social variables common to all chronic conditions (Jessop & Stein, 1983).

An example of an evaluation that examined input, process, and outcome aspects of a program is contained in a report on the implementation of the SSI/DCP in nine states (Pratt & Bachman, 1979). The SSI/DCP was a program designed to ensure that individual service plans were developed by Crippled Children's Service agencies for children enrolled in the SSI program. The evaluation was carried out two years after the enabling legislation was passed, before the program was firmly established in all states. Among other findings, the evaluation revealed that, in many instances, the necessary staff were hired very slowly and the bureaucratic base for the program was quite weak. These findings (part of the input aspects of the program) underscored the problems in the conceptualization, design, and initial implementation of the program. The process aspect of the evaluation focused, in part, on the competencies of the program's staff. It found that many of the staff in the state programs were inadequately trained in developing and writing individual service plans. Finally, the report noted that the program was reaching only a small portion of its target population—a measure of the program's impact or outcome. In addition to these negative findings the evaluation pinpointed positive aspects of the program, including the establishment of formal interagency agreements and the likelihood of a continued increase in completed individual service plans.

SUMMARY

This chapter has provided an overview of selected topics in the field of evaluation that are especially pertinent to programs serving children and youth with diverse handicaps. Evaluation is defined as a systematic gathering of evidence—a task that requires careful planning. The pragmatics of developing such a plan include the selection of a project manageable with available resources; the identification of relative strengths, weaknesses, and potential solutions to problems; and recognition of values that may bear on the problem. Goals for a particular evaluation may include assisting in the development of a new program (formative evaluation); helping to decide how an existing program might change (summative evaluation); or obtaining evidence to justify a program's existence.

Various approaches may be used to gather evidence, from informal testimony to rigorous experimental studies. The best approach emerges from the needs and resources within a particular situation. Whatever the choice, evaluation projects can focus on any or all of three aspects of a program: the input factors, which refer to the elements necessary for a program to exist; the process elements, which refer to the activities that enable a program to achieve its goals; and the output aspects, which refer to the products or effects of a program. For any evaluation, measures are needed. Within the chapter we specify several approaches to identifying appropriate measures, including generic and categorical methods.

The record of service delivery programs for children and youth with chronic illnesses and disabilities has been impressive. The task for these programs is now to match their achievements in delivering care with the quality of their evaluation efforts.

REFERENCES

Anderson, S., & Ball, S. (1983). *The profession and practice of program evaluation*. San Francisco: Jossey-Bass.

Attkisson, C., Hargreaves, W., Horowitz, M., & Sorensen, J. (1978). *Evaluation of human services programs*. New York: Academic Press.

Boston Children's Hospital. (1984). *Collaborative study of children with special needs: Report of findings*. Boston: Author.

Campbell, D., & Kimmel, A. (1985). *Guiding preventive intervention research centers for research validity*. Washington, DC: National Institute of Mental Health, Center for Prevention Research.

Cook, T., & Campbell, D. (1979). *Quasi-experimentation: Design and analysis for field settings*. Boston: Houghton Mifflin.

Haggerty, R. (1978). Summing up. In S. Bosch & J. Arias (Eds.), *Evaluation of child health services: The interface between research and medical practice*. (DHEW Publication No. 78-1066). Washington, DC: U.S. Department of Health, Education and Welfare.

Haggerty, R., Roghman, K., & Pless, I. (1975). *Child health and the community*. New York: Wiley Interscience.

Hobbs, N. (1982). *The troubled and troubling child*. San Francisco: Jossey-Bass.

Ireys, H. (1980). *The Crippled Children's Service: A comparative analysis of four state programs*. Mental Health Policy Monograph Series, Number 7. Nashville, TN: Vanderbilt Institute for Public Policy Studies.

Jessop, D., & Stein, R. (1983). A noncategorical approach to psychosocial research. *Journal of Psychosocial Oncology, 4*, 61–64.

Magrab, P., & Ireys, H. (April 1985). *Outcome measures in Crippled Children's Services*. Abstract for workshop conducted at 12th Annual Conference on Maternal and Child Health, Family Planning, and Crippled Children's Services, Chapel Hill, NC.

Pless, I. (1978). Child health and the community: The Rochester child health studies, 1967–1977. In S. Bosch & J. Arias (Eds.), *Evaluation of child health services: The interface between research and medical practice* (DHEW Publication No. 78-1066). Washington, DC: U.S. Department of Health, Education and Welfare.

Pratt, M., & Bachman, G. (1979). *Evaluation of the implementation of the supplemental security income program for disabled children, 1977–1979*. Silver Spring, MD: Information Sciences Research Institute.

Price, R., & Smith, S. (1985). *A guide to evaluating prevention programs in mental health* (Publication No. (ADM) 85-1365). Washington, DC: U.S. Department of Health and Human Services.

Rogers, D., Blendon, R., & Hearn, R. (1981). Some observations on pediatrics: Its past, present and future. *Pediatrics, 67*, 776–784.

Starfield, B. (1974). Measurement of outcome: A proposed scheme. *Millbank Memorial Fund Quarterly*, 52, 39–50.

Stein, R. K., & Jessop, D. J. (1984). Does pediatric home care make a difference for children with chronic illness? Findings from the Pediatric Ambulatory Care Treatment Study. *Pediatrics, 73*, 845–853.

Struening, E., & Guttentog, M. (Eds.). (1975). *Handbook of evaluation research*. Beverly Hills, CA: Sage Publications.

Suchman, E. (1976). *Evaluative research*. New York: Russell Sage.

Van Dyck, P.C., & Nangle, B. (November 1983). *Feasibility study for collecting outcome data for the MCH block grant*. Paper presented to the American Public Health Association, Dallas, TX.

Wallace, H., Siffert, R., Tobis, J., Losty, M., & Elledge, C. (1956). Evaluating care of the orthopedically crippled. *Children, 3* (4), 139–144.

Yavorsky, D. (1984). *Discrepancy evaluation: A practitioner's guide*. Charlottesville, VA: University of Virginia, Evaluation Research Center.

Part IV

COMMON HANDICAPPING CONDITIONS IN CHILDREN AND YOUTH

Chapter 25

CLEFT LIP AND PALATE

Hughlett Morris

DEFINITION

Cleft lip and palate is one of the most frequently occurring major human birth defects, affecting about 1 in 650 live-born babies. The term *cleft lip and palate* is descriptive. There is division of the parts of the upper lip and the roof of the mouth (the palate). As indicated later, there is considerable variance in type and extent of clefting, and the cleft may be an isolated birth defect or may occur in conjunction with other birth defects (Ross & Johnston, 1972). In the latter case, there may be evidence of a previously recognized syndrome (Cohen, 1978). In addition, an individual occasionally demonstrates a disorder (such as nasalized speech) or structural abnormality (such as congenitally missing upper incisor teeth) that suggests a microform of clefting or a disorder related to clefting. For example, nasalized speech usually is evidence of a structural deficiency of the soft palate (the posterior portion of the palate, a muscular "curtain" of tissue that can be seen at the back of the throat) or of the pharynx (the upper part of the throat) (McWilliams, Morris & Shelton, 1984). These deficiences result in a failure of adequate partitioning, during speech, between the mouth and the nasal cavity, such as is seen in patients with cleft palate. Sometimes this disorder (called congenital palatal incompetence) is not detected until after adenoidectomy. Presumably, the adenoidal pad had successfully compensated for the deficiency.

Generally, then, we speak of cleft lip and palate and related disorders to indicate this variability in the clinical picture.

INCIDENCE, PREVALENCE, DEMOGRAPHICS

A large number of factors have been investigated for possible importance in determining rate of occurrence of cleft lip and palate, but only one factor, skin color, has emerged with predictable significance. In general, highest occurrence rates are predicted for red skin-color groups, then yellow, then white and tan, then brown and black. The range appears to be in the neighborhood of 1 in 350 (red) to 1 in 1,200 (black) (Stevenson, Johnston, Stewart & Golding, 1966). No satisfactory explanation for these differences has yet been provided. Other factors, such as maternal age, may be important but have not been so demonstrated in a clear fashion.

ETIOLOGY, CONTRIBUTING FACTORS, PREVENTIVE TECHNIQUES

Without much doubt, genetic factors are highly important in accounting for etiology. The significance of heredity can be easily demonstrated in the following clearly oversimplified but clearly substantiated statement: the occurrence rate for the general population (1 in 650) rises significantly (1 in 20) when there is one occurrence in the family, and dramatically higher still (1 in 5) when there are two! These ratios must be regarded carefully because obviously there are a number of other factors (such as cleft type or the presence of a suspected syndrome) to be considered in making predictions about any single family. Further, giving such information in such simplified terms to any single family may be misleading. They may take the 1-in-20 ratio to indicate that 19 more normal babies could be born of the sexual union before another baby would be affected. Obviously, that is not so. However, the trend is unmistakable and cannot be denied. Parents who have a baby with a cleft must consider in their family planning that the cleft is likely to be genetic and that the genetic forces, so to speak, are still operative. That is also the case when a parent (or some other member of the family) has a cleft.

The difficult part here is that the trait is clearly not dominant, and so a negative family history cannot be interpreted to indicate absence of a genetic tendency. Neither is it a chromosomal aberration that can be diagnosed by available measures. Therefore, the family must rely solely on information about their family history and the most conservative interpretation of that information.

It is certainly the case that there are reliable indications that a wide range of factors influencing early fetal development in *research animals* can result in cleft palate. These seem to include vitamin and nutrition deficiencies, hormonal imbalances, diseases, drugs, and (perhaps) radiation. However, there is almost no evidence that these factors are influential in humans. It seems likely that the lack of evidence is highly related to the difficulties in research design that are encountered in studying the problem. As a consequence, it seems wise to remain suspicious about any factor—disease, drugs, nutrition–that could affect a woman in the early stages of pregnancy, specifically week 6 through week 12. It follows that women who may be pregnant should maintain the best of health and clearly should avoid any type of drugs except in time of urgent need. Even medications for morning sickness should be avoided as an extra precaution.

Many geneticists favor an explanation for the etiology of cleft lip and palate that is multifactorial in nature. Such an explanation includes the notion of a threshold of sensitivity (genetic) to the trait, interacting with any one of several possible intrauterine factors. Such a notion seems highly plausible and could account for the observed variability in findings. However, it may be equally difficult to "prove."

All of this is rather difficult to convey in any meaningful way to the public, yet we must find ways to do so. A reasonable approach, in the absence of information to the contrary, is to suggest strongly the probability of a genetic factor, with the possibility of other undetermined intrauterine factors as well.

In most affected families, discussions about the etiology of cleft lip and palate are continued over a period of time, and so every opportunity should be used to encourage the family members to ask questions, seek information from a clinical geneticist, and certainly express feelings about this complicated subject. Of particular concern in this regard is the adolescent with a cleft who is beginning to consider issues of marriage and children.

CLINICAL DESCRIPTION

As indicated earlier, cleft lip and palate shows considerable variance, ranging from a partial cleft lip or a partial cleft palate to a complete cleft lip and palate to a cleft that extends through both structures. Determination of severity of defect is based on several factors. An obvious factor is number of structures affected (sometimes referred to as the length of the cleft): a cleft lip and palate is more severe than a cleft lip only, and a partial cleft lip (or palate) is less severe than a cleft that extends through the entire structure.

The width of the cleft is also an important gauge of severity; a wide cleft (of either lip, alveolus, or palate) probably indicates also a greater degree of tissue deficiency than does a narrow one. This tissue deficiency is important in surgical repair because the surgeon has less material (tissue adjacent to the cleft) to work with in the reconstruction (Millard, 1980).

Briefly, the effects on the patient and family are several (McWilliams, Morris & Shelton, 1984). The newborn has problems feeding, particularly when there is cleft palate. With some guidance, however, the parents usually find an acceptable feeding method, and typically there are no feeding problems of a serious or permanent nature. A cleft lip results in facial deformity that will require expert surgical assistance in infancy and possibly later in the life of the child. Cleft palate leads to distortions of speech, typically in control of nasalization but frequently in other aspects of speech and language also. When the cleft extends through the gum (the alveolar ridge) there will most likely be significant deformities of dentition, occlusion, and general growth and development of the midthird of the face. Typically, the young child has considerably more episodes of middle ear disease than other children, so earaches and some hearing loss (usually mild but sometimes persistent) are part of the clinical picture until the age of six or eight years. Many parents and families experience problems in adjusting to the reality of the congenital cleft and the implications for care, nurture, family relationships, future family planning, educational impact, and use of financial resources. Frequently these factors are regarded as "psychosocial" aspects of cleft lip and palate. They vary in nature, extent, and severity from one family to another, but they are important and must not be ignored.

Finally, it is important to observe that, in many patients, cleft lip and palate is not an isolated birth defect but appears in the context of several other congenital anomalies. These other anomalies may be minor and of interest primarily to the pediatric or clinical geneticist. Or they may be highly significant clinically, and indeed their treatment may take precedence over the cleft(s) to ensure the well-being of the child.

MANAGEMENT

The clinical description above of cleft lip and palate and related disorders indicates the complexity of the disorder and dramatizes the need for a wide range of specialists, at various points in the life of the child (and adult), working in concert with equally important community resources (Morris, 1980; Morris, Jakobi & Harrington, 1978). Together, the two teams (local and specialty) can expect to make it possible for the child and family to see the problem through to a satisfactory conclusion.

Typically, the baby with a cleft is born in a community hospital, so local personnel—mainly the delivery physician, attending nursing staff, and the family doctor—enter the scene first. Theirs is the task of telling the family about the problem and about resources for treatment (the specialty team) and assisting the family in use of those resources (making appointments, discussing the options, etc.).

After referral, the specialty team provides a substantial amount of the specialized care needed, but the local practitioners have an important continuing role. They provide primary medical and dental care from infancy, and the local speech pathologists may provide early speech therapy (either directly or through the parents). Depending on the circumstances, otologic and orthodontic treatment may be provided locally also. Local social service workers are key to resolving any financial or family problems that interfere with effective treatment. When the child is of school age, school personnel, including the speech pathologist and the psychologist, may have major contributions to make.

Meanwhile, members of the specialty team are proceeding with treatment for specific aspects of the problem. These include identification of any other deformities; assistance with feeding; treatment of any special health problems; discussions with the family about the nature of clefting and its etiology; cleft lip surgery at about 10 weeks of age; observation of dental and speech development, with appropriate guidance to the parents; observation and treatment of any upper respiratory infections and middle ear disease; and cleft palate surgery at about 12 months.

During preschool and early school years the emphasis is on speech production and the decision as to whether the initial palate surgery will be satisfactory for normal speech, so the speech pathologists on the specialty team must follow the patient closely. There may be other kinds of speech, language, and voice problems also. If the initial palatal surgery proves unsatisfactory for normal speech, additional palatal surgery may be performed by the plastic and reconstructive surgeon, probably between the ages of six and eight years.

The orthodontist and other dental specialists on the team need to observe the patient over a period of time to estimate the nature and severity of any midfacial growth problems and to decide about proper treatment. Typically, an important portion of orthodontic therapy is delayed until adolescence, when the orthodontist can better determine the status of the adult face. However, therapy may be begun much earlier than that.

When cosmetic surgery is indicated, and it frequently is, it also may be delayed until adolescence for the same reasons. Here also the plastic and reconstructive surgeon needs to study the patient over time to determine developmental trends and predicted adult status.

It should be apparent from this discussion that (a) each team has an important role to play, (b) each team can be maximally effective by coordinating efforts among members, and (c), most important, there must be sufficient exchange of information between the two teams so that the patient and the family has the desired advantage. Certainly, to the degree possible, the working relationships among the members of each team and between the two teams ought to be developed so that the patient and the family are not caught in the middle of philosophical or procedural differences about what constitutes "proper" treatment. Indeed, there likely will be differences, but these should be considered, and resolved if possible, in discussions before the patient is called upon to make a decision. However, sometimes this is wishful thinking because there are clearly several satisfactory methods for dealing with almost all issues in cleft lip and palate treatment, and some differences among practitioners are bound to arise. When that happens, the two (or more) sides of the question must be put squarely to the patient with the supporting rationales so that the patient can make the decision with the most and best information that is available.

The patient and the family who have the benefit of two groups of people such as those described above can be expected to emerge from the treatment process in pretty good shape: a nice-looking, if not entirely normal face; normal or near normal speech; a nice smile and good dental occlusion for speech and deglutition; good health; a good education and vocational potential; and, very important, a good self-image!

UNMET NEEDS

The discussion above about clinical management of cleft lip and palate ended on a positive note, with the assertion that if the patient and family have access to contemporary care, at both local and specialty levels, they have the right to expect a satisfactory outcome. That certainly is the case, yet there still is much to be done in the improvement of both the quality of care and the efficiency of the delivery system.

Following are brief descriptions of some improvements to be made. The list is not intended to be inclusive but rather to indicate examples of need.

1. Clearly, we have far to go in understanding the mechanisms by which clefts occur, how they may be detected and predicted even before birth (maybe before conception) and how they may be prevented.

2. Our surgical methods are nothing short of miraculous, when one considers cosmetic appearance and speech patterns before and after surgery, yet 30 percent of cleft-palate patients may need a second surgery for better speech, and maybe twice that percentage of cleft patients can benefit, cosmetically, from a second or third revision surgery. It seems probable that both of those success rates could be improved.

3. We really ought to be better at identifying potentially serious speech problems at an early age and at devising methods by which they can be more efficiently and effectively treated. Many patients seem to develop relatively normal speech production and require little special assistance except for excellent palatal surgery. However, others have considerably more difficulty and require as much as three or four years of extensive and expensive therapy. We need better prognostic tests that are noninvasive and that assist us to identify potential behavioral (learned?) problems as well as to identify deficiencies in oral structures.

4. The search continues for methods by which severe midfacial growth deformities, including dental defects and malocclusion, can be avoided or lessened in severity. Conventional orthodontic therapy is time-consuming, expensive, and of limited effectiveness. Surgical orthodontics appear useful for some patients at older ages (adolescence), but results are sometimes dis-

appointing, in part because of the complicated interactions between well-established patterns of oral function and the newly obtained oral structure relationships. There remains much to be done.

5. As is true with understanding human nature in general, there still is inadequate information about the mechanisms by which some people cope well with adversity and others do not. If these differences could be better identified and predicted, the psychosocial aspects of cleft lip and palate, as well as other similar problems, could be better and more efficiently addressed.

6. One emphasis in this discussion is on aspects of delivery of care to the patient and family with cleft lip and palate as provided by practitioners in the local community and those from a specialty team at a tertiary health care facility such as a teaching hospital. Very specialized services are required from a variety of specialists if best results are to be obtained. Clearly, cleft lip surgery or any other kind of treatment of cleft lip and palate should not be performed by anyone who is not sufficiently well trained and well experienced and who does not perform such treatment on a regular basis. Yet these specialists rarely can provide comprehensive care for all the needs of the patient, so the skills and services of the general practitioner (medical, dental, speech pathology) is also greatly in demand. These requirements call for a delicate balance between the specialist and the general practitioner and certainly a delivery system that supports, economically and otherwise, both types of services. The economic side of this picture is improving rapidly for families with health insurance, particularly if they had insurance before the affected baby was born. However, the family without such protection is in pretty deep trouble financially because the resources for public assistance have been dwindling fast since the early 1970s and are now practically nonexistent in many communities and states (Morris & Tharp, 1978). This is indeed a very important unmet need.

REFERENCES

Cohen, M. M. (1978). Syndromes with cleft lip and cleft palate. *Cleft Palate Journal, 15,* 306–328.

McWilliams, B. J., Morris, H. L., & Shelton, R. L. (1984). *Cleft palate speech.* Toronto: B. C. Decker.

Millard, D. R. (1980). *Cleft craft* (3 vols.). Boston: Little, Brown.

Morris, H. L. (1980). The structure and function of interdisciplinary health teams. In C. F. Salinas & R. J. Jorgenson (Eds.), *Dentistry in the interdisciplinary treatment of genetic diseases.* (pp. 105–110). New York: Alan R. Liss.

Morris, H. L., Jakobi, P., & Harringotn, D. (1978). Objectives and criteria for management of cleft lip and palate and the delivery of management services. *Cleft Palate Journal, 15* 1–5.

Morris, H. L., & Tharp, R. (1978). Some economic aspects of cleft lip and palate treatment in the United States in 1974. *Cleft Palate Journal, 15,* 167–175.

Ross, R. B., & Johnston, M. C. (1972). *Cleft lip and palate.* Baltimore: Williams and Wilkins.

Stevenson, A. C., Johnston, H. A., Stewart, M. P., & Golding, D. R. (1966). Congenital malformations. *Bulletin of the World Health Organization, 34.*

Chapter 26

CEREBRAL PALSY

Lawrence T. Taft

DEFINITION

Cerebral palsy (CP) is a disorder of movement and/or posture, the result of a static encephalopathy with the insult to the brain occurring prenatally, perinatally, or during early childhood. Inherent in this definition of CP is that it cannot be used if the motor disorder is the result of a progressive central nervous system disorder, as may be the case with cerebral dysfunction secondary to neurodegenerative diseases or tumors. Furthermore, a disorder of movement due to extracranial pathology cannot be classified as CP. Consequently, spinal cord lesions of the meningomyelocele type and peripheral nerve lesions, an example of which would be a brachial palsy, or muscle diseases in pseudohypertrophic muscular dystrophy cannot be considered CP.

Classification of subtypes of CP has been unsatisfactory. The ideal would be to have a classification based on etiology, pathology, clinical symptoms, and prognosis. However, our present state of knowledge precludes the use of a comprehensive nosology (Bax, 1964). Currently used is a clinical classification based on the type of movement disorder (Table 26-1).

The clinical classification of CP has its limitations. The varying types of muscle tone and involuntary movements that are utilized for classification purposes may not be fully manifest until one to two years of age in spite of the fact that the insult to the brain may have occurred prenatally or peri-

Table 26-1. Table of Classification

Type	Frequency (%)
Spastic	70–80
Hemiparesis (monoparesis)	20–25
Perinatal 50%	
Postnatal 50%	
Diplegia	25–35
Quadriparesis (double hemiplegia)	25–30
Dyskinesis	
Athetosis	10–12
Dystonia	3–5
Chorea	Rare
Ballismus	Rare
Tremor	Rare
Rigid	4–5
Atonic (hypotonic)	Rare
Mixed	10–20
Spastic athetoid	10–15
Spastic ataxic	Rare
Spastic-rigid	3–5

From Molnar, G. E. *Pediatric rehabilitation*. Baltimore: Williams & Wilkins, 1985.
Reprinted by permission of author and publisher.

natally. Furthermore, many patients have a mixed neuromotor disorder, making it a difficult clinical decision as to the specific types of movement disorders that are present.

INCIDENCE, PREVALENCE, AND DEMOGRAPHICS

The incidence and prevalence of CP has been undergoing changes since the early 1960s, at which time technological advances available in neonatal intensive care units were utilized. Mortality of "at risk" infants has declined dramatically, but of concern is that this has resulted in an increase in morbidity, especially of cerebral dysfuntion syndromes. In spite of the fact that incidence of CP is on the decrease (the number of babies born who develop CP out of 1,000 live births) (Hagberg, Hagberg, & Olow, 1976), the prevalence of CP (number of CP cases in the community) may be on the rise. Because many more babies are being kept alive who, prior to 1966, would have succumbed during the neonatal period, the pool of living infants increased. Although the percentage of such infants who will develop cerebral palsy has decreased, it is of concern that in the near future an increase in the total population of cerebral palsied individuals may occur.

For the last two decades there has been a change in the frequency of the different types of CP. Spastic hemiparesis CP at one time was the most common type, but now spastic diparesis and quadriparesis prevail. The recent success in preventing death in severely anoxic or extremely premature infants has been responsible for this change. Prematurely born infants are prone to develop a spastic diplegia. Anoxic infants are prone to develop quadriparetic and/or dyskinetic abnormalities.

There is a high incidence of CP among the black population. This probably reflects poor prenatal care and increased incidence of prematurity, as is the case in the black community.

ETIOLOGY, CONTRIBUTING FACTORS, PREVENTIVE TECHNIQUES

There are many causes of CP. Any adverse influence on the developing brain may affect the integrity of the neuromotor components and result in a motor dysfunction (see Table 32-2).

Gross malformation of the brain may occur if the insult is active during embryogenesis in the first few weeks of pregnancy. Chromosomal abnormalities, toxic drugs, maternal infections such as toxoplasmosis, cytomegalic virus, rubella, or herpes, or exposure to X-ray radiation may be etiological factors. Later in pregnancy adverse influences may cause problems in differentiation of specific cerebral areas or sometimes actual destruction of brain tissue.

Of major significance prenatally is insufficient oxygen or blood reaching the brain. Toxemia, with its associated hypertension and vasoconstriction of placental blood vessels, and placenta previa with excessive placental bleeding may cause insufficient blood supply to the brain.

During parturition the fetus is at risk for suffering ischemic–anoxic insults due either to prolonged labor or compression of the umbilical cord.

During the neonatal period complications of prematurity are a common cause of CP. Very low birth weight infants, those under 1,500 g, are especially vulnerable. They are prone to develop bleeding into the subependymal area of the lateral ventricles of the cerebrum. The hemorrhage may be primarily into the ventricular system but often extends into the subependymal area and then into the adjacent white matter of the cortex. The white matter juxtaposed to the ventricles are the pyramidal tract fibers destined for the lower extremities. Their destruction will cause a spastic diplegia in which the legs are involved more than the arms. If the hemorrhage extends further laterally, the pyramidal tracts destined for the upper extremities are then involved, with spastic quadriparesis the likely result.

Neonatally, a static encephalopathy may be the end result of intracranial infection. Streptococcal meningitis is an example of an infectious disorder. Respiratory distress syndrome, cardiac abnormalities, and shock can cause anoxic–ischemic encephalopathy.

Postnatally, head trauma, environmental toxins such as lead, and infections such as meningitis and encephalitis are frequently pathogenically responsible for CP.

Prevention of CP is directed toward the known etiologies. Currently these are being addressed by rubella immunizations, development of vaccines for other infectious agents known to be teratogenic (e.g., cytomegalic virus), improving maternal nutrition, and educating mothers about the adverse effects of smoking and alcohol consumption, the need for early and continuous prenatal medical care, the risk of using non-prescription drugs during pregnancy, and the value of amniocentesis in women over thirty-five and when one suspects the possibility of a fetus with a chromosomal abnormality. Mothers who are at risk for having complications of delivery and/or having a baby at risk for developing neonatal complications are being referred to tertiary-care perinatal centers, where there are available highly specialized obstetricians and obstetrical nurses and where there exists a neonatal intensive care unit. Promoting good nutrition for infants, accident prevention programs, and appropriate and timely immunizations also can prevent some cases of CP. The recent influenza bacillus vaccine should decrease the incidence of influenza meningitis and therefore the incidence of cerebral dysfunction syndromes. Decrease in environmental toxins, especially lead, will significantly decrease the incidence and prevalence of CP.

CLINICAL DESCRIPTION

The clinical manifestations of damage to the neuromotor integrity of the brain may not be evident during the first few months of life, and there may be continuing changes in the clinical picture for the first year or two (Taft, 1982). For a full-term newborn, movements, tone, and posture are the result of primitive reflexes, with the highest level of the reflex arc being subcortical. Extensive damage to the cortex, therefore, may not be clinically evident. For example, an infant born with hydranencephaly, a condition in which the cortex has not developed, but with the diencephalon and the caudal parts of the brain intact may not show neuromotor abnormalities neonatally. An infant with extensive damage to one cerebral hemisphere will rarely show asymmetry of tone, movement, or reflexes during the first few months of life. In fact, when a newborn infant is found to have decreased tone and movement of the extremities, the lesion is rarely of central origin but usually peripheral in origin. That is, the pathology would be either in the anterior horn cell, peripheral myoneural junction, or muscle.

Types of Cerebral Palsy

Hemiparesis.   Infants who have unilateral damage to the motor cortex will rarely reveal manifestations of a motor disability at birth (Bobath, 1966; Taft, 1982). At approximately four months of age, it will be noted that the uninvolved hand will no longer be fisted, in contrast to the persistent fisting and cortical thumb of the involved extremity. At this point, if the infant is passive during the examination, one might be able to demonstrate an asymmetry in tone of the upper extremities evidenced by tightness of the elbow flexors and pronators of the wrists. Also, for the first time a reflex asymmetry may be present with exaggerated reflexes on the abnormal side. Examination of the low extremities may not reveal evidence of dysfunction until the latter half of the first year.

At approximately six months of age, preferential use of one hand may be evident. A cover placed over the face of the infant will be removed singlehandedly. As protective reflexes come into play at around 6 to 7 months, such as lateral propping and anterior propping (parachuting) (Fig. 26-1), the asymmetry of response of the extremities will be quite evident. In fact, these tests are valuable because if such abnormal protective reflexes can be confirmed on repeat testing, one must consider hemiparesis present even though at this early stage tone or reflex changes may not exist.

Figure 26-1. Parachuting.

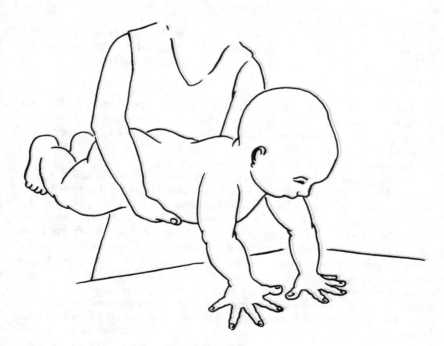

PARACHUTING

When the infant crawls, there will be a tendency to push off solely with the uninvolved extremities. There usually will be a slight delay in walking, and when it is accomplished, the infant will usually assume an equinovarus position of the involved lower extremity and will circumduct the leg. Fully manifest antigravity spasticity could be delayed until two to three years of age. If intelligence is normal or mildly impaired, practically all infants with hemiparesis will ambulate independently.

Spastic diparesis.   If the lower extremities are spastic and the upper extremities are grossly normal, the term *spastic diparesis* is used. Most diparetics will present with a delay in sitting, crawling, and standing. Early, there will often be hypotonia of the trunk and lower extremities. The clue that the hypotonia is not due to a lower motor neuron lesion will be the finding of exaggerated deep-tendon reflexes and unsustained clonus. One may be able to demonstrate that there is a tendency toward increased extensor tone of the trunk and hypertonus of the lower extremities. When the baby is picked up from the supine position, there will be the tendency for the hips and knees to assume an extended position, with plantarflexion of the ankles, so that the infant assumes an erect standing position instead of the expected sitting position. When held in vertical suspension, the spasticity of the hip adductors will cause scissoring of the lower extremities (Figure 26-2).

At approximately 10 to 24 months there will be a gradual change from hypotonia to hypertonus of the spastic type. Spasticity of the antigravity muscles will gradually increase and may only reach its maximum at around two to three years of age.

Spastic quadriparesis.   When all four extremities are involved, the term *spastic quadriparesis* is used. However, if the upper extremities show more dysfunction than the lower extremities and there is asymmetry between sides, the term *double hemiplegia* is frequently assigned.

In early infancy an infant who will go on to develop a spastic quadriparesis may show evidence of either hypertonus or hypotonia (Ellenberg & Nelson, 1981). If hypertonus is the initial problem, it is usually of the extensor type. However, even in babies who are hypotonic certain positions of the body in space will stimulate the tonic labyrinth reflexes and may result in intermittent extensor posturing. For example, such infants may have increased tendency to extension of the neck and trunk. A normal infant in the prone position will demonstrate a tonic labyrinth reflex that increases flexor posturing. That is why a normal infant appears to be in a so-called fetal position when lying prone. In the same infant, when placed in the supine position, modifying the tonic labyrinth reflex, a slight increase in extensor posturing will occur although the flexor position will still predominate. However, with damage to the neuromotor tracts of the brain there is a change in the sensitivity of the tonic labyrinth reflexes so that the supine position results in a more than normal increase in the amount of stimuli going to the

Figure 26-2. Scissoring.

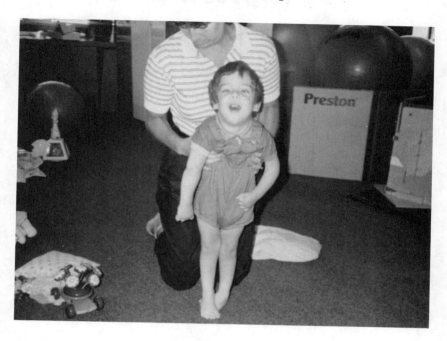

extensors. What ensues is extensor posturing. Infants with this tone disorder may appear to be precocious in motor development. When they are lying in the prone position, head control may be consistent with that of an older infant. The deception will be further enhanced when these same infants are noted to roll over from prone to supine at an early age. What is happening is a mechanical advantage for the purpose of rolling over when there is hyperextension of the trunk and neck. The rolling over is accidental, not voluntary. Proof that this early rolling over is not a manifestation of precocious normal development can be ascertained by pulling the supine infant up by the forearms. There will be head lag and not the expected voluntary control of the head and neck so that they rise in line with the trunk.

Deep-tendon reflexes and ankle clonus will be exaggerated in the hypertonic as well as the hypotonic infant. An obligatory asymmetrical tonic neck reflex (ATNR) can be expected (Figure 26-3) (Taft & Cohen, 1961). Passively turning the head to one side results in posturing of the arms and legs in a fencing position that, if obligatory, will persist in spite of the baby's crying for at least 30 seconds.

When the infant is lying supine, the lower extremities may assume a frog position, that is, the hips will be slightly flexed, abducted, and externally ro-

Figure 26-3. Asymmetrical tonic neck reflex.

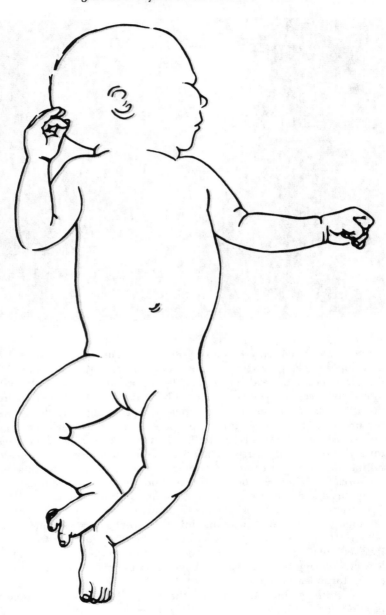

tated, with the knees partially flexed. If the infant is picked up and placed in a vertical position, there will be an exaggeration of internal rotation and adduction of the hips, so much so that scissoring may occur. If the infant's soles are placed on the examining table, a positive supporting reaction may be elicited that normally should have disappeared by four to six months.

Beginning around the second half of the first year and continuing through the second year of life, the hypotonic infant will gradually begin to show signs of spasticity. However, some hypotonic infants remain with diminished tone throughout their lives. These infants with "atonic" CP are usually severely motor- and intellectually disabled.

Dyskinesis.   A classic example of the changing pattern of tone and posture associated with maturation of the brain has been well documented in infants who develop an encephalopathy due to hyperbilirubinemia. A full-term infant who has had a toxic level of bilirubin due to blood incompatability will develop, at approximately three to five days, a symptom complex known as kernicterus. At this stage the infant will be opisthotonic due to increased tone of the neck and trunk, will have a high-pitched cry, will be irritable, will have an obligatory tonic neck reflex, and may convulse. Many infants with these symptoms of bilirubin encephalopathy die. However, if the infant survives, there will be a gradual change noted over the first months of life from the hypertonic state to what appears to be normal tone. One may suspect that an abnormality exists because the tone will vary depending on the state of activity of the infant. Crying will result in exaggerated extensor posturing. A further clue would be the persistence of an obligatory ATNR. Deep-tendon reflexes are frequently normal even though no dyskinetic movements will be noted at this stage.

At two to three months the previous normal tone is gradually replaced by hypotonus. The decrease in tone will persist for the first year of life.

At around ten months the post-kernicteric infant will be demonstrating immature motor patterns but no involuntary movements. For example, when the baby reaches out, instead of having a pincer grasp appropriate for a ten-month-old, there will be a raking grasp more like that of a five- to 6-month-old. At about one to one and a half years of age, a further change in tone and movement eventuates. The hypotonic state is replaced by hypertonus of the rigid type, and concomitantly slow, writhing, athetoid movements begin to appear. The extent of the hypertonicity and the dyskinetic movements may not be fully evident until two to three years of age. The involuntary movements are usually of the athetoid type, but either choreoathetosis or dystonia may be the type of dysfunction that predominates.

Other types.   In the rigid type of CP the involuntary movements are inconsequential although skilled movements are difficult to perform. Pure ataxic CP reveals itself in early infancy by the presence of hypotonia. It is usually difficult to diagnose until ambulation when truncal ataxia becomes evident or there is actually appendicular ataxis with dysmetria noticed on reaching out. Ataxic cerebral palsies tend to show improvement in motor control as they get older.

ASSOCIATED HANDICAPS AND COMPLICATIONS

Although CP is defined primarily in terms of a motor handicap it may not be the most disabling problem. Most individuals with CP are multiply handicapped (Ellenberg & Nelson, 1981). Of the associated handicaps the most serious in terms of independent functioning is mental retardation. It is estimated that more than 50 percent of individuals with CP are mentally retarded. Many non-retarded cerebral palsied individuals may have learning difficulties, attention deficit disorders, impulsivity, and hyperactivity.

Visual handicaps are quite frequent. Nearsightedness and strabismus are seen in more than 75 percent of children with CP. Hearing deficits of the sensorineural type have been estimated to occur in more than 75 percent of infants with CP whose etiology was bilirubin encephalopathy. Bilirubin is especially toxic to the eighth nerve. However, in all types of CP, sensorineural hearing deficits may be present. Epilepsy occurs in about 30 percent of individuals with CP. The age of onset varies but often is around school age. The types of seizures also vary. Hemiparetics usually have focal seizures affecting the spastic extremities. They may have hemianopsia and trophic growth disturbance of the extremities (Holt, 1961). Shortening of an extremity will be quite evident in the first few years of life but rarely will a leg discrepancy be greater than 2 inches.

Extremely carious teeth are often seen in the CP population. Poor dental hygiene secondary to the motor handicap is not the only cause of excessive number of caries. Individuals with CP are prone to have enamel hypoplasia that is an additional consequence of the insult that originally caused the CP (Cohen & Diner, 1970). If this insult occurred at a time of enamelogenesis and/or odontogenesis, teeth malformations may occur.

The complications of CP include joint contractures resulting from hypertonicity, scoliosis, amblyopia, less than optimal cognitive functioning, and emotional problems.

If an infant is delayed in voluntary motor control and is not given opportunities for gaining sensory experiences, his cognitive development may be permanently impaired.

Psychological disorders are quite common in individuals with CP. Some behaviors may be physiologically based, such as the hyperactivity and impulsivity. However, many are of environmental origin. From early infancy normal maternal-infant interactions may be at risk because of aberrant responses of the dysfunctional infant that cause maternal misunderstanding, insecurity, and anxiety.

MANAGEMENT

Because most individuals with CP are multiply handicapped, many disciplines are necessary to ensure adequate and comprehensive care (Taft, Matthews & Molnar, 1983). An interdisciplinary health team with expertise in CP is the ideal.

The overall philosophy of care should include optimizing all areas of functioning, helping the child achieve as much independence in activities of daily living as is possible within the constraints of the existing handicap, maintaining the child's self-esteem and motivation for achievement, and assuring that proper educational, social, and recreational resources are utilized. Of prime importance is attention to the maintenance of family integrity and aid to family members in coping with the additional stresses of life that the presence of a handicapped loved one is bound to cause.

Early Intervention

As soon as the diagnosis is made, the family should be so informed in a supportive but compassionate way. They should be told that early-intervention programs are available to infants with CP and that if parents participate in these programs, they will gain a better understanding of cerebral palsy and the infant will be given the chance to develop in a functionally optimal manner. No claim should be made that early intervention will dramatically change the natural course of the disorder.

In many states early intervention centers are mandated by law and are the responsibility of the education health systems. In 1975 Public Law 94-142, a bill of rights for the developmentally disabled (DD), was passed. This law mandated that states make available free and appropriate education for the DD from the age of three years to twenty-one years. It encouraged states to develop early-intervention programs for infants from birth to three years.

These early-intervention programs are multidiscipline and usually include a social worker, nurse physical therapist, occupational therapist, language therapist, and in an increasing number of centers, early infant educators (Soboloff, 1981). Other professionals, such as orthopedists and neurologists, are available as consultants. The programs are either home-based, center-based, or include both of these services. For the home-based programs, a team of health professionals visit the home, evaluate the child, and make recommendations to the parents regarding intervention modalities. These are implemented by the parents or team members in the home. In the center-based programs, the mother or guardian brings the infant to the program, where an assessment and recommendations are made for parental intervention. Successful programs are oriented toward the parents as the therapists. The parents are taught the techniques to improve the function of their infant. Usually only one visit per week is required.

Research as to the effectiveness of early-intervention programs has been limited, and research designs have been criticized. However, on the basis of experience, many clinicians see the value in the programs (Denhoff, 1981; Soboloff, 1981). They report earlier adaptation and improved coping abilities of parents. Infants are believed to experience less frustration because of their motor limitations, and their emotional and cognitive development is enhanced.

When an infant is registered in a program, focus is initially on parental education and support. During the grieving period this is accomplished through individual counseling or by utilizing educational or psychoeducational therapeutic group sessions. Demystifying the infant's abnormal reaction patterns is helpful for improving parents' coping abilities. It is very difficult for parents of a handicapped infant, whether cerebral palsied or retarded, to "read" an infant's responses because they are often not the routinely expected ones. Infants with CP may have difficulty with bottle or breast feeding and may literally appear to spit out the nipple. This type of response reduces a pleasurable experience that infant and mother should have during a feeding sequence. Many infants with CP are stiff and therefore are considered cold and not cuddly. They may appear to be backing away from the caretaker when being held. Their cries are undifferentiated, which makes interpretation of whether the crying represents pain or hunger impossible. Therapists aid parents to understand these aberrant reflex responses of their infants, thus minimizing abnormal maternal– and paternal–infant interactions that might have developed because of parental ignorance as to cause and effect.

After observing the infant, the therapist may recommend specific postural changes in the way the mother holds the infant in order to minimize any feeding difficulties (Finnie, 1970). For example, an infant with a very obligatory ATNR and a tendency toward extensor posturing will frequently have extreme difficulty in feeding. This infant, when held by the mother in a semi-supine position to feed, will often have an overreactive tonic labyrinth reflex and begin to arch the back as if voluntarily backing away from the mother. When the head is turned toward the breast or the bottle, an exaggerated ATNR may ensue, which results in extension of the upper extremities on the same side the face is turned toward. This simulates straight-arming of the mother as if to push her away. If in spite of these responses the mother is successful in getting the nipple of her breast into the baby's mouth, a tongue thrust may ensue that literally appears as if the infant is spitting out the nipple. This may have a dramatic and adverse effect on the infant as well as the mother and interfere with normal maternal–infant bonding. A physical therapist and/or a speech and language therapist assessing an infant with these problems would be able to recommend to the mother certain positions that would minimize the tonic labyrinth reflex so that the baby no longer hyperextends, and also techniques of holding the jaw forward that decrease the tongue thrust. These simple explanations to the mother may make for more pleasurable interactions.

Improving Functional Control

One of the main objectives of therapeutic exercise in relation to CP is to improve functional control. To achieve this it is not necessary to normalize tone or diminish or abolish involuntary movements, as desirable as these changes would be. Much can be done to permit an individual with CP to improve his functional ability without significantly changing the neuromotor abnormalities imposed by the damaged central nervous system.

There are many doctrinaire physical therapy regimens for diminishing motor disability. Unfortunately, they have not been subjected to rigid scientific assessment, so the validity of their success as claimed by their adherents remains in doubt. Most treatment regimens attempt to influence sensory input systems such as proprioception and touch to modify hypertonus and to improve motor control.

One of the more widely accepted treatment regimens is the Bobath technique (Molmar, 1982; Taft et al., 1962). This approach is based on normal neurodevelopmental sequences and utilizes primitive reflexes to achieve reflex postural changes that allow for better functional control of movement. For example, if an infant tends to have extensor posturing, the therapist will attempt to maintain the infant in a flexor position. This will usually allow for better hand control because of the influence of persistent symmetrical tonic neck reflexes. In these infants trunk flexion will cause arm flexion and therefore permit coordinated eye-hand movements.

In addition to the value of stabilization of the trunk and proximal joints, optimal fine motor performance requires voluntary practice at a specific task. Improving motor skills requires repetitive attempts to do the same specific task. There is continual feedback to the nervous system of visual, tactile, proprioceptive influences, which involuntarily refines a specific motor movement until maximum efficiency is reached. When this occurs, performance becomes automatic and does not require any forethought as to "how it should be done." A child with CP benefits less from practice than a child with an intact nervous system because there may be abnormal sensory feedback signals as well as sensorimotor integration difficulties. Notwithstanding these interferences, a therapist will attempt to break down a gross skilled movement pattern into discrete units and through the use of facilitation and/or inhibition techniques simplify the voluntary acquisition of a more skilled performance. If the child is cooperative and perseveres, successful repetition of these movement patterns may lead to more refined and skilled movements with better functional control. Unfortunately, practice with a successful outcome in accomplishing a specific motor task does not generalize into improved performance on other tasks (Kottke, Halpern, & Easton, 1978).

Orthoses

Orthoses or bracing are used to prevent deformities and to help improve motor function (Molnar, 1980). If a spastic diplegic walks on his toes because of a spastic gastrocnemius muscle, an ankle-foot orthoses could minimize that tendency. As regards the upper extremities, the use of a cock-up wrist splint to prevent spastic wrist flexion, plus an opponens splint to prevent "cortical thumb," will place the hand in a more functional position and allow more successful hand use.

Bracing also has been utilized to prevent or delay soft-tissue contracture. It provides constant stretching of the muscle around the joints. Bracing is frequently used to maintain a joint in an appropriate position after surgical correction of a contracture.

Orthopedic Surgery

Orthopedic surgery is frequently of benefit for the spastic type of CP (Black, 1979; Samilson, 1975). It is used to prevent or correct deformities. It also may be utilized as a means of improving motor function. Examples would include heel cord lengthening operations to decrease a spastic equinus, thereby improving gait and preventing a fixed ankle contracture. Adductor tenotomies to abolish the instability of gait caused by scissoring of the lower extremities due to spastic hip adductors frequently improves ambulation. Adductor tenotomies also are done to prevent or treat subluxation of the hip.

Orthopedic surgery is of infrequent benefit for dyskinetic CP, such as athetosis. Orthopedic surgery is rarely prescribed before the age of three to four years because prior to that time maturation of the nervous system is incomplete and the extent of the motor dysfunction may be still evolving.

Neurosurgery

In the past decade attempts to modify hypertonus through neurosurgical techniques have been tried (Gornall, Hitchcock & Kirkland, 1975). Cerebellar or spinal cord implants that stimulate the inhibitory fibers and posterior spinal cord rhizotomies have been done in a few major centers. There is no consensus as to the value of these techniques and which types of CP would benefit the most. These procedures are considered experimental at present.

Medication

Diazepam, a tranquilizer, and baclofen, a gamma-aminobutyric acid–like agent, act through the central nervous system. They have been used to decrease spasticity in order to improve functional motor control (Young & Delwaide, 1981). These drugs rarely result in significant improvement because sedation often occurs before there is an effect on tone. Dantrolene, which acts directly on the muscle, has a less sedative effect, but is hepatotoxic. Additionally, dantrolene may cause profound weakness which, in spite of the decreased tone, further limits mobility.

These medications frequently prove to be of more value for patients with severe hypertonus, especially those with spastic quadriparesis or dystonic athetosis. Minor relief of the hypertonus will make the patient more comfortable and allow for easier care.

A 4- to 6-month decrease in spasticity of local muscle groups can be achieved by the injection of phenol or alcohol directly into the motor end points of a muscle or into the peripheral nerve (Easton, Ozel & Halpern, 1979). This procedure may improve function and carry the patient to a point in time that is more suitable for orthopedic correction. In addition, the technique may permit the surgeon to preoperatively gain knowledge of the functional results that would occur with tenotomizing a muscle.

Prevention of Complications

Contractures. Unequal pull between agonist and antagonist muscles across a joint will result in soft-tissue contracture. The resulting deformities limit motor and postural control. The use of passive stretching or active assistive movements of the joints through a full range of motion may prevent or at least delay the onset of contractures. The mother can be taught these exercises and, when the child is older, he may be able to perform many of them by himself.

Visual disorders.. An infant or child with CP should be routinely examined every 6 months for the presence of strabismus and/or problems with visual acuity. If the strabismus is allowed to persist for more than a year, there is risk of the development of amblyopia–exanopsia. The child becomes cortically blind, and even though the eyes may be placed in line surgically, vision in the deviating eye may not improve.

Scoliosis. Curvature of the back is not uncommon in CP. It may develop at any age. A hemiplegic child with a shortened lower extremity may develop a pelvic tilt and secondarily develop a curvature of the spine. Also, the unequal pull of the back muscles in spastic dystonic individuals may result in a spinal distortion.

General Health Maintenance

The primary care physician must maintain his normal role in routine health maintenance and in the care of any acute or chronic illness that might develop. However, he has the additional responsibility of routinely assessing for potentially complicating factors that youngsters with CP are prone to. He also should monitor the psychosocial, educational, vocational, and recreational needs of his patient. He should interview the siblings to find out how they are dealing with the problem and also educate them as to what CP is, its causes and its genetics. Many siblings are troubled by (a) the parents spending too much time with their handicapped brother or sister and not giving them enough attention; (b) fantasies that they did something wrong that caused their sibling to have a handicap; and (c) worry that they may have children of their own with CP.

Inquiries should be made to see if respite care is needed so that parents can get some time off from their care of their child with cerebral palsy.

Finally, the primary care physician has the responsibility to coordinate care and to be an advocate for the child to obtain those rights available to every child, disabled or not.

REFERENCES

Bax, M. C. O. (1964). Terminology and classification of cerebral palsy. *Developmental Medicine and Childhood Neurology, 6,* 295.

Bleck, E. E. (1979). *Orthopedic management of cerebral palsy.* Philadelphia: W. B. Saunders.

Bobath, K. (1966). *The motor deficit in patients with cerebral palsy* (Clinics in Developmental Medicine Series No. 2 and 3). Philadelphia: Lippincott.

Cohen, J. H., & Diner, H. (1970). The significance of developmental dental enamel defects in neurological diagnosis. *Pediatrics, 46,* 737.

Denhoff, E. (1981). Current status of infant stimulation or enrichment programs for children with developmental disabilities. *Pediatrics, 67,* 32.

Easton, J. K. M., Ozel, T., & Halpern, D. (1979). Intramuscular neurolysis for spasticity in children. *Archives of Physical Medicine and Rehabilitation, 60,* 155.

Ellenberg, J., & Nelson, K. B. (1981). Early recognition of infants at high risk for cerebral palsy: Examination at four months. *Developmental Medicine and Childhood Neurology, 23,* 703.

Finnie, N. R. (1970). *Handling the young cerebral palsied child at home.* New York: E. P. Dutton.

Gornall, P., Hitchcock, E., & Kirkland, I. S. (1975). Stereotaxic neurosurgery in the management of cerebral palsy. *Developmental Medicine and Childhood Neurology, 17,* 279.

Hagberg, G., Hagberg, B., & Olow, I. (1976). The changing panorama of cerebral palsy in Sweden, 1954–1970. *Acta Paediatrica in Scandinavia, 65,* 403.

Holt, K. S. (1961). *Growth disturbances: Hemiplegic cerebral palsy in children and adults* (Clinics in Developmental Medicine Series No. 4). London: Spastics Society/ Heinemann.

Kottke, F. H., Halpern, D., & Easton, J. K. M. (1978). The training of coordination. *Archives of Physical Medicine and Rehabilitation, 59,* 567.

Molnar, G. E. (1980). Orthotic management of children. In J. Redford (Ed.), *Orthotics Etc.* Baltimore: Williams & Wilkins.

Molnar, G. E. (1982). Intervention for physically handicapped children. In M. Lewis & L. T. Taft (Eds.), *Developmental disabilities, theory, assessment and intervention.* Jamaica, NY: Spectrum Publications.

Samilson, R. L. (Ed.). (1975). *Orthopaedic aspects of cerebral palsy* (Clinics in Developmental Medicine Series Nos. 52, 53). Philadelphia: Lippincott.

Soboloff, H. R. (1981). Early intervention—Fact or fiction. *Developmental Medicine and Childhood Neurology, 23,* 61.

Taft, L. T. (1982). Neuromotor assessment of infants. In M. Lewis & L. T. Taft (Eds.), *Developmental disabilities, theory, assessment and intervention.* Jamaica, NY: Spectrum Publications.

Taft, L. T., & Cohen, H. J. (1961). Neonatal and infant reflexology. In J. Helmuth (Ed.), *Exceptional infant* (Vol. 1, pp. 81–120). Seattle: Special Child Publications.

Taft, L. T., Delagi, E. F., Wilkie, O. L., & Abramson, A. S. (1962). Critique of rehabilitative techniques in treatment of cerebral palsy. *Archives of Physical Medicine and Rehabilitation, 43,* 238.

Taft, L. T., Matthews, W. S., & Molnar, G. E. (1983). Pediatric management of the physically handicapped child. In L. A. Barness (Ed.), *Advances in pediatrics.* Chicago: Year Book Medical Publishers.

Young, R. R., & Delwaide, P. J. (1981). Drug therapy: Spasticity. *New England Journal of Medicine, 304,* 96.

Chapter 27

NEURAL TUBE DEFECTS

Mark L. Wolraich

DEFINITIONS

Neural tube defects are embryologic malformations of the central nervous system and its bony support structures. The most common malformation is a meningomyelocele defect involving the spinal cord and bony spines. This type of spine defect has been detected even in mummified remains from Egyptian tombs, although meningomyelocele defects were not described until the seventeenth century by Tulp. (Brocklehurst, 1976). Figure 27-1 shows the types of lesion and their locations in the central nervous system.

A defect involving the total maldevelopment of the brain is referred to as anencephaly. If they are born alive, children with this malformation rarely survive beyond a few months of age. A defect involving an outpouching of malformed brain tissue through the skull is referred to as an encephalocele. Defects involving the spinal cord are of three types as shown in Figure 27-2.

The most common and most debilitating defect is meningomyelocele, an outpouching of malformed spinal cord tissue through split or *bifid* spines. This is also referred to as spina bifida cystica or aperta (frequently shortened to spina bifida). If only the meninges, or covering around the spinal cord, pouches out, without any spinal cord involvement, the defect is referred to as a meningocele. If there are only several bifid spines, with no spinal cord or meningeal involvement, it is referred to as spina bifida occulta.

Figure 27-1.

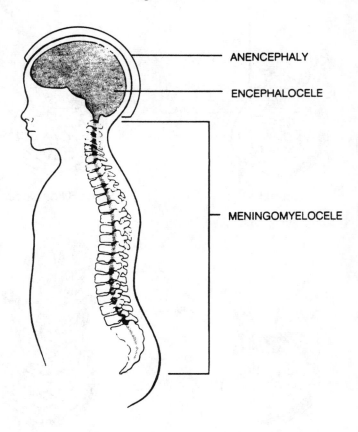

ANENCEPHALY

ENCEPHALOCELE

MENINGOMYELOCELE

INCIDENCE, PREVALENCE, AND DEMOGRAPHICS

Meningomyelocele and anencephaly occur in about equal frequencies at about 1 per 1,000 live births in the United States. For reasons as yet undetermined, the rates of these disorders are gradually declining, and the incidence in many areas of the country is now about 0.8 per 1,000 live births (Windham & Edmonds, 1982). The incidence has been considerably higher in the British Isles, particularly in Ireland and South Wales, with rates as high as 5 per 1,000 live births; but the frequency there also has declined in recent years. In the United States, couples of English and Irish extraction have a slightly higher incidence than couples of other ethnic origins, but their rates are less than the rates in the British Isles (Naggan & MacMahon, 1967).

The incidence of encephalocele defects is 5 to 10 times less frequent than

Figure 27-2.

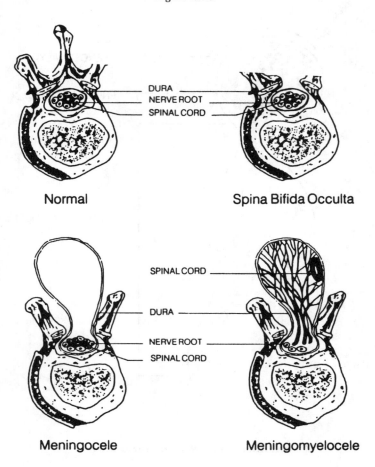

Normal

Spina Bifida Occulta

DURA
NERVE ROOT
SPINAL CORD

SPINAL CORD
DURA
NERVE ROOT
SPINAL CORD

Meningocele

Meningomyelocele

meningomyelocele or anencephaly, occuring about once in 10,000 live births. The simple bony defect of spina bifida occulta occurs frequently (5 to 10 percent of the population). It is usually of no medical import and needs no further discussion except to say that there is evidence to suggest that spina bifida occulta occurs more frequently than expected in parents of children with meningomyelocele. It has yet to be determined if this makes individuals with spina bifida occulta at greater risk for having children with neural tube defects. The meningocele lesion itself rarely poses any significant long-term problem once the defect is surgically corrected during infancy.

ETIOLOGY, CONTRIBUTING FACTORS AND PREVENTIVE TECHNIQUES

The cause of neural tube defects remains elusive and is most likely multifactoral in nature. In terms of embryologic development, the abnormality occurs early in fetal development, between the 19th and 31st days of gestation. One animal model has demonstrated a relationship between maternal fever and the defect in the offspring, but this has not been confirmed by human experience (Clarren, Smith, Harvey, & Ward, 1979). Recent research in England suggests that a recurrence of the defect in subsequent offspring can be prevented if high-risk mothers take large doses of vitamins both prior to conception and during pregnancy (Smithells et al., 1980). The research completed to date has some methodologic problems (Toriello, 1982); confirmation research is currently being undertaken in both the British Isles and the United States. Any more definitive statement about the efficacy of vitamin therapy in preventing neural tube defects must await the results.

Whatever the cause, it is known that certain couples are more predisposed to having a child with a neural tube defect. In couples who have had a previous child with a neural tube defect, the risk of having a second child is 20 per 10,000 live births, a 20-fold increase in risk over the general population. If the parents have had two children with neural tube defects, the risk goes up to 100 per 1,000 live births.

Neural tube defects can be detected *in utero*. Since most of the defects entail leakage of central spinal fluid into the amniotic fluid, through amniocentesis it is possible to detect the presence of the defect by measuring a substance found predominantly in fetal spinal fluid. The most frequently monitored substance has been alpha-fetal protein. This test can accurately detect a neural tube defect at about 16 weeks gestation. Amniocentesis is recommended because it makes possible either the therapeutic termination of the pregnancy or the appropriate planning of care for the child during the birth and neonatal period for couples who do not wish to terminate the pregnancy. Ultrasonography also can detect certain spinal cord defects. This has become increasingly possible as refinements in this technology have improved the quality of the resolution of the pictures. However, it is important to note that ultrasound is not as accurate nor as sensitive as amniocentesis, particularly during the early phases of the pregnancy.

Within the past few years, a technique for testing maternal blood levels of alpha-fetal protein to detect neural tube defects has been developed. It is not as accurate as amniocentesis and is very dependent on the gestational age of the fetus. However, it has been used successfully as a method to screen large numbers of women, since amniocentesis is indicated only for women at a higher than usual risk. The serum or blood alpha-fetal protein test has been successful as a screening procedure when undertaken in a systematic manner, with amniocentesis available as a confirmatory test (Macri & Weiss, 1982).

Clinical Description

The main focus of the clinical description is meningomyelocele because it is the most common and the most complex abnormality in children who survive with neural tube defects. Children with encephalocele generally have hydrocephalus and mental retardation and may have motor involvement similar to that seen in cerebral palsy. For children with meningomyelocele, the two major underlying problems are spinal cord dysfunction and hydrocephalus, usually secondary to a brain defect called an Arnold–Chiari malformation.

Spinal Cord Dysfunction

Spinal cord dysfunction results from the abnormal development of the spinal cord at the level of the exposed lesion. This can be anywhere along the axis of the spinal cord. The higher the lesion on the spine, the greater the involvement, because rarely is any of the spinal cord below the defect connected to the upper spinal cord and brain. This means that nerves are not able to transmit messages *from* the brain to control muscle activity, nor messages *to* the brain to convey sensation. The former results in flaccid paralysis in the lower extremities; the latter results in loss of sensation in the same areas. The extent of involvement is dependent on the location or level of the lesion on the spinal axis. Figure 27-3 demonstrates how the various vertebral levels are labeled.

Any lesions above the lumbar region result in total paralysis of the lower extremities. Upper extremity function in terms of paralysis does not occur unless the high thoracic and low cervical vertebrae are involved, and this is rare. Figure 27-4 demonstrates the extent of leg movement for each of the spinal levels below the thoracic level.

Nerves required for providing voluntary control of urination and defecation are located in the lowest spinal sections (sacral levels three and four). For this reason, at least 90 percent of patients with meningomyelocele do not have bowel and bladder control. This deficit is referred to as a neurogenic bowel and bladder.

Hydrocephalus

Hydrocephalus, referred to in lay terminology as "water on the brain," results from an obstruction within the spaces in the central part of the brain and spinal cord that prevents the appropriate reabsorption of the central spinal fluid. If untreated, the continued production of this fluid results in a buildup of cerebrospinal fluid that can cause brain damage and an enlargement of the head size in infants. In children with meningomyelocele, the hydrocephalus is the result of a brain malformation called Arnold–Chiari

Figure 27-3. Regions of the spine.

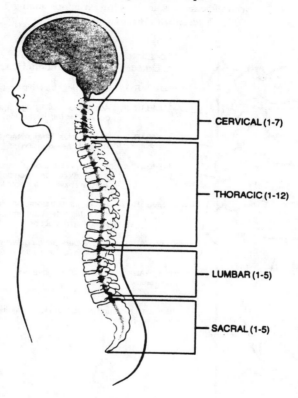

CERVICAL (1-7)

THORACIC (1-12)

LUMBAR (1-5)

SACRAL (1-5)

malformation. Eighty percent of children with meningomyelocele will have hydrocephalus.

Associated Conditions

The paralysis of the lower extremities can lead to joint contractures and bony malformation. *Scoliosis,* a lateral curvature of the spine, can develop over time; and a congenital anterior/posterior spine curvature, *kyphosis,* may be present from birth. A neurogenic bladder may cause repeated urinary tract infections, resulting in kidney damage and ultimately in kidney failure. A neurogenic bowel may cause severe constipation and even bowel obstruction secondary to the constipation. The lack of sensation in the lower extremities makes patients at high risk for the problem of pressure sores. Hydrocephalus can cause brain damage resulting in mental retardation, learning disa-

Figure 27-4. Relationship between level of defect and leg movement—
Incomplete lesions account for variations among
children with myelomeningocele.

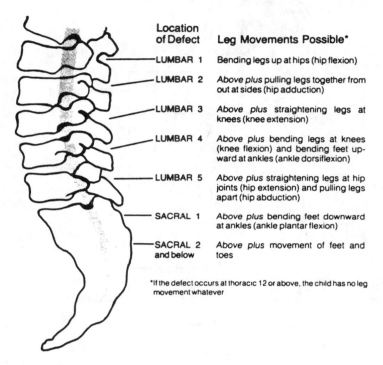

Location of Defect	Leg Movements Possible*
LUMBAR 1	Bending legs up at hips (hip flexion)
LUMBAR 2	*Above plus* pulling legs together from out at sides (hip adduction)
LUMBAR 3	*Above plus* straightening legs at knees (knee extension)
LUMBAR 4	*Above plus* bending legs at knees (knee flexion) and bending feet upward at ankles (ankle dorsiflexion)
LUMBAR 5	*Above plus* straightening legs at hip joints (hip extension) and pulling legs apart (hip abduction)
SACRAL 1	*Above plus* bending feet downward at ankles (ankle plantar flexion)
SACRAL 2 and below	*Above plus* movement of feet and toes

*If the defect occurs at thoracic 12 or above, the child has no leg movement whatever

bilities, and poor fine-motor coordination. In a small percentage of children, the brain stem, which controls the coordination of breathing and swallowing, can be affected and even can cause death during infancy from respiratory problems.

MANAGEMENT

Initial management entails surgical closure of the defect and treatment of the hydrocephalus. Until the defect is closed, the infant is susceptible to severe central nervous system infections such as meningitis and ventriculitis. Once the defect has been closed, a ventriculoperitoneal shunt is surgically placed to treat hydrocephalus if it is present. The shunt is a tube connected to a one-way valve and most commonly runs from a ventricle in the center of the brain to the peritoneal cavity in the abdomen. (Another shunt is one that runs from the ventricle in the brain to the heart. It is referred to as a ventriculocaval or ventriculoatrial shunt and is now rarely used). The ventriculoperitoneal shunt effectively prevents hydrocephalus from progressing but cannot repair brain damage that has already occurred *in utero* if the hydrocephalus was extensive prior to birth. Some *in utero* treatments of hydrocephalus have recently been tried on an experimental basis.

Most of the long-term management of children with meningomyelocele entails efforts to minimize the disability and to prevent secondary problems. This requires a coordinated effort by professionals from a number of medical, allied health, and educational professionals. Table 27-1 presents a list of some of these professionals and their role in the management of children with meningomyelocele.

Orthopedic and physiotherapeutic care consists of exercises, bracing, and surgery to minimize lower extremity joint contractures, prevent bony deformities, and enhance ambulation. New types of bracing encourage ambulation in children with little lower extremity function; many braces are now made of formed plastic so that they are lightweight and less visible. However, most patients with little lower extremity control will use wheelchairs as

Table 27-1. Professionals and Responsibilities

PEDIATRICIAN: coordination of medical care; triage when the nature of the medical problem is unclear; care for associated health problems, such as seizure disorders; primary contact for general health care

UROLOGIST: management of urinary tract infections and programs to achieve continence

ORTHOPEDIST: management of bracing, and problems associated with scoliosis; joint and extremity surgery

NEUROSURGEON: closure of open spine; management of shunt surgery; management of hydrocephalus

NEUROLOGIST: management of seizures; may be involved in monitoring shunt function or infections

PSYCHOLOGIST: educational testing, counseling; behavior management programs

NURSE: skin care, bowel and bladder management, counseling; work with local care provider; training child and local care providers in intermittent catheterization techniques

SOCIAL WORKER: consultation and help with financial management; support counseling; coordinating care with local providers

PHYSICAL THERAPIST: bracing; exercise routines to help improve mobility; training to help child use devices to aid ambulation

OCCUPATIONAL THERAPIST: management techniques for child's daily routines, such as feeding, dressing, and play activities

NUTRITIONIST: dietary management to prevent obesity, to help recovery after surgery, to promote skin healing, and to help with bowel and bladder management

adults. Orthopedic and physiotherapeutic management also closely monitor spinal growth to prevent, delay, or, if needed, surgically treat scoliosis.

Urologic care focuses on the prevention of urinary tract infections and kidney damage, as well as the provision of a means for managing urinary incontinence so that the patients are socially acceptable. At present the mainstay of treatment for this problem is clean intermittent catheterization, in which the patients or their care givers pass a tube into the bladder several times a day, under clean but not sterile conditions. For many children this can prevent urinary tract infections as well as provide social continence. Nurses play a key role in this therapy by instructing the families and facilitating the process. Placement of an artificial sphincter is an option for patients who are not able to become socially continent on intermittent catheterization alone. Pediatric and nursing staff assist with bowel management to attain social continence and also monitor skin care to prevent pressure sores. Pediatricians also deal with associated problems, such as seizure disorders, which occur more frequently in this population.

Neurosurgical care primarily involves the initial surgical closure of the back defect and shunt placement if hydrocephalus is present. Subsequent neurosurgical care involves the maintenance of the child's status. Occasionally, the shunt requires revision or replacement because of the child's growth needs, shunt malfunction, or shunt infection. Occasional scarring at the site of the back surgery can cause tension on the spinal cord during a child's rapid-growth phase. This is referred to as a tethered cord and requires neurosurgical correction.

Cognitive impairment also may be present in the form of mental retardation, learning disability, or fine motor incoordination. Special educational, psychological, and/or occupational therapeutic services may be required. The multiple aspects of disability caused by meningomyelocele also place heavy psychological and financial demands on the children and their families. Counseling for patients, parents, and siblings is an important but not always recognized need. Both psychologists and social workers must be involved. As children grow, counseling also must address the issue of their sexuality. Excessive weight gain is an additional and often serious problem. Children with meningomyelocele frequently have lower than average caloric needs; an excessive weight gain can have serious functional as well as cosmetic consequences. Preventive nutritional counseling for parents and children needs to be provided to prevent excessive weight gain before it becomes a significant problem.

It becomes clear that the services required by children with meningomyelocele are extensive, complex, and interrelated, and that they involve a large number of health and education professionals. In many communities it has not been possible to provide these services in an effectively coordinated way. Often, effective coordination requires an agency or individuals who are willing and able to provide this coordination. The other professionals involved also must cooperate in the endeavor, a factor that is complicated

NEURAL TUBE DEFECTS 307

by the various expectations of the organizational structures that define how professionals relate to the families.

SPECIFIC PROGRAMS AND RELATED LEGISLATION

Meningomyelocele has been one of the conditions receiving support under Crippled Children Services, and in many states coordinated clinics have been set up under their auspices. For a period of time, services also were provided through birth defect clinics established with March of Dimes or federal grants, but a number of these programs have been terminated. Several other private agencies have provided limited services. Orthopedic care is available through hospitals sponsored by the Shriners, and the Easter Seal Society has provided support for orthopedic equipment, adult living arrangements, and recreational activities such as summer camps.

Educational programs and some therapeutic services related to education are covered under the federal Education for All Handicapped Children Act (PL 94-142). Specifically relevant to meningomyelocele and PL 94-142 is a recent Supreme Court ruling in the case of Tartro versus California, which requires school staff to aid in clean intermittent catheterization therapy so that the children needing this service can attend public school even if they cannot independently manage the catheterization themselves. The federal legislation and regulations to ensure neonatal care for severely handicapped infants were enacted, in part, in response to the Baby Jane Doe case, which involved an infant with a meningomyelocele defect.

UNMET NEEDS

Coordination of services is still probably the greatest unmet need of children with neural tube defects. Even where coordination is provided, it is frequently not extensive enough to meet all of the interrelated needs of these patients. For example, orthopedic surgery for scoliosis can significantly impair a patient's ability to do self-catheterization, and excessive weight gain can reduce the ambulatory abilities of a patient. Professionals not only need to provide their specific services, but they need to prioritize and sequence those services in cooperation with other professionals. There have been cases in which the patient's medical needs are met, but despite having the physical and intellectual capabilities to become independent, the patient cannot, because of psychological needs that remain unmet. Because the overall needs of each patient are interrelated and extensive, someone must consider the entirety of the patient, prioritize the patient's needs, and coordinate the services required to meet those needs. Such programs are costly and time-consuming but essential if we are to assist individuals with meningomyelocele to reach their full potential.

REFERENCES

Brocklehurst, G. (1976). The nature of spina bifida. In G. Brocklehurst (Ed.), *Spina bifida for the clinician* (Clinics in Developmental Medicine, No. 57). Philadelphia: J. B. Lippincott Co.

Clarren, S. K., Smith, D. W., Harvey, M. A. S., & Ward, R. H. (1979). Hyperthermia—A prospective evaluation of a possible teratogenic agent in man. *Journal of Pediatrics, 95,* 81–83.

Macri, J. N., & Weiss, R. R. (1982). Prenatal serum alpha-fetaprotein screening for neural tube defects. *Obstetrics and Gynecology, 59,* 633–639.

Naggan, L., & MacMahon, B. (1967). Ethnic differences in the prevalence of anencephaly and spina bifida in Boston, Massachusetts. *New England Journal of Medicine, 277,* 1119–1123.

Smithells, R., Sheppard, S. Schoral, C., Seller, M., Nevin, N., Harris, R., Read, R., & Fielding, D. (1980). Possible prevention of neural tube defects by periconception vitamin supplementation. *Lancet,* 339–340.

Toriello, H. V. (1982). Periconceptual vitamin supplementation for the prevention of neural tube defects: A review. *Spina Bifida Theraphy, 4,* 59–62.

Windham, G. C., & Edmonds, L. D. (1982). Current trends in the incidence of neural tube defects. *Pediatrics, 79,* 333–337.

Chapter 28

MUSCULAR DYSTROPHY

Alfred J. Spiro

The term *muscular dystrophy* is used generically to describe a heterogeneous group of genetically determined disorders involving muscle. Virtually all of the entities in this group are progressive, and some are severely disabling (Brooke, 1976; Dubowitz, 1978; Walton, 1981).

Original accounts of clinical and pathological aspects of various types of muscular disorders appeared in the literature more than a century ago, but it is only in the past two to three decades in which these entities have been classified and delineated and the hereditary patterns clarified.

One useful greatly simplified schema would classify the muscular dystrophies as follows:

1. X-linked muscular dystrophy:
    Duchenne type
    Becker type

2. Generally autosomal recessive type (limb-girdle muscular dystrophy)

3. Autosomal dominant: facioscapulohumeral muscular dystrophy

4. Myotonic dystrophy:
    Childhood and adult form
    Infantile form

There are several other types of disorders generally listed under the grouping of muscular dystrophies but they are beyond the scope of this chapter.

INCIDENCE AND PREVALENCE

Muscular dystrophy affects all ethnic groups. This group of disorders contains uncommon entities, but because of the protracted nature of some of the individual diseases, e.g., Duchenne X-linked muscular dystrophy, they are common handicapping conditions despite the rather low prevalence. Some estimates of incidence and prevalence are as follows:

Dystrophy	Incidence	Prevalence
X-linked form (Duchenne)	13–33/100,000 live-born males	1.9–3.4/100,000 population
Facioscapulohumeral form	0.4–5/100,000	0.2/100,000
Myotonic dystrophy	13.5/100,000 at birth	4.9 to 5.5/100,000

ETIOLOGY

The pathogenesis of the various types of muscular dystrophy is unknown. In X-linked muscular dystrophy of the Duchenne type a leading postulate is that there is a defect in the sarcolemmal membrane that permits a substance or several substances, one of which is probably calcium, to enter the muscle cell freely. This leads to muscle fiber necrosis by a complex process of events.

CLINICAL DESCRIPTION

X-linked Duchenne Type

This disease occurs virtually always only in boys. The earliest complaints of the parents at the onset of independent walking frequently are those of gait abnormalities, such as toe walking or flat-footed gait. At about the time at which the child should be able to run, the parents may be aware that the child has a waddle "like a duck." They may also note, somewhat later, that when he attempts to climb stairs he lurches one leg at a time forward and assists himself by pulling inordinately hard on the banister. When getting up from the floor, he either assists himself by holding onto furniture or other objects or by climbing up on his own body using his arms, the Gower's maneuver. In early childhood enlargement of the calves is noted; less commonly other muscles are enlarged, and occasionally virtually all of the limb and torso muscles are enlarged, producing a herculean appearance. In early childhood the only manifestation of upper extremity involvement may be proximal hypotonicity; if the examiner puts his own hands in the child's axillae and tries to lift him, there is a diminished resistance. An increasing lumbar lordosis also is observed.

The disease is relentlessly progressive, and *overt* symmetrical weakness of the legs and arms is apparent by age five or six years. Because of progressive weakness and wasting, walking eventually (always by twelve years of age) becomes no longer possible despite adaptive devices, and the boy becomes wheelchair-bound. Weakness of the arms and legs progresses in the wheelchair state, and this is very frequently coupled with contractures of all joints, making performance of activities of daily life impossible, with the exception of manipulating the control of a motorized wheelchair or holding a pen or pencil.

Weakness of neck extensor muscles may occur in the late teenage period, making sitting in a wheelchair even more difficult. By the early or mid-twenties all patients with this type of muscular dystrophy die, generally from cardiac or respiratory involvement.

A significant percentage of children with X-linked muscular dystrophy of the Duchenne type function subnormally intellectually; the mean IQ is about 20 points below a normal control group. In early childhood patients with muscular dystrophy tend to be hyperkinetic and infantile compared with their peers; they also tend to have shortened attention spans. In addition to the weakness and personality and intellectual problems, once they become wheelchair-bound they frequently develop scoliosis and increased contractures in all joints. Obesity, occasionally extreme, also may be present, although some wheelchair-bound patients become extremely wasted and literally appear to be "skin and bone."

Even prior to becoming wheelchair-bound, children with Duchenne muscular dystrophy (and other muscle-wasting disorders) are subject to increased complications of otherwise insignificant respiratory disorders. Overt evidence of cardiac involvement is rare, but electrocardiographic changes reflect the involvement of cardiac musculature. Boys with muscular dystrophy are also subject to increased risks during general anesthesia.

Diagnosis can be established when the rather typical clinical pattern is couples with the results of studies usually employed to diagnose children with weakness, namely, (a) genetic studies; (b) studies of serum muscle enzymes (CK, SGOT, SGPT, and LDH); (c) electrodiagnostic studies; and (d) histological and histochemical studies of properly performed muscle biopsies.

Genetic studies consist of assessment of an accurate family pedigree; at least three CK determinations should be obtained on female family members to attempt to define the X-linkage, but it should be recognized that significant CK elevations are seen in only about one-half of obligate carriers, and approximately one-third of cases of Duchenne type of muscular dystrophy are the result of spontaneous mutations. More refined genetic studies using DNA probes have become available.

Studies of serum muscle enzymes are crucial in affected boys, in that every boy with muscular dystrophy of the Duchenne type will have a CK value more than 10 times the highest normal value of the particular laboratory in which it is performed. These values are markedly elevated very early in infancy prior to the onset of signs or symptoms of disease. The other serum muscle enzymes are also markedly elevated.

Electromyography is also helpful in establishing the diagnosis of a myopathy. Motor and sensory nerve conduction velocity studies are normal in this disease.

A muscle biopsy, when correlated with the clinical and other laboratory and genetic studies, can readily confirm the diagnosis. Some of the features include marked variability of fiber size, large "hyalinized" fibers containing excessive calcium, degenerating fibers and regenerating fibers, and increased endomysial connective tissue and fat.

Becker Type of X-linked Muscular Dystrophy

This disease occurs only in males, but the onset generally is not until school age (eight to ten years) or may not occur until significantly later. Symmetrical weakness of the proximal muscles of the legs may manifest itself with difficulty in climbing stairs, riding a bicycle, or arising from a low chair. The patient also may exhibit a tendency to walk on his toes. Large calves may be striking but generally are not in themselves part of the patient's complaint. The progression of weakness in the legs, and later in the proximal arm muscles, is very variable but always slow and painless and never precipitous. However, after two to three decades, lower extremity weakness may become so severe that the patient becomes wheelchair-bound. Patients with this type of muscular dystrophy will frequently be able to marry and have children.

A significant portion of individuals with the Becker type of muscular dystrophy will be mentally subnormal. Scoliosis and joint contractures may become problems when these patients become wheelchair-bound.

Diagnosis can be established in a manner similar to that of the Duchenne type of muscular dystrophy, in that results of genetic, biochemical, pathological, and electrodiagnostic studies are similar. More refined genetic studies, which will probably be available in the near future, will be able to determine if the disease is a continuation of the spectrum of variation in Duchenne muscular dystrophy or a separate genetically defined entity.

Limb-girdle Type of Muscular Dystrophy

This type of muscular disorder consists of several subgroups, with the mode of inheritance being either autosomal recessive or autosomal dominant. There is a great deal of variability in age of onset, which may be child-hood to middle age, and progression, which may be slow and insidious, more rapidly progressive, or stepwise progressive. A precipitous increase in weak-ness is generally not observed. Both sexes are involved. Initially, weakness is generally present in the proximal muscles of the legs, followed by weakness in the proximal muscles of the arms. The patient's or parent's complaints usually include the following: difficulty running or "duck-like" waddle while running; difficulty in climbing stairs or getting out of a low chair; difficulty in holding the arms above the head or in carrying packages. Examination (manual muscle testing) confirms the patient's functional complaints and also may reveal an increased lumbar lordosis. Enlargement of the calves is un-common. Although the disease is very variable, weakness may progress to the degree that the patient becomes wheelchair-bound, and distal muscles also may become weak. Intellectual subnormality and cardiac abnormalities are not generally features of limb-girdle syndromes.

Diagnosis can be established by correlating the clinical pattern with re-sults of genetic, biochemical, electrodiagnostic, and pathological studies. As noted, the genetic patterns are variable, but they should be assessed in every case. This may be difficult because serum muscle enzyme values are less use-ful for carrier detection in this group of disorders. Results of patient's serum muscle enzymes usually reveal elevated values but are not as constant as in the X-linked dystrophies.

Electromyography may be very helpful in establishing the presence of a myopathy. Pathological studies of muscle biopsies are also helpful, but the patterns are much more variable than those observed in X-linked disorders.

Facioscapulohumeral Type

In this autosomal dominant disorder expression, onset and progression are extremely variable. Onset can be in childhood to adult life, but the initial abnormalities consist of facial muscle weakness, and patients may be una-ware that inability to close the eyelids against the examiner's attempt to open them, inability to whistle with pursed lips, inability to blow up a balloon or puff one's cheeks may be abnormal. This may be the only abnormality pres-ent for the patient's entire life, but slow progression also may ensue, result-ing in weakness of muscles around the scapulae and upper arms, as the name implies. The patient may develop a round-shouldered appearance (resulting frequently in his being accused of having poor posture), winging of the scapulae, and difficulty in raising the arms over the head. In some cases lower extremity weakness follows, occasionally severe enough to force the patient to become wheelchair-bound.

Intellectual and cardiac functions are not generally impaired in this disorder.

Diagnosis can be strongly suspected in a patient with the typical pattern of weakness and a positive family history. Because of the possibility of min-

314   HANDICAPPED CHILDREN AND YOUTH

imal asymptomatic involvement of other family members, as many family members as possible should be examined and a negative verbal family history should not be sufficient. This syndrome encompasses a group of disorders that clinically appear similar although the pathology is quite different; it therefore can be expected that the serum muscle enzymes, the results of electromyographic studies, and muscle biopsies are quite variable, and this is the case. One cannot rely singularly on a normal CK to exclude the presence of this disease. The pathology may help define the underlying etiology, but the clinician must be aware of the variability of changes, including a severe inflammatory myopathy, that may be observed in this group of disorders.

Myotonic Dystrophy

Childhood and adult form (Harper, 1979).   In this autosomal dominant disease, onset may be difficult to date but may be observed from school age to middle adult life. The patient's early complaints may be associated with muscle weakness or stiffness, primarily of the hands. He also may complain of inability to open his hand muscles after grasping an object. In a typical case, examination may reveal weakness of the intrinsic muscles of the hands and the wrist extensor muscles, the facial musculature, the sternocleidomastoid muscles and the temporalis muscles. Reflex and percussion myotonia in the thenar mass can be elicited. Myotonia is the inability to relax muscles promptly after a voluntary or induced contraction. The natural course of the disease is strikingly variable; in some patients minimal involvement is present throughout their lifetime; in others global weakness over years or decades follows, in some cases resulting in wheelchair existence.

In myotonic dystrophy the skeletal muscles are one of many organ systems involved. Following are some of the *possible* accompanying features that may occur in addition, or even aside from weakness and myotonia: mental subnormality, presenile lenticular cataracts, testicular atrophy, frontal balding and alopecia, gall bladder disease, diabetes.

Diagnosis generally can be strongly suspected when the patient's facial appearance, pattern of weakness, and presence of myotonia are typical. The results of electromyographic studies can readily confirm the clinical suspicion. A careful family history and/or examination of members of the immediate family can generally substantiate the autosomal dominant genetic pattern. Serum muscle enzymes may be normal or moderately above normal. Muscle biopsies are generally unnecessary for diagnostic purposes alone.

Infantile myotonic dystrophy syndrome (Harper, 1979).   This disorder may be recognized immediately at birth in that the newborn is *extremely floppy* and may have respiratory distress, swallowing and sucking difficulties, and club feet. Examination also reveals muscle weakness with a "tented" upper lip (carp mouth appearance) and areflexia. Neither electromyographic nor clinical myotonia can be detected at this stage, but the diagnosis can be established if the affected infant's mother has myotonic dystrophy. Even though myotonic dystrophy is an autosomal dominant disease, in the *infantile* form the mother is always the affected parent. She may be asymptomatic and her neurological abnormalities, e.g., weakness of the facial muscles and wrist extensors, may be slight. The diagnosis of the mother can be confirmed electromyographically.

The natural course of the infantile myotonic dystrophy is one of lessening hypotonicity with eventual improvement in the ability to suck and swallow. Increase in strength also follows, but there generally is delay in attaining all developmental landmarks, with language development being the most severely affected. These children subsequently develop manifestations of myotonic dystrophy as seen in the adult form of the disease.

MANAGEMENT

There is no specific drug treatment that will appreciably alter the course of any of the diseases listed under the category of muscular dystrophy. Patients can be reassured that an enormous amount of research is in progress in this direction. Modes of therapy, which have to be tailor-made in each individual, currently include (a) realistic reassurance; (b) rehabilitative efforts; (c) surgery, when needed (for example, for scoliosis or severe equinovalrus); (d) genetic counseling; and (e) multidisciplinary management of multiple ancillary problems.

Rehabilitative efforts include active and passive range-of-motion exercises when indicated; appropriate bracing and application of devices to assist the patient with the activities of daily life; occupational, respiratory, and speech therapy; and education of the patient in the appropriate use of conventional and/or motorized wheelchairs if and when needed. It is beyond the scope of this chapter to detail various modes of therapy, but in any case of muscular dystrophy realistic goals must be set, and the patient and his parents must understand that therapy alone does not reverse the basic natural course of the disease.

Patients should be evaluated for surgery, for example, when scoliosis is present, when equinovarus is severe, and when flexion contractures are present. In some cases surgery can be extremely helpful to the patient, but each patient must be evaluated as an individual.

Ongoing genetic counseling should be an integral part of the management of patients with muscular dystrophy and their families, since all of the diseases are genetically determined. Optimally, this counseling is provided by an individual trained and experienced in the genetics of muscular disorders. The genetic counselor must be experienced in obtaining an accurate and precise family history, which, in diseases like myotonic dystrophy, may be extremely difficult to extract. The genetic counselor also must be familiar with the modern use of amniocentesis, chorionic villi biopsies, DNA probes, and muscle enzyme determinations in assessing prenatal diagnosis and probability of involvement in a family.

Because patients with muscular dystrophy frequently have multiple problems, care is best provided in a setting in which multiple specialists can function with their services coordinated by a knowledgeable individual. In many cases, at some time in the course of the disease, the services of neurologists, psychiatrists, pediatricians, internists, orthopedic surgeons, psychologists, genetic counselors, and physical, occupational, and respiratory therapists must be available for optimum patient management. Specific programs that, in general, provide these services include the more than 200 clinics set up by the Muscular Dystrophy Association (MDA) for this purpose. These are found throughout the United States and Puerto Rico, and they provide services at no cost to the individual patient. MDA services include diagnostic examinations, muscle biopsies, electrodiagnostic and laboratory studies, gentic counseling, physical therapy, transportation to and from clinics, orthopedic aids, respiratory equipment, camp programs and recreational facilities, and others.

There are many unmet needs in muscular dystrophy. The most critical need is a specific medical cure for these disorders or a drug that will halt or delay the progression. At this writing no such drug exists. A better and more precise genetic understanding of these disorders is also critical.

From the adult patient's standpoint better job opportunities and better methods of transportation for handicapped individuals appear to be two of the most prominent unmet needs.

REFERENCES

Brooke, M. H. (1976). *A clinician's view of neuromuscular diseases*. Baltimore: Williams & Wilkins.

Dubowitz, V. (1978). *Muscle disorders in childhood*. Philadelphia: W. B. Saunders.

Harper, P. S. (1979). *Myotonic dystrophy*. Philadelphia: W. B. Saunders.

Walton, J. (1981). *Disorders of voluntary muscle*. Edinburgh: Churchill Livingstone.

Chapter 29

LEARNING DISABILITIES

Melvin D. Levine

The term *learning disabilities* is used to describe a wide range of frequently subtle dysfunctions of the central nervous system. Collectively, these also have been referred to as the "low severity–high prevalence" disabilities of childhood. These disorders are considered to be of low severity when compared with mental retardation and other extreme handicapping conditions. They are of high prevalence in that they are extremely common when compared to prevalence rates for the various severe disabilities. These often indolent developmental delays exact a heavy toll on academic performance, self-esteem, behavioral adjustment, and social competency (Bryan & Bryan, 1977). Their effects are likely to endure beyond childhood and detract significantly from the quality of adult life.

Although "learning disabilities" have been recognized for several decades, there has been little agreement with regard to a universally acceptable and applicable definition. The "classical" formulation was compiled by the national Advisory Committee on Handicapped Children in their annual report to Congress in 1968 (Lerner, 1985):

> Children with special learning disabilities exhibit a disorder in one or more of the basic psychological processes involved in understanding or using spoken or written languages. These may be manifested in disorders of listening, thinking, talking, reading, writing, spelling, or arithmetic. They include conditions which have been referred to as perceptual

handicaps, brain injury, minimal brain dysfunction, dyslexia, developmental aphasia, etc. They do not include learning problems which are due primarily to visual, hearing or motor handicaps, to mental retardation, emotional disturbance, or to environmental disadvantage.

The definition above has been remarkably widely quoted. However, it has serious shortcomings. First, it is too exclusionary. Children frequently harbor both emotional difficulties *and* learning disabilities (Levine, Brooks, & Shonkoff, 1980). Environmental disadvantage and developmental dysfunctions are by no means mutually exclusive. It can be difficult or impossible to distinguish between "mild" mental retardation and "severe" learning disability; such arbitrary line drawing may be misleading and harmful. The emphasis on language in this definition is also inappropriate. Children with certain motor problems may have difficulty with writing, for example. Attention deficits are not well covered and yet are the most common of all the low-severity disabilities (Levine & Melmed, 1982).

Some definitions of learning disability have emphasized discrepancies between achievement and potential. This requires the documentation of a disparity between intelligence testing and achievement scores. Such definitions are likely to exclude the many children whose day-to-day performance impediments may not be reflected in traditional multiple-choice achievement tests as well as those whose learning disabilities tend to be in areas directly tapped by IQ subtests. In the latter case a child's intelligence (or "potential") may appear spuriously low simply because his learning disability happens to be in cognitive areas that influence strongly an intelligence test score. The diminished IQ effectively abolishes the discrepancy required to "qualify" as having a learning disability.

Children with learning disabilities are an extremely heterogeneous group. It is likely that no uniform definition will cover all of them. Instead, the most justifiable practice is one in which children are identified as having learning disabilities by proving the existence and relevance of specific handicaps that impede information processing and/or academic productivity. Often such students have more than one developmental dysfunction. In fact, there is now evidence to suggest that *clusters* of disabilities are more likely to lead to serious failure and major social consequences than are isolated neurodevelopmental delays (which can be encountered in many normally achieving youngsters) (Karniski, Levine, & Clark, 1982). Ultimately, to determine that a child is being adversely affected, it is necessary to describe accurately that youngster's personal ledger of developmental strengths and weaknesses and to advance a stringent argument for the relationship between his discrete developmental deficits and poor academic performance.

In part due to the confusion over definitions, precise figures regarding the incidence or prevalence of learning disabilities are unavailable. Various studies have suggested that anywhere from 5 to 20 percent of school-age youngsters exhibit these dysfunctions. The lack of agreement results from the lack of universally accepted diagnostic criteria. In most studies males outnumber females. Epidemiological investigations suggest that learning disorders exist at every socioeconomic level, although prognosis is significantly influenced by social class (Eisenberg, 1966).

PREDISPOSING FACTORS

It is likely that learning disabilities represent a final common pathway of multiple predispositions. Among these varied etiological influences are genetic factors, perinatal stresses (such as low birth weight or smallness for gestational age), early health problems (such as meningitis or recurrent otitis media), environmental agents (such as low-level lead intoxication), family stresses (such as domestic turmoil or cultural deprivation), temperamental aberrations, and educational shortcomings (such as schools that misinterpret, mismanage, or overlook indicators of developmental dysfunction). For many youngsters with learning problems, multiple contributing factors are operative. Such a realization has substantial preventive implications. Professionals caring for young children need to be alert for evolving "risk factor complexes" or combinations of predisposing factors that make school failure a highly likely outcome (Levine & Karniski, 1985). For example, a preschool child with a compelling family history of academic difficulty, one who has also had multiple episodes of otitis media and is in a suboptimal home environment, must be considered at high risk for school difficulties. Such a child should be monitored carefully throughout the toddler and preschool years. Early intensive educational experience, some parent counseling, additional preparation for educational readiness, informing of preschool and early school teachers, and targeted remediation for developmental delays (such as language disability) could minimize the degree of school failure and secondary emotional injury.

CLINICAL DESCRIPTION

For a child with learning disabilities, the best prescription invariably derives from the most accurate description. The goal is to generate a "functional profile," an account of a child's strengths and deficits in those developmental areas most germane to academic success and productivity. For purposes of this discussion, five of the major categories of developmental competency can be elucidated. The clinical description of a child should include specific accounts of strengths and weaknesses in each of these domains and their subcomponents. The broad areas to be considered are selective attention, information processing, memory, higher cognition, and output.

Selective Attention

Attention deficits constitute probably the most common form of learning disability. Affected children have difficulty with sustained attention to detail. They tend to be distractible, impulsive, extremely inconsistent in their learning and productivity, poor at self-monitoring, and generally impersistent when it comes to school work (Levine & Melmed, 1982). Such students may or may not be overactive (Ross & Ross, 1982). Most have no difficulty concentrating and working effectively under *high motivational conditions* but have enormous trouble focusing at more moderate motivational levels (such as in the classroom). These children are often restless, difficulty to satisfy, and unpredictable. Some have equivalent social inattention, making it hard for them to form and sustain relationships with peers.

Information Processing

Information processing weaknesses present themselves in a variety of forms. Three principal subtypes are *simultaneous processing weaknesses, successive processing deficiencies,* and *language disabilities.* Simultaneous processing refers to a child's capacity to appreciate a set of stimuli the components of which enter the central nervous system all at the same time. The challenge is to understand relationships between such stimuli and to distinguish their features clearly. Most frequently, such simultaneous processing occurs through visual pathways. The capacity to differentiate clearly letters and other symbols, to recognize faces, and to appreciate a range of perceptual qualities in space, are examples of simultaneous processing demands. Youngsters with deficiencies of simultaneous processing may experience problems acquiring good reading and spelling skills, especially during the early grades.

Successive processing entails the ability to appreciate, store, retrieve, and apply information that is delivered to the central nervous system in a coded sequence or serial order. As children progress through school, they are able to master larger and larger "chunks" of such sequential data. Following multistep directions, performing complex mathematics operations, and assimilating time concepts (such as days of the weeks and months of the year) are examples of successive processing activities. Children with weaknesses in this area may encounter problems with organization, with following directions in school, and with certain aspects of mathematics and writing (Levine, 1982).

Language abilities are the third component of information processing. The capacity to interpret language accurately and easily is a critical requisite for academic success in our society. Children with language disabilities therefore are at a distinct disadvantage. Such dysfunctions constrain reading comprehension, writing ability, the capacity to follow and understand verbal instructions, and the acquisition of a foreign language (Wallach & Butler,

1984; Wiig & Semel, 1984). Language difficulties can also compromise social skill development.

Memory

There is increasing recognition that certain children harbor specific deficits of memory. There are many subtypes of memory dysfunction in childhood. Included are modality-specific memory problems (such as weakness of visual or auditory recall), pervasive deficits of retrieval memory, and disabilities impairing active working memory or the capacity to hold in mind part of a task while completing some other aspect of it. Memory deficiencies can impair performance in mathematics, reading comprehension, and most content area subjects. These disorders become increasingly incapacitating as students approach and enter secondary school, a period when accelerated demands on memory grow exponentially.

Higher Cognition

Higher cognitive abilities include a child's overall conceptual strengths, the ability to reason (verbally and nonverbally), the capacity to apply and understand rules, the use of effective and flexible strategies to solve problems, and the development of formal logical systems. Children with specific learning disabilities are prone to having discrete areas of deficit on this level (Meltzer, 1978). For example, some youngsters may have specific problems with verbal reasoning. They may be quite good at figuring out spatial or mechanical relationships but have substantial trouble interpreting metaphors, verbal analogies, and linguistic rules.

Output

Many youngsters with learning disabilities also have working disabilities (Levine, Oberklaid, & Meltzer, 1981). That is, they have as much, if not more, difficulty transmitting information as they have interpreting it. Students who have "developmental output failure," in particular, have trouble conveying thoughts on paper. Specific fine motor weaknesses may make it hard for them to write and think or write and remember simultaneously. They may be overwhelmed by the demands for productivity in late elementary and junior high school. Combinations of weaknesses of motor output, organization, retrieval memory, expressive language, and attention predispose to output insufficiency.

Gross motor function constitutes another important output channel (Cratty, 1979). Facility in sports and overall body image can be determined by a child's gross motor coordination. Therefore, this aspect of development, while not directly relevant to learning, needs to be accounted for.

The five broad areas described above should not be construed as mutually exclusive or isolated. There are multiple interactions between them. Attention influences memory, and strong memory can strengthen attention. Good language abilities facilitate the development of good auditory memory and good verbal cognition. Sustained attention enhances output functions. Thus, while describing individual elements of strength and weakness, it is equally important to observe their dynamic interrelationships. Furthermore, no clinical description is complete without accounting for associated findings, such as a child's behavior, style of coping with stress, general health, neurological status (including neuromaturational level), and the presence or absence of any concomitant or secondary emotional difficulties. Finally, a good description should include some estimate of the past and current impact (either positive or negative) of peers, siblings, parents, domestic conditions, and the educational system.

MANAGEMENT

Because learning disabilities are so varied, it is difficult to describe any uniformly applicable treatment program. In general, however, the following steps are most helpful to most affected youngsters:

1. *Demystification.* Children, parents, and teachers can benefit from exposure to an accurate description of a child's functional profile. This helps to alleviate guilt, reduce feelings of inadequacy, and suggest a measure of consistency of approach.

2. *Special education.* Special help in school can be critically important for treatment and for the prevention of complications. Tutorial programs, resource rooms, and learning centers are the mainstays of such intervention. Therein students can receive specific help to overcome their developmental weaknesses and (perhaps more important) to make some gains on their academic lags. Within the special educational setting interventions can be customized to conform to a youngster's patterns of developmental function. For example, a child with relative strengths in language can be taught mathematics through a highly verbal/linguistic approach.

3. *Regular educational management.* Most children with learning disabilities can participate in regular classrooms for a substantial portion of each school day. However, the regular classroom teacher must be knowledgeable and sympathetic to the child's difficulties. There must be a willingness to employ *bypass strategies* or methods of circumvention that can minimize the daily effects of a child's learning problems. Children with certain kinds of output failure might be allowed to write less, to type, or to submit shorter assignments. A child with a language disability may need heavy visual reinforcement, frequent repetition of directions, and short sentences of input.

One with attention deficits may require preferential seating as close to the teacher as possible.

The regular classroom teacher must strive not to humiliate the young-ster before the tribunal of his peers. For example, a child who has word-finding difficulties should not be called on to generate a long complex an-swer to a question in the classroom. A yes–no response should suffice. A child with significant fine motor weaknesses should not have his papers corrected by peers. Such sensitivity within the regular classroom can do a great deal to minimize the profound and desperate feelings of inadequacy that frequently invade this childhood population, resulting commonly in secondary behav-ioral maladaptations.

4. *Special services.* Depending on the individual requirements of a child, more highly specialized interventions may be called for. Options include speech and language therapy, occupational therapy, social work, recreation therapy, and various prototypes of mental health services.

5. *Home management.* Parents need to be provided with guidelines to manage a child's learning problems at home. These are sometimes offered by a mental health professional. Alternatively, the child's physician or a professional in the school may communicate this critical input. Optimal home management of maladaptive or reactive behaviors can be especially impor-tant. In addition, parents need help in assisting their children with home-work as well as with other aspects of their learning difficulties.

6. *Medical therapies.* Any medical needs of the child need to be met as part of an overall treatment program. Therapies for allergies, various somatic symptoms (such as headaches and abdominal pain), seizures, or sensory problems are examples of possible needs. In addition, certain youngsters are good candidates for psychopharmacological intervention (Ottenbacher & Cooper, 1983). Most commonly, this involves the use of stimulant medica-tions in those with attention deficits. Such drugs need to be prescribed by an experienced physician and monitored closely.

7. *Advocacy and follow-up.* Children with learning problems benefit from strong advocacy. Their difficulties run a tortuous course, like that of a chronic disease; long-range continuing follow-up is therefore critical. A physician can play a vital role as a continuing source of information, advice, and unbiased support. As part of this advocacy, it is important to help parents distinguish between possible interventions that are scientifically unjustified and those that are more responsible. Such scientific consumer advocacy must be built into any child therapeutic and monitoring program.

SPECIFIC CATEGORICAL PROGRAMS

Children with learning disabilities qualify for services under Public Law 94-142. Each is entitled to an individualized educational plan. There is considerable variation from state to state with regard to what it takes to qualify as having a learning disability. There appears to be widespread fear of the numbers of children that might be so classified, thereby creating an alarming drain on resources. Consequently, it is not unusual for relatively antiquated or unnecessarily narrow criteria to be applied. Such standards often exclude children with attention deficits, organizational problems, and writing difficulties that may not be detectable on standardized, multiple-choice achievement tests. Clinicians need to work on behalf of these disadvantaged students, striving to fit them into categories that will make them eligible for the kinds of services described above. Furthermore, every effort should be made to ensure that they receive services *before* they reach a point at which they are so delayed that they, their parents, and their teachers feel fatalistic or hopelessly pessimistic. Children display limited tolerance for failure. When they have been too frustrated for too long, they are apt to become amotivational. Intervention must always precede the onset of this complication. Regrettably, there are few categorical programs allowing for the treatment of mild or early failure, whose victims may be some of the most needy and vulnerable youngsters in our society.

Unmet Needs

The field of learning disabilities is young. Future research should be oriented toward a more precise characterization of the elements of development, those functional cogs whose impairments lead to chronic underachievement and lack of fulfillment. There must evolve a generally agreed on taxonomy. This can then form the basis for legislation to guarantee services for these youngsters.

Future studies should enrich our understanding of the natural histories of various clusters or combinations of dysfunctions. We need to be able to differentiate between those learning disabilities that are relatively benign and self-limited and those that are likely to cause lifelong underachievement and social maladjustment. Therapeutic programs need to address the needs implicit in these patterns. There need to be new service prototypes that are cost-effective, that maintain affected youngsters within the educational mainstream, and that address their individual needs.

Future critiques of the American education system must take into consideration the interests of this substantial portion of the student population. While calling for competency testing, for more mathematics and science, for better-trained teachers, and for rigorous education in general, it is essential also to acknowledge the compelling requirements of this vulnerable segment of the student body. In the future, the training of all teachers should include courses in child development and developmental dysfunction, highlighting the implications of that subject matter for day-to-day classroom management. Greater knowledge of this varied group of handicapping conditions will go far in minimizing their malignant effects on evolving life adjustment and fulfillment.

REFERENCES

Bryan, T. H., & Bryan, J. H. (1977). The social-emotional side of learning disabled children. *Behavioral Disorders, 2,* 141.

Cratty, B. J. (1979). *Perceptual and motor development in infants and children.* Englewood Cliffs, NJ: Prentice-Hall.

Eisenberg, L. (1966). Reading retardation: I. Psychiatric and sociologic aspects. *Pediatrics, 37,* 352.

Karniski, W. M., Levine, M. D., & Clarke, S. (1982). A study of neurodevelopmental findings in early adolescent delinquents. *Journal of Adolescent Health Care, 3,* 151.

Lerner, J. (1985). *Children with learning disabilities* (3rd ed.). Boston: Houghton Mifflin.

Levine, M. D. (1982). The low severity-high prevalence disabilities of childhood. In L. Barness (Ed.), *Advances in pediatrics* (p. 529). Chicago: Year Book Publishers.

Levine, M. D., Brooks, R., & Shonkoff, J. (1980). *A pediatric approach to learning disorders.* New York: John Wiley.

Levine, M. D., & Karniski, W. M. (1985). Risk factor complexes in early adolescent delinquents. *American Journal of Diseases in Childhood, 139,* 50.

Levine, M. D., & Melmed, R. (1982). The unhappy wanderers: Children with attention deficits. *Pediatric Clinics of North America, 29,* 105.

Levine, M. D., Oberklaid, F., & Meltzer, L. J. (1981). Developmental output failure: A study of low productivity in school children. *Pediatrics, 67,* 18.

Meltzer, L. J. (1978). Abstract reasoning in a specific group of perceptually impaired children, namely the learning disabled. *Journal of Genetic Psychology, 132,* 185.

Ottenbacher, K., & Cooper, H. (1983). Drug treatment of hyperactivity in children. *Developmental Medicine and Childhood Neurology, 25,* 358.

Ross, D. M., & Ross, S. A. (1982). *Hyperactivity: Current issues, research and theory.* New York: Wiley Interscience.

Wallach, G. P., & Butler, K. G. (1984). *Language learning disabilities in school-age children.* Baltimore: Williams & Wilkins.

Wiig, E., & Semel, E. (1984). *Language disabilities in children and adolescents.* Columbus, OH: Charles E. Merrill.

Chapter 30

HEARING IMPAIRMENT IN CHILDHOOD

Hiroshi Shimizu

Comparing deafness with blindness, Helen Keller, who was deaf as well as blind, said that deafness is the much worse misfortune for it means the loss of the most vital stimulus—the sound of the voice that brings language, sets thoughts astir, and keeps us in the intellectual company of man. We are able to communicate or exchange our thoughts by speech. This unique ability distinguishes us from the rest of the mammalian world, and its loss, whatever the cause, can easily be perceived as the worst tragedy of mankind. This tragedy takes place whenever a child is born deaf, hard of hearing, or when hearing loss develops during the early period of life, for hearing plays a basic role in language, speech, and intellectual and emotional development. Reis (1973) reported that the highest average language comprehension obtained by a large number of nineteen-year-old deaf and hard-of-hearing students was equivalent to the normal fourth-grade level. Acquisition of syntax also remains delayed for most hearing-impaired children, and the reading ability of the average deaf person is at the fifth-grade level or below (Bess, 1985). Even children with a mild to moderate degree of hearing loss, when taught in regular classes, are usually behind in their academic achievement. Despite these catastrophic consequences, the seriousness of early childhood hearing impairment has not been widely recognized. The object of this chapter is to describe the variety of presentations of this invisible ailment and emphasize the importance of early identification and immediate remediation.

CLASSIFICATION AND DEFINITION

Hearing impairment is commonly classified as conductive, senorineural, or mixed type, depending on location of the lesion in the external and/or middle ear, cochlea and/or auditory nerve, or both areas. The most common cause of conductive hearing loss in children is serous otitis media or middle ear effusion. The main functional problem of conductive hearing loss lies in the softness of sound heard. Loud speech can be understood without difficulty. The majority of moderate to profound early childhood hearing loss is sensorineural and is usually accompanied by added difficulty in discriminating and processing speech signals, called dysacusis.

For many years the term *deafness* was used for all hearing loss regardless of degree. Recently, a more precise definition has gained acceptance because of its value in addressing social, educational, and medical objectives. The Education of the Handicapped Regulations (34 Code of Federal Regulations, Part 300) define deafness as hearing impairment that is so severe that the child is impaired in processing linguistic information through hearing, with or without amplification, which adversely affects educational performance, and *hard of hearing* as hearing impairment that is not included under the definition of *deaf*. The concept of differentiating deaf from hard of hearing is useful when appropriate resources are available. However, in deprived communities many who might be categorized as hard of hearing must be considered deaf for all practical purposes, as they lack otologic and audiologic services that would permit effective use of their residual hearing (Wilson, 1985). Finally, so wide a range of auditory capacity lies between the totally deaf and mild hearing impairment that even these terms do not clearly convey true pictures of each handicap, and individual functional description becomes necessary.

PREVALENCE

There are about 450 million disabled people in the world, 80 percent of whom live in the poorest communities of Asia, Africa, and Latin America. Hearing loss is one of the major disabling conditions.

In the United States, approximately 8 percent of the noninstitutionalized population now experience some degree of difficulty in hearing or understanding speech. Approximately 1 percent of these are considered deaf (Punch, 1983). The prevalence rate of all hearing impairments is reported as 0.63 percent in children younger than five years of age and 1.63 percent in the age group between five and fourteen years. Based on 1982 Census Bureau estimates, the number of children who become deaf prior to age nineteen is about 0.2 percent and those with prelinguistic-onset deafness about 0.1 percent (Punch, 1983). These figures from the United States do not differ significantly from those reported from Europe and other industrialized countries (Martin, 1982). However, the estimated prevalence of hearing impairment in developing countries and among Eskimo and American Indian children is much greater and seems to be the result or high incidence of chronic otitis media in those populations (Nelson & Horn, 1984). It should be kept in mind that prevalence and incidence estimates are influenced by definitions and classifications of hearing impairment as well as by the age of the study group. Unfortunately, criteria vary widely from one source to another, making comparison of data difficult.

ETIOLOGY

The reported causes of hearing impairment in children and their relative importance as etiologic factors vary greatly depending on the source. This variability stems from differences in the size and nature of the specific study population, methodology, and criteria used for identifying their causative factors. Most published epidemiologic reports have been based on data from narrowly selected populations, such as children in deaf schools, children with prelinguistic deafness, and so on. Despite this, consensus exists concerning the importance of many causative factors (Table 30-1).

Identifying specific etiology is not always easy. In many cases the patient has a history of two or more possible etiologic factors, e.g., low birth weight, perinatal hypoxia, and meningitis in early infancy. Some parents are not good reporters or do not have the information needed. In some cases of adopted children, no prenatal record or family history is available. Therefore, the "etiology unknown" group in many reports contains not only those cases with obscure etiology but also those of undetermined cause due to insufficient information (Shimizu, 1980). The incidence of "etiology unknown" ranges from 28 to 50 percent (Martin, 1982; Taylor, Hine, & Brasier, 1975).

Marcus (1970) reported a reduced incidence of congenital and prelinguistic deafness associated with rubella, Rh-incompatibility, prematurity, and ototoxicity and cited reduced birth rate, improved medical care and widespread vaccination as contributing factors. However, a recent review of 2,157 patients with pre-linguistic hearing impairment, conducted at the Johns Hopkins Hospital Hearing and Speech Clinic, revealed a dramatic decrease only in cases of rubella deafness during the past two to three decades.

A common problem that has recently become a controversial issue is recurrent or chronic middle ear effusion. Despite the mildness of the hearing loss produced by serous otitis media, serious adverse effect on language development of young children has been reported (Bess, 1985; Wilson, 1985). This is of such concern that Friedel-Patti has proposed that language screening be added to routine pediatric management as otitis-prone children approach their second birthday (Friedel-Patti, Finitzo-Hieber, Conti, & Brown,

**Table 30-1. Reported Causative Factors of
Childhood Hearing Impairment**

Prenatal
  Genetic
  Intrauterine viral infection
  Deformity of the ear of unknown etiology
  Chromosomal anomalies
  Ototoxic drugs
  Congenital hypothyroidism
  Congenital syphilis
Perinatal
  Premature birth (low birth weight)
  Hyperbilirubinemia
  Hypoxia
Postnatal
  Otitis media
  Systemic viral or bacterial infections
    Meningitis
    Mumps
    Measles
    Influenza
    Unspecified
  Trauma
    Fracture of the temporal bone
    Traumatic disconnection of the ossicles
    Barotrauma
    Head blow
    Noise-induced
  Ototoxic drugs

1982). Not all are convinced, however, and these reports have not remained unchallenged (Allen & Robinson, 1984).

IDENTIFICATION AND EVALUATION

The role of parents in early identification of their child's hearing impairment is significant. Parving (1984) demonstrated that parents were the first to suspect hearing loss in 59 percent of cases. The same report, however, showed that delay in testing hearing was caused by health personnel in 59 percent. Physicians not infrequently dismissed the parental concerns about the child's hearing or felt the child was too young to test, delaying the discovery of the child's hearing impairment (Shimizu, 1980). The idea that any child is too young to be tested is no longer true, owing to the advancement of audiologic technology. Appropriate audiological services are now available in hospitals, rehabilitation centers, colleges and universities, health departments, community clinics, and many private practices.

Because of the importance of early detection of hearing impairment and the high incidence of hearing loss among infants with certain characteristics, high-risk registries have been recommended. The Joint Committee on Infant Hearing Screening (1982) has recommended that hearing of infants with a history of childhood hearing impairment in the family, congenital parental infection, anatomic malformations in the head and neck, birth weight less than 1,500 g, hyperbilirubinemia at levels exceeding indications for exchange transfusions, bacterial meningitis or severe asphyxia be identified and screened within three to six months of birth by means of behavioral observation audiometry or electrophysiologic measures. Several states have already implemented a state-wide high-risk registry and several more states are in the process of bringing about such a program. Three states (Georgia, Tennessee, Utah) utilize the birth certificate as the basis for their registry and follow-up program. Seven states (Arkansas, Colorado, Florida, Massachusetts, New Jersey, Oklahoma, and Oregon) utilize a form of maternal hospital questionnaire. Many of those programs are tightly centralized operations.

The diagnostic workup (Figure 30-1) should begin with a detailed history that includes family history, prenatal-perinatal-postnatal history, motor development, speech and language development, response to sounds, behavior, learning ability, and school experience. Although the pathology of hearing impairment lies within the ear and/or retrocochlear auditory pathway, general physical and neurological examination is important as a means of identifying those syndromes that associate hidden impairments with more obvious markers in other organs. The physical and neurological examination also will identify associated disabilities that could impact on later management. Special laboratory tests may be required to clarify etiology and plan management, and the hearing impairment must then be confirmed audiologically.

Audiological evaluation must include the entire auditory, cognitive, and feedback system (Figure 30-2). It should be kept in mind that hearing, language, and speech cannot be separated. We hear not with the ear but with the brain. The primary task is to find what part of the system has been impaired. A breakdown can exist in any one or more of those parts. Three types of procedures are available to assess the hearing of children: (a) behavioral response audiometry (behavioral observation audiometry, conditioned orienting response audiometry, visual reinforcement audiometry, tangible reinforcement operant conditioning audiometry, play audiometry); (b) instrument recording audiometry (Crib-O-Gram, heart rate response audiometry, acoustic reflex measurement, evoked potential audiometry); and (c) speech audiometry (Mahoney, 1984). The choice of procedure will be influenced by the age of the child, the degree of disability, other associated problems, and the expertise of the examiner.

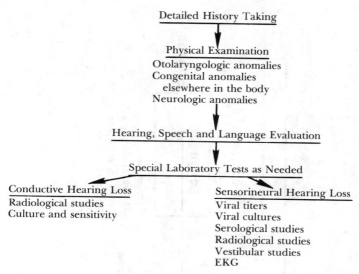

Figure 30-1. Protocol for workup of a hearing impaired child.

MANAGEMENT

Team Approach

The development of communicative skills or the ability to function with a hearing loss is influenced by many factors: basic intellectual capacity, age of onset, degree and type of hearing loss, visual perception, central nervous system interference, behavioral and emotional factors, access to appropriate educational programs, availability of properly fitted hearing aids, counseling for patients, and socioeconomic factors. As all of these factors are interrelated, hearing impairment in children cannot be treated as an isolated disorder. The child is best helped by a multidisciplinary approach.

Amplification

Once the condition is determined not to contraindicate the use of amplification, the child should be fitted with an appropriate hearing aid. Even for children with severe to profound hearing impairment, amplification serves as a tool to bring them to the sound world, as an attention device and as an aid to improve speech-reading (lipreading) ability. Audiologists are responsible for selecting the proper gain, frequency characteristics, maximal deliverable sound pressure level, style of the aid, number of aids (monaural or

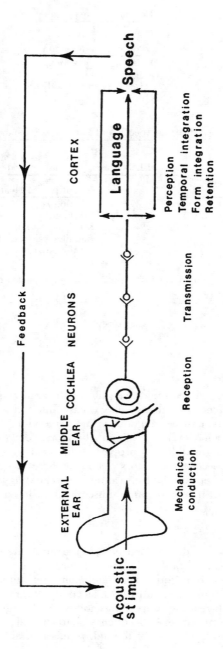

Figure 30-2. The simplified system of audition

binaural), and type of earmolds. But treatment does not end with fitting of a hearing aid. It must be followed by intensive auditory training and active parental involvement. School personnel also must monitor the function and fit of individual hearing aids frequently. Random inspections of hearing aids worn by school-age children reveal that 40 to 60 percent of the aids are inadequate or not properly operating (Riedner, 1978).

In addition to individual hearing aids, various other amplification systems, such as induction loop systems, FM radio frequency systems, infrared listening systems, and portable desk auditory trainers, can be used to assist auditory training. For more detailed information about amplification, readers are referred to a book written by Bess, Freeman, and Sinclair (1981).

Cochlear Implant

In 1960 the House Ear Institute in Los Angeles began to develop cochlear implants for patients whose hearing loss is so profound that an ordinary hearing aid is of no use. The device is designed to stimulate auditory neurons using an electrode inserted into the scala tympani. Sound, received by a microphone, is converted to electrical signals by a signal processor and transmitted to the electrode. Two cochlear implant systems, single and multichannel, have been approved by the Food and Drug Administration. Increased awareness of sounds and improvement of lipreading skills have been the major reported benefits. The devices have been used experimentally with some success in young, profoundly deaf children (Mecklenburg, 1986).

Appropriate Special Education

Training should be started as early as possible. The primary goal is to help the child achieve maximal communication skill through whatever means possible. The prerequisites for achieving this goal are (a) parental understanding and acceptance of the problem with which they are faced, (b) motivated interactive involvement, and (c) a training method that best fits the needs of the child. The choice of method—whether aural/oral approach (Pollack, 1982), total communication method (Jordan, Gustason, & Rosen, 1976), or mainstreaming program (Brackett & Schine)—depends on the child's age, degree of loss, learning potential, care giver's attitude, socioeconomic situation, geographic location, and availability of supportive services at school.

FUTURE NEEDS

1. Congenital and early childhood sensorineural hearing impairments are medically incurable. Future emphasis therefore must be placed on the prevention of conditions that cause hearing impairment. Prevention of rubella

deafness through the widespread use of rubella vaccine has been highly successful and serves as an excellent example of the potential impact of primary prevention on this problem.

2. Secondary preventive programs utilizing high-risk registries and early examination of high-risk infants and young children are very important. All states should mandate these programs and provide the necessary support to ensure their success.

3. Primary health care workers must be informed about the existence and availability of newer diagnostic and treatment resources. Appreciation of the probable success of early intervention and the significant damage caused by delay in diagnosis must be part of the training of all health care professionals.

4. Much of the handicap of hearing impairment results from public misunderstanding of the problems faced by those impaired. Programs designed to educate the public to promote understanding and acceptance of the hearing-impaired in schools and the work place are essential.

REFERENCES

Allen, I. M., Robinson, D. O. (1984). Middle ear status and language development in preschool children. *Asha, 26,* 33–37.

Bess, F. H. (1985). The minimally hearing-impaired child. *Ear Hear, 6,* 43–47.

Bess, F. H., Freeman, B., & Sinclair, J. B. (1981). *Amplification in education.* Washington, DC: A. G. Bell.

Brackett, D., & Schine, R. (1984). Evaluation for educational planning. *Seminars in Hearing, 5,* 393–403.

Friel-Patti, S., Finitzo-Hieber, T., Conti, G. & Brown, K. C. (1982). Learning delay in infants associated with middle ear disease and mild, fluctuating hearing impairment. *Pediatric Infectious Diseases, 1,* 104–109.

Joint Committee on Infant Hearing. (1982). Position statement. *Asha, 24,* 1017–1018.

Jordan, I. K., Gustason, G., & Rosen, R. (1976). Current communication trends at programs for the deaf. *American Annals of the Deaf, 121,* 527–532.

Mahoney, T. (Ed.). (1984). Early identification of hearing loss in infants. *Seminars in Hearing, 5,* 1–99.

Marcus, R. E. (1970). Reduced incidence of congenital and prelingual deafness. *Archives of Otolaryngology, 92,* 343–347.

Martin, J. M. (1982). Aetiological factors relating to childhood deafness in the European community. *Audiology, 21,* 149–203.

Mecklenburg, D.J. (Ed.) (1986). Cochlear Implants in Children. *Seminars in Hearing,* Vol. 7, No. 4, November.

Nelson, S. M., & Horn, R. M. (1984). Ear disease and hearing loss among Navajo children: A mass survey. *Laryngoscope, 94,* 316–323.

Parving, A. (1984). Early detection and identification of congenital/early acquired hearing disability: Who takes the initiative? *International Journal of Pediatric Otorhinolaryngology, 7,* 107–117.

Pollack, D. (1982). Amplification and auditory/verbal training for the limited hearing infant 0 to 30 months. *Seminars in Speech, Language and Hearing, 3,* 52–67.

Punch, J. (1983). The prevalence of hearing impairment. *Asha, 25,* 27.

Reis, P. (1973). *Academic achievement test results of a national testing program for hearing impaired students.* Washington, DC: Gallaudet College, Office of Demographic Studies.

Riedner, E. D. (1978). Monitoring of hearing aids and earmolds in an educational setting. *Journal of the American Audiology Society, 4,* 39–43.

Shimizu, H. (1980). Medical aspects of hearing evaluation in children. *Audiology: An Audio Journal for Continuing Education, 5*(10).

Taylor, I. G., Hine, W. D., & Brasier, V. J. (1975). A study of the causes of hearing loss in a population of deaf children with special reference to genetic factors. *Journal of Laryngology and Otolaryngology, 89,* 899–914.

Wilson, J. (1985). Deafness in developing countries. *Archives of Otolaryngology, 111,* 2–9.

Chapter 31

EPILEPSY AND CONVULSIVE DISORDERS

Eileen P. G. Vining
John M. Freeman

A *seizure* is a sudden paroxysmal electrical discharge of neurons within the cerebral cortex. To become manifest, this electrical discharge must recruit sufficient neurons to alter function or behavior. The clinical manifestations of a seizure depend on where the electrical discharge starts in the cortex, how rapidly it recruits sufficient additional neurons, and the direction and rapidity of spread throughout the nervous system. *Epilepsy* is merely recurrent unprovoked seizures, seizures that do not have a clear precipitating cause (fever, infection, trauma, etc.).

INCIDENCE, PREVALENCE, AND DEMOGRAPHICS

Seizures are among the most prevalent of handicapping conditions. They occur in 0.5 to 1 percent of the general population. Seventy percent of epilepsy begins in childhood. Epilepsy is more common in children in whom there is other evidence for damage to the central nervous system (mental retardation, cerebral palsy).

ETIOLOGY, CONTRIBUTING FACTORS, AND PREVENTIVE TECHNIQUES

A seizure does not occur simply because there is abnormal firing of a cell

Table 31-1. Effect of Cortical Maturation on Seizures

Age Group	Cortex	Seizure Manifestations
Newborn	Mainly inhibitory influences Poorly myelinated Neuronal interconnections not fully established	"Subtle," fragmentary, poorly sustained Many are "subcortical"
Infancy & childhood	Lower "threshold" Control mechanisms developing Complexity of interconnection developing	Febrile seizures Specific age-dependent types (absence, benign rolandic, juvenile, myoclonic, etc.)
Older child & adolescent	Threshold reaches adult level Complexity of interconnections increasing	Some age-specific types disappear Classification as in adults

or even a group of neurons. This is evident in observing the EEG between seizures when it is often possible to record considerable amounts of abnormal electrical activity. Epilepsy requires the recruitment and firing of a sufficient population of cells to produce the alterations in function or behavior called seizures. There is a "threshold" that must be exceeded for a seizure to occur. The threshold for firing of individual cells is dependent on transport of ions into and out of cells or portions of cells. This transport in turn is dependent on pore size, intrinsic cell recovery processes, and the inhibitory and excitatory modulation acting on the cell. The threshold involved in producing a clinical seizure is dependent on these factors, as well as many others, including the developmental state of the cortex (Schwartzkroin, 1984). Some of these factors and their impact on seizure manifestations are shown in Table 31-1. Genetic influences and external factors such as fever, excitement, anxiety, and lack of sleep also may play a significant role in producing an "environment" in which a seizure can occur.

Underlying these influences is often damage to the brain that may not be apparent. Clearly, developmental abnormalities of the brain, perinatal damage to the brain sufficient to produce cerebral palsy, trauma at a latter age, infarction, infection, and tumors may all produce localized lowering of threshold. It should be noted, however, that most children who have these types of damage to the brain do *not* develop epilepsy, and most children with epilepsy have no defined cause. It is the presumed interaction of "damage" and the influences mentioned that permit a seizure to occur.

Apart from preventing these known causes of cerebral damage, there is no method of preventing epilepsy. The usual approach to preventing seizures is through the use of medication. Although the mechanism of action of anticonvulsants is, in general, unknown, they serve to increase the threshold for individual or groups of cells and prevent spread of firing to other cells.

CLINICAL DESCRIPTION AND CLASSIFICATION

Many people classify seizures as grand mal or petit mal. "Grand" (big) is when a child falls down and jerks, and "petit" (small) is used to describe anything else. A more accurate classification is important, however, and it may aid in identifying etiology, in choice of the appropriate anticonvulsant, and in prognostication.

Most classification now divide seizures into those that began locally or focally (termed partial) and those that are generalized at onset. The classification currently in use (Commission on Classification, 1981) is shown in Table 31-2.

Since seizures are rarely witnessed by the physician, a meticulous, detailed history of the event is necessary to differentiate it from non-seizure events as well as for appropriate classification. This history should include the initial events (aura, focality), what occurred during the seizure, whether it generalized, and a description of the postictal period. Events surrounding, or perhaps precipitating, the seizure also must be clarified.

Perhaps it is spells during which the child stops and stares that remain most confusing to the observer. Absence seizures and partial complex seizures require different therapies and have different prognoses. *Absence* seizures (previously called petit mal) are staring spells, usually lasting less than 15 seconds, that involve essentially no movement. The child then returns abruptly and unimpaired to his previous activity. Spike-and-wave activity can usually be found on the EEG. These spells can easily be elicited in the office by hyperventilation.

Atypical absence seizures have other clinical manifestations , such as automatisms or clonic, atonic, or autonomic components. The EEG usually shows somewhat faster or slower spike–wave abnormalities. *Partial complex seizures* (previously called psychomotor seizures) often include an aura, last 30 seconds to minutes, and have some postictal confusion. The characteristics of these seizures are shown in Table 31-3.

EVALUATION

The evaluation depends on a careful history, as indicated above, and a careful neurologic exam looking for focal neurologic deficits. The examination also establishes a baseline should neurologic deficit evolve. The procedures and tests used in the initial and chronic evaluation of a child with seizures are shown in Table 31-4.

In the evaluation of seizures (or epilepsy), the EEG is useful as a baseline and for assistance in corroborating the seizure classification. On rare occasions it may lead to further diagnostic workup. However, *the diagnosis of epilepsy is never based on the EEG*. A patient may have seizures and a normal EEG. A child may have an abnormal EEG and never have seizures. Diag-

Table 31-2. Seizure Classification

International Classification	"Old Terms"
Partial seizures	Focal or local seizures
Simple partial seizures (consciousness not impaired)	Focal motor
With motor symptoms	Jacksonian seizures
With somatosensory or special sensory symptoms	Focal sensory
With autonomic symptoms	
With psychic symptoms	
Complex partial seizures (with impairment of consciousness)	Psychomotor seizures
Simple partial onset	Temporal lobe
With impairment of consciousness at onset	seizures
Partial seizures which secondarily generalize	
Generalized seizures (convulsive or nonconvulsive)	
Absence	Petit mal
Absence	
Atypical	
Myoclonic	Minor motor
Clonic seizures	Grand mal
Tonic seizures	Grand mal
Tonic–clonic seizures	Grand mal
Atonic seizures (astatic)	Akinetic, drop attacks

Adapted from Commission on Classification and Terminology, International League Against Epilepsy, 1981.

nosis is based on the history of the event(s) and the physician's interpretation of that history (Lewis & Freeman, 1977).

A CT scan is rarely a necessary part of the initial workup of a child with a seizure. Tumors make themselves manifest through neurological signs or by slowing on the EEG. Persistent focal seizures or changing seizure patterns also should lead to a CT scan. Unlike seizures in adults, tumors are a rare cause of seizures in childhood (Bachman, Hodges, & Freeman).

MEDICAL MANAGEMENT

Seizures should not be treated *just* because they are there. They should be treated if and when they interfere with function or risk interfering with function. Decisions to initiate therapy must include consideration of such factors as the age of the patient and the type of seizure, frequency of occurrence of seizures, predisposing factors, and the psychological and social consequences of further seizures. The chance of recurrence of further seizures also should enter into the decision.

Some studies indicate that an individual with a single seizure has only a 30 percent chance of having a further seizure. This is independent of the presence of other neurologic problems and independent of the EEG, unless the EEG shows a spike-and-wave pattern (Hauser, Anderson, & Loewenson, 1982). Even if the risk of recurrence is considerably higher (Hirtz, Ellen-

Table 31-3. Seizures that Impair Consciousness

Characteristics	Absence	Atypical Absence	Complex Partial
Age	Childhood	Childhood	Any age
Onset	Abrupt	Slightly less abrupt	Frequently an aura
Automatisms	None (?eye-blinking)	Simple movements	Complex
Duration	Usually <15 sec	Usually >15 sec.	Usually >30 sec.
Postictal	Immediate recovery	Immediate recovery	Slow recovery (seconds to minutes)
EEG-ictal	Usually 3/s spike-wave, symmetrical	Usually irregular spike-wave, asymmetrical	Diffuse or focal temporal or frontal-temporal discharges
Interictal	Usually normal	Usually abnormal	Diffuse or focal temporal or frontal-temporal discharges

Table 31-4. Evaluation of Seizure Disorders in Children

Procedure/Test	Acute Onset	Chronic
History		Yes
Ictal event	Yes	Yes
Precipitating factors	Yes	Yes
Family history	Yes	Yes
Past intercurrent medical history	Yes	Yes
Evidence for other changes (?deterioration)	Yes	
Examination		Possibly
Complete physical exam	Yes	Yes
Careful attention to neurologic exam (?focality)	Yes	
Test		
Fasting glucose	Yes	Possibly
Ca, PO$_4$, Mg, Na	Yes	Possibly
Lumbar puncture	Consider	Not routine
Skull X-ray	No	No
CT	Not routine	Consider
EEG	Yes	Yes

berg, & Nelson, 1984), it may not always be necessary to treat a first seizure. The data on recurrence after a second seizure in children are less clear, but the recurrence rate after a second seizure may be as high as 75 percent. There is no evidence that seizures beget further seizures or that untreated electrical activity worsens the epilepsy.

Tonic-clonic seizures. A child who has had two or more generalized tonic–clonic (grand mal) seizures should be considered for therapy, but it should be understood that the primary reason for treating seizures is their psychosocial risks, not the risk of status epilepticus nor of worsening epilepsy. The three most commonly used antiepileptic drugs for tonic–clonic seizures are phenobarbital, phenytoin, and carbamazepine. Table 31-5 indicates the commonly used anticonvulsants, their indications, dosage, side effects, and therapeutic range (Johnston & Freeman, 1981). Phenobarbital, while cheap, safe, and effective, clearly has major effects on behavior, and probably on learning (Wolf & Forsythe, 1978; Vining, Mellits, & Dorsen, 1983). Phenytoin (Dilantin), while also safe and effective, may have some effects on learning. Our concern about the common side effect of gingival hyperplasia and hirsutism makes this drug slightly less desirable in our opinion than carbamazepine. Carbamazepine (Tegretol) is more expensive; the *Physicians' Desk Reference* lists significant side effects involving the white count and the risk of aplastic anemia and recommends frequent white cell counts, serum iron and platelet counts. While neutrapenia is common (Hart & Easton, 1982), we usually find it to be transient and not of great significance. Despite these published warnings, we find carbamazepine to be effective and safe. This safety has been verified recently in the Veteran's Administration Comparative Study (Mattson, Cramer, & Collins, 1985). Carbamazepine appears to have less effect on learning and behavior than other drugs. We consider this drug to be our first choice in the treatment of tonic–clonic seizures. Re-

Table 31-5. Anti-Epileptic Drugs in Children

Drug	Indications	Usual Dosage mg/kg/day	T½ (hrs.)	Usual Dosage	Side Effects	Therapeutic Range
Carbamazepine	F, C, G	10–40	8–12	BID–QID	Headache, drowsy, dizzy, diplopia, blood dyscrasia	5–14 mg/ml
Clonazepam	M, A	0.05–0.3	24–36	QD–TID	Drowsy, ataxia, secretions	
Ethosuximide	A (?C)	20–40	30	QD–BID	GI distress, rash, drowsy, dizzy, SLE, blood dyscrasia	40–100 mg/ml
Phenobarbital	F, C, G, S	2–8	48–100	QD–BID	Drowsy, rash, ataxia, behavior	10–35 mg/ml
Phenytoin	F, C, G, S	4–8	6–30	QD–BID	Drowsy, gums, rash, anemia, ataxia, hirsute	10–20 mg/ml
Primidone	F, C, G	12–25	6–12	BID–QID	Drowsy, dizzy, rash, anemia, ataxia, diplopia	6–12 mg/ml
Valproate	F, C, G, M, A	30–60	6–18	BID–QID	GI distress, liver, platelet, alopecia, drowsy, ataxia	50–100 mg/ml

F, focal (partial-simple); G, generalized (tonic–clonic); C, Partial-complex; A, absence; M, minor motor (akinetic, atonic, myoclonic); S, status.

cently, sodium valproate has been shown to be effective in preventing tonic–clonic seizures, but because of concerns regarding hepatic toxicity (especially in young children) we would not choose it as initial therapy.

Partial complex seizures respond well to carbamazepine and often to sodium valproate. Because of the rare hepatic side effects, sodium valproate is our drug of second choice.

Absence seizures respond well to both ethosuximide and sodium valproate. We prefer to use ethosuximide as our initial therapy, especially in classical absence seizures. Sodium valproate may be more effective in atypical absence seizures. If a child has both absence and tonic–clonic seizures, sodium valproate would be our drug of choice because it provides the potential for monotherapy. Atonic and myoclonic seizures usually require sodium valproate or one of the benzodiazepines for control.

MONITORING

The principal role of the physician taking care of patients with epilepsy is adequate monitoring: monitoring of seizure control, of blood drug levels, of the major and subtle side effects of medication, of the psychosocial issues associated with epilepsy, and of the patient's progress with appropriate education and ultimately independent productive experience (Vining & Freeman, 1985) (See Table 31-6).

Ideally, a patient should have no seizures. Although a single recurrent seizure is unlikely to do physical harm, recurrence clearly represents a psychological threat to the patient and the family. For the young child it may well result in continued overprotection by the family, for the older child it may cause continued restrictions in increasing independence, and for the adolescent it may impose limitations on the ability to drive.

The most common reason for recurrence of seizures in a patient who has been doing well is lack of compliance. Seizure recurrence should lead to a careful assessment of compliance as well as a search for exogenous factors such as excitement, fever, and infection, which may alter threshold, and questioning about other medications that may affect blood levels. These potential reasons should be explored before medication is automatically increased. The medication should be increased if blood levels indicate a subtherapeutic level as long as compliance is not an issue. For the young child or the adolescent, an occasional seizure may be preferable to over-medication; however, in general, infrequent seizures should not be tolerated if they can be controlled without significant side effects. This issue of tolerating some seizures may be particularly important to the child with other neurologic handicaps. Occasionally, the quest for control leads to sedation or further motor impairment from the medication.

In addition to monitoring seizure control, blood levels, and both manifest and subtle side effects of medication, perhaps the most important role

Table 31-6. Monitoring the Total Patient

Areas to Monitor	Importance
Seizure control	May need to adjust medication, evaluate compliance or precipitating factor
Side effects of medication	May need to lower dose or change to another drug
Psychosocial issues	May need to re-counsel or refer to agency such as EFA
Educational progress	May need psychological testing, assistance in obtaining appropriate placement, evaluation of medication
Progress toward independent productive existence	May need vocational/living skills guidance

for the physician is the monitoring of the psychosocial issues. These issues are often as important as seizure control in determining the long-term outlook of children with seizures (Hirtz et al., 1984). Unlike the more stable problems, such as mental retardation and cerebral palsy, the unpredictability of seizure recurrence leads to overprotection (Hermann, Black, & Chabria, 1981). The manifestations of this overprotection vary with the age of the child. Independence *must* be allowed, especially as seizures come under control, and they do in the vast majority of cases. Even with continued seizures, independence must be fostered within the realistic limitations of the type and frequency of the seizures. If family and the child are to be expected to foster and achieve this growth, they must be informed. Both must understand what seizures are and what they aren't. They also must understand realistic limitations on independence.

There is an increased prevalence of impaired intellectual function and learning problems in children with seizures. The physician should therefore monitor the child's school performance to assure that education is appropriate and optimal. He should be aware that anticonvulsant overdosage and side effects may also impair learning. Both the physician and the school should be aware that absence seizures may be subtle and may also impair learning. Ideally, the teacher and physician should work in partnership to note changes in performance and behavior that might indicate either seizures or drug toxicity.

There are few specific categorical programs for people with epilepsy although the children are eligible for all programs for chronic handicapping conditions (PL 94-142). They may be eligible under specific programs should they have mental retardation, cerebral palsy, or other learning disabilities. One model program, originated in the Baltimore city school system, is specifically targeted at adolescents with epilepsy. This program, which has sought to assure that the child is in the appropriate educational program, has provided counseling for the student and his parents, and after school and summer work programs. The program has documented that children enrolled in the program have half the non-promotion rate and only half the dropout rate of children in the school system as a whole. Children enrolled are only half as likely to be unemployed two years out of school. The cost of this program is less than $1,000 per year, per student, and its cost-effectiveness has been documented (Jacobs, Vining, & Rabin, 1984).

UNMET NEEDS

Perhaps the greatest unmet need in the field of epilepsy is physicians' lack of knowledge of the appropriate use of anticonvulsants. These drugs are both underused, allowing continued seizures, and overused, with consequent toxicity. Careful choice of drugs and the monitoring of seizure frequency, drug levels, and function can result in improved control and improved performance.

The second greatest unmet need is lack of continued counseling for children and families about epilepsy. There are clear correlations between knowledge about epilepsy, compliance, and general performance (Jacobs et al., 1984). Often we discuss epilepsy at the time of the first visit and then assume that the family and child understand. At the time of diagnosis, probably little of the information we provide is heard, and it must be repeated on subsequent visits. Ample time should be allowed to answer questions. This must be done on repeated occasions. Parent groups and groups for older children are also useful avenues for coping with problems.

The third unmet need is for the more severely handicapped child, often those with cerebral palsy or mental retardation. Their seizures frequently are more difficult to control. These patients should often be referred to a specialist in epilepsy where new drugs and less common treatment, such as the ketogenic diet, may prove to be of major benefit.

With appropriate management, seizure control should be achieved in 80 percent of individuals. For the remainder, decrease in the number of seizures without consequent toxicity should be a realistic aim.

REFERENCES

Bachman, D. S., Hodges, F., & Freeman, J. M. (1976). Computerized axial tomography in chronic seizure disorders of childhood. *Pediatrics, 58,* 828–832.

Commission on Classification and Terminology of the International League Against Epilepsy. (1981). Proposal for revised clinical and electroencephalgraphic classification of epileptic seizures. *Epilepsia, 22,* 489–501.

Hart, R. G., & Easton, J. D. (1982). Carbamazepine and hematological monitoring. *Annals of Neurology, 11,* 309–312.

Hauser, W. A., Anderson, V. E., & Loewenson, A. B. (1982). Seizure recurrence after a first unprovoked seizure. *New England Journal of Medicine, 307,* 522–528.

Hermann, B. P., Black, R. B., & Chabria, S. (1981). Behavioral problems and social competence in children with epilepsy. *Epilepsia, 22,* 703–710.

Hirtz, D. G., Ellenberg, J. H., & Nelson, K. B. (1984). The risk of recurrence of non-febrile seizures. *Neurology, 34,* 637–641.

Jacobs, H. E., Vining, E. P. G., & Rabin, C. (1984). School intervention can improve outcome for adolescents with epilepsy. *Epilepsia, 25,* 438–442.

Johnston, M. V., & Freeman, J. M. (1981). Pharmacologic advances in seizure control. In S. N. Cohen & R. E. Kauffman (Eds.), *Pediatric Clinics of North America, 28*(1), 179–194.

Lewis, D. V., & Freeman, J. M. (1977). The use and abuse of the electroencephalogram in pediatrics. *Pediatrics, 60,* 324–330.

Mattson, R. H., Cramer, J. A., & Collins, J. F. (1985). Comparison of carbamazepine, phenobarbital, phenytoin, and primidone in partial and secondarily generalized tonic–clonic seizures. *New England Journal of Medicine, 313,* 145–151.

Schwartzkroin, P. A. (1984). Epileptogenesis in the immature central nervous system. In P. A. Schwartzkroin & H. Wheal (Eds.), *Electrophysiology of epilepsy.* London: Academic Press.

Vining, E. P. G., & Freeman, J. M. (1985). Epilepsy in children. *Pediatric Annals, 14,* 695–770.

Vining, E. P. G., Mellits, E. D., & Dorsen, M. M. (1983). Effects of phenobarbital and sodium valproate on neuropsychological function and behavior. *Annals of Neurology, 14,* 360.

Wolf, S. M., & Forsythe, A. (1978). Behavior disturbance, phenobarbital, and febrile seizures. *Pediatrics, 61,* 728–731.

Chapter 32

MENTAL RETARDATION

Herbert J. Cohen

DEFINITION

The definition of mental retardation has changed in recent years, as has the classification system used to define the types and/or degrees of mental subnormality. According to the current manual, *Classification in Mental Retardation* of the American Association for Mental Deficiency (AAMD) (Grossman, 1983), mental retardation is defined as "Significantly subaverage general intellectual functioning existing concurrently with deficits in adaptive behavior and manifested during the developmental period."

According to the AAMD:

Significantly subaverage intellectual functioning is defined as approximately IQ 70 or below.

Adaptive behavior is defined as the effectiveness or degree with which individuals meet the standards of personal independence and social responsibility expected for age and cultural group.

The developmental period is defined as the period of time between birth and the 18th birthday.

Therefore, the current definition places an emphasis on functional level, irrespective of etiology. This requires an assessment of both intellectual and adaptive functioning, using standardized tests developed specifically for those

Table 32-1. Level of Retardation by IQ Range

Term	IQ Range or Level
Mild mental retardation	50–55 to approx. 70
Moderate mental retardation	35–40 to 50–55
Severe mental retardation	20–25 to 35–40
Profound mental retardation	Below 20–25

purposes. IQ tests are used to measure intelligence. Adaptive behavior is assessed using scales to determine whether skills in self-help, academic performance, and social functioning as applied to everyday activities are at the appropriate levels for age expectations.

The classification of the degrees of mental retardation has changed in the past few decades (Grossman, 1983). Until 1959 anyone testing below an IQ of 85 was considered at risk of mental subnormality. From 1959 to 1973 children testing between about 70 to 84 on standardized IQ tests were called borderline. Currently, all those above an 80 IQ are considered to be in the average range. There is still some disagreement as to what to call the group whose test scores range from an IQ of 70 to 79. Most label this group as borderline, even though this term was eliminated in 1973 from the AAMD classification system. Now only those testing below 70 on standardized IQ tests are considered mentally retarded.

Table 32-1 illustrates the current AAMD classification system for levels of retardation based on IQ tests (Grossman, 1983). This table recognizes ranges of test performance that may vary with the types of tests administered. However, as noted, particularly for older children and adults, adaptive behavior scales are considered essential to confirm the actual level of retardation.

INCIDENCE, PREVALENCE, AND DEMOGRAPHICS

The incidence and prevalence of mental retardation have been a subject of considerable controversy and discussion. Because in the past IQ test performance has been the key accepted indicator of intellectual deficit, all those who scored 2 standard deviations below the mean on standardized testing were considered to be mentally retarded. This led to the wide acceptance of a 3 percent prevalence figure because the estimated mentally retarded population was supposed to encompass all individuals who tested 2 standard deviations below the mean. Actual prevalence studies have been few and far between, and none have supported a prevalence as high as the 3 percent figure. To complicate matters, recent reports from Scandinavian countries have indicated prevalence rates of around 0.5 percent as the total for all degrees of retardation (Dupont, 1980; Gruenwald, 1979; Hagberg et al., 1981). It is evident, however, that the Scandinavian data do not reflect the results of formal testing performed on all children or adults suspected of being mentally retarded. In addition, because there is greater acceptance of disabled individuals within these countries than is evident in the United States, under-identification is a likely possibility. Many experts feel that the actual prevalence of mental retardation in the United States is between 1.0 and 1.5 per 100 people.

There is no adequate method of determining the incidence of mental retardation because it is impossible to detect all new cases at birth or at any other time, given the wide range of disability, the multiple etiologies, and the variation in test procedures. Nevertheless, it is estimated that the incidence of mental retardation in the United States may be as high as 150,000 births per year (President's Committee on Mental Retardation, 1980).

It is clear that the prevalence of moderate to severe mental retardation is more uniform irrespective of the characteristics of the community or location that is studied. In general, a prevalence figure of 3 to 4 per 1,000 is widely reported (Abramowicz & Richardson, 1975). Related to this are consistent reports that children with IQs of less than 50 are generally equally distributed among all social classes (Abramowicz & Richardson, 1975; Birch et al., 1970). It has been hypothesized that the types of biological accidents that cause moderate to severe mental retardation have a similar distribution, resulting in the even social class distribution. In contrast, mild mental retardation is found primarily among the lower social classes, a phenomenon that has led to much speculation about possible etiologies (Birch et al., 1970).

ETIOLOGY

There is no single cause of mental retardation. Biological, environmental, genetic, and psychological influences may all produce intellectual deficits either alone or in combination. As noted, epidemiological studies have revealed a striking correlation between mild mental retardation and lower socioeconomic status. What is less clear is how factors such as poor nutrition, high rates of exposure to toxic substances or substance abuse, smoking, less frequent use of or the availability of prenatal care, higher frequencies of illness and low birth weight, or nurturing in an impoverished environment, individually or in combination, contribute to the higher prevalence of mild mental retardation among the poor. Economic disadvantage and discrimination also may contribute to educational disadvantage, with potential decreased availability of preschool programs or overall educational programs that may be of poorer quality. These factors, coupled with potentially less stimulating or less motivating home environments, could contribute to poor test performance when standardized measures are applied to all social classes. Some proponents claim that the tests themselves have a cultural bias, and that this may lead to segregation of poorer and disadvantaged children into special educational programs, especially those for the mildly mentally retarded (Mercer, 1973; 1979).

Specific biological factors leading to mental retardation are easier to identify. Table 32-2 lists many of the biological factors known to cause mental retardation, categorized by their occurrence in either the prenatal, perinatal, or postnatal period. However, less than half of the cases of moderate, severe, and profound mental retardation, the degrees of subnormality usually attributed to biological causes, have a clearly identifiable etiology (Taft & Cohen, 1977).

Prevention of mental retardation has two major components: those that are related to *primary prevention*, which involves the prevention of the occurrence of the condition, or to *secondary prevention*, which aims at ameliorating the condition or mitigating its adverse effects (President's Committee on Mental Retardation, 1980).

The extensive list of causes in Table 32-2 are predominantly ones that are amenable to primary prevention efforts. This could be accomplished either through genetic counseling; improved prenatal care, particularly for high-risk situations; a reduction in the incidence of asphyxia, anoxia, trauma, and infections during the prenatal and perinatal periods; and attempts to minimize and reduce the occurrence of accidents, poisonings, infections, and exposure to toxins affecting the central nervous system in the postnatal period. All of the factors contributing to a higher incidence of low-birth-weight infants concomitantly increase the risk of mental subnormality (Crocker, 1982). Efforts to decrease prematurity rates, as well as the frequency of intrauterine growth retardation, would be beneficial in reducing the occurrence of mental retardation.

In the area of secondary prevention, early intervention during the postnatal period for medical conditions such as infections of the central nervous system, hydrocephalus, and toxic encephalopathies could in some cases reduce the degree of disability resulting from the condition. The major focus of secondary prevention is on early identification and early educational, habilitative, and rehabilitative interventions for infants and young children with existing disabilities. These programs should help both the parent and the child. The objective is to maximize the child's ability to reach his full potential.

CLINICAL DESCRIPTION

Because mental retardation is a disorder with a wide variety of causes, the clinical findings are quite variable, ranging from an entirely normal physical appearance to grossly abnormal physical characteristics and/or numerous stigmata. Generally, but not always—Down syndrome being one notable exception—those with the most abnormal physical characteristics are more severely impaired from a neurodevelopmental standpoint. More reliable from a clinical standpoint is the likelihood that the more severely impaired will be identified at a younger age than those with milder degrees of retardation. The major reason for this finding is that more severely re-

Table 32-2. Biologic Factors in the Causation of Mental Retardation

Prenatal factors
  Chromosomal anomalies
     Autosomes; nondisjunction (trisomies), translocation, deletion or partial deletion of chromosome material, mosaicism
     Sex chromosome abnormalities
  Effects of abnormal genes
     Homozygous genes: produce identifiable recessive disorders of metabolism of amino acids (PKU, nonketotic glycinemia), lipids (leukodystrophies, lipidoses), carbohydrates (galactosemia, mucopolysaccharidoses), purines (hyperuricemia)
     Heterozygous genes: carrier states (maple syrup urine disease, Tay–Sachs disease), dominant disorders (some anencephalies, osteogenesis imperfecta)
     X-linked recessive disorders
     Unknown causation: identifiable syndromes of unknown etiology
  Deleterious intrauterine influences
     Maternal illness, infection, nutritional deficiency, hormonal imbalance
     Teratogens: maternal drug ingestion, including alcohol, phenytoin, cocaine antimetabolites, nicotine, quinine, environmental toxins (lead, cadmium), radiation
     Uterine disease, malformations, dysfunction
     Multiple pregnancy
     Placental dysfunction, malimplantation
     Isoimmunization
     Trauma: foreign body in uterus; direct blow or accident
     Prematurity (resulting from intrauterine problems but also associated with perinatal difficulties)
Perinatal factors (including those associated with trauma or hypoxia)
  Prolonged labor due to malpresentation of fetus, cephalopelvic disproportion, uterine inertia, placental abnormalities, placenta previa, abruptio placentae
  Umbilical cord prolapse, torsion, looping around neck
  Maternal hypotension: hemorrhage, anesthesia
  Neonatal sepsis or meningitis
  Asphyxia neonatorum and respiratory distress
  Kernicterus
Postnatal factors
  Anoxia (drowning, plastic bag over head)
  Cerebrovascular accidents: hemorrhage, thrombosis, embolism
  Degenerative diseases: leukodystrophies, Tay-Sachs disease
  Encephalopathies: postimmunization, associated with common childhood infections, secondary to toxins; metabolic (e.g., hypoglycemia)
  Endocrine disorders (e.g., hypothyroidism)
  Head trauma: falls, auto accidents, child abuse
  Central nervous system infections: meningitis, encephalitis
  Severe nutritional deficiencies
  Poisons and environmental toxins: lead or mercury ingestion, carbon monoxide, other contaminants of food, water, or air
  Space-occupying lesions: neoplasms, abscesses, subdural hematomas
  Anatomic factors: premature synostosis, hydrocephalus

Modified from Taft & Cohen, 1977. Used by permission.

tarded children have greater delays in attaining developmental milestones than do those with lesser degrees of retardation. The major exceptions are children whose disability is primarily due to a motor disorder such as cerebral palsy. There are other neuromuscular disorders or muscle diseases that may cause only motor problems but still give the impression of a significant overall delay in development in the first few years of life. However, some of these conditions are also associated with global retardation in all areas of the functioning.

Table 32-3 lists the common presenting characteristics for children with mental retardation in different age groups. Table 32-4 describes the prognosis and expected functional level based on the degree of retardation, including the probable eventual achievements in the academics sphere, the expected ability to perform activities of daily living, the travel capacity, and the possible vocational potential (Cohen, 1982a).

In order to confirm the diagnosis of mental retardation, sequential assessments are often necessary to assess the rate of development over a period of time. Therefore, particularly in young children and those with milder degrees of developmental delay, there is a need to follow them over a period of time and to retest the children periodically in order to determine more accurately the degree of mental retardation, if any, and to be more certain about the prognosis.

MANAGEMENT

Once the diagnosis is established and the degree of mental retardation is verified, the first step in management is to be certain that the parents or caretaker(s) have a clear understanding of what can be expected of the child and how to help the child achieve his maximum potential. The process of informing parents of a diagnosis with significant negative lifelong implications is a very difficult one and fraught with serious problems in communications (Doernberg, 1982). These include potentially misleading statements or vague remarks by physicians, often prompted by the desire to soften the blow to the family and/or the professional's discomfort in the role as the bearer of bad news. On the parent's side is the strong potential to misinterpret what is said, to retain only certain information out of context, to cease listening after the use of certain "trigger" words (e.g., brain damage, mental retardation), or to relate what is said to their own erroneous perception of what the diagnosis actually means.

Whenever possible, the communication process should occur over a period of time in order to clarify the nature and implications of the child's problem.

In the past few decades, attitudes and management strategies for the mentally retarded have change considerably (Begab & Richardson, 1975; Cohen, 1982b). Institutional care, a common choice in the past for families

Table 32-3. Common Presenting Characteristics Among the Mentally Retarded

Age	Common Presenting Problems	Milestones of Development	Neurological Findings	Other Findings
0–1 year	Delayed motor milestones	Delayed head control, delay in rolling over, sitting, crawling or standing; limited response to language, especially mimicry	Increased or decreased muscle tone; abnormal patterns of primitive reflexes including delayed disappearance; delayed appearance of adaptive reflexes	Failure to recognize familiar people or display stranger anxiety; stigmata in those with a genetic or prenatal etiology
1–3 years	Delayed expressive language	Subtle differences in milestones among the mildly retarded; general delays in all areas which vary with the degree of retardation	None except if associated with a neuromuscular disorder, hydrocephalous or overt brain damage	Some with CNS deficits have hyperactivity; with autistic features, have behavioral abnormalities
3–5 years	Delayed language development; failure to acquire skills in activities of daily living	Obvious delays in milestones only in the more severely involved; motor clumsiness in some others. Delays in dressing, self-feeding, toilet training and in expressive language	None except as noted in the 1–3-year-olds	Social skills may be delayed or vary with the amount of stimulation
5–7 years	Failure to acquire academic skills for the mildly retarded or self-care for the more severely involved	Milestones often normal for the mildly retarded, but mild language problems may be evident	Some "soft signs" may be present	Social skills may be deficient; secondary behavior problems may be present
7–14 years	Failure to acquire academic skills in some mildly retarded not detected at earlier ages	Milestones often normal or only slightly delayed in the mildly retarded	Some "soft signs" may be present	Possible speech articulation or subtle language problems; secondary behavior problems possible

Table 32-4. Prognosis and Expected Functional Level Based on Degree of Retardation

Level	Academic Potential	Activities of Daily Living (ADL)[a]	Travel Capability	Vocational Ability
Borderline	Educable, with potential up to about 6th-grade level	Fully independent	Independent	Employable without special help though may need vocational training for competitive employment
Mild	Educable to 4th- or 5th-grade level (or less): capable of reading and writing	Relatively independent in all areas; some training might be required	May require travel training to use public transportation	Employable but often needs some special training if competitive employment is feasible
Moderate	May read or write but very limited (1st- or 2nd-grade level)	Trainable for all ADL; can dress, be toilet-trained, prepare food	Travels only with special training; usually requires special transport	No real competitive employment except in restricted setting; sheltered employment likely with specialized training
Severe	Very unlikely to read or write	Partially trainable; should acquire most ADL skills; is toilet trainable, can dress, but may require assistance	Very limited independent-travel potential	Sheltered employment only, special training required
Profound	None	May sometimes be toilet-trained and dress with assistance; generally very dependent	May or may not be ambulatory; requires special transport	Very limited trainability for vocational functions

[a]Dressing, feeding, bathing, routine self-care, toileting.

From Cohen, 1982a. Used by permission.

and one that was frequently recommended by physicians, is no longer a serious option. In the United States and most of the Western world, large institutions are being phased out or gradually depopulated. Few, if any, children are being admitted to large congregate-care facilities. The only exceptions tend to be multiply handicapped, profoundly impaired children, many from homes with social stresses or disruptions for whom some nursing-care type of facility is available.

In the 1980s the vast majority of children with mental retardation live at home. The objective for these children is to provide a range of services to meet their own and their family's needs. Comprehensive medical diagnostic and follow-up services are required, including primary care, developmental and neurological assessments, and, when needed, consultations with psychiatrists, rehabilitation medicine specialists, ophthalmologists, and otolaryngologists. The services of psychologists, audiologists, social workers, physical therapists, occupational therapists, and speech therapists also may be required.

Other important requirements, in addition to residential care, include counseling for families on management issues, specialized educational programs, recreation and after-school programs, special transportation, travel training, vocational planning and training, and advocacy services (Cohen & Kligler, 1980). Families often need respite care, special baby-sitting, or homemaker services in order to be relieved of the constant strain of having to provide 24-hour care for a mentally retarded child or relative. Families also may require direct financial support to relieve them of the extra financial burden inherent in the care of a child or a relative living at home who may need special equipment, special diets, and other modifications of physical environment. Psychosocial support also may be helpful in view of the considerable psychological stress resulting from the responsibility or burdens of caring for a child with a disability.

Small community residences, primarily called group houses, are increasingly acceptable alternative to both institutional placement and care by the affected individual's own family (Cohen & Kligler, 1980; Kugel & Shearer, 1976). Foster care and adoption also are used to a considerable extent in some localities. There is a growing number of communities in the United States that have group homes in their midst. The intent is to provide a small living accommodation for the mentally retarded in residential areas where people normally live in order to promote normalization. This term signifies the intent to permit the mentally retarded a more normal existence in a normal living environment both to improve social adaptation and functional capabilities and to enhance the acceptance of disabled people within communities (Wolfensberger, 1972). This approach has generally proved successful. Mentally retarded people living in group homes appear to have better behavior and a higher level of achievement than do their institutionalized peers. However, not all of the mentally retarded easily adapt to community residences. Those with significant behavior or emotional problems may be discharged from such settings when staff are unable to cope with or manage aberrant behavior. More intensive treatment programs are required for such individuals.

In general, community residential programs have provided a successful approach to the care and treatment of the mentally retarded. Property values have not declined when group homes are placed in communities, and the mentally retarded have shown improvement when placed in these settings.

SPECIFIC CATEGORICAL PROGRAMS AND RELATED LEGISLATION

Since 1935 there has been a substantial growth in federal programs that assist children and adults with mental retardation. PL 74-271, the Social Security Act, provided the initial impetus to develop and expand state programs for crippled children, including the mentally retarded. In the 1950s, federal legislation enhanced support for special education. The most rapid changes have occurred since the early 1960s. In 1963 legislation recommended by President Kennedy that resulted in the passage of PL 88-164, the Mental Retardation Facilities and Community Mental Health Centers Construction Act, gave an impetus to the development of programs for the mentally retarded. This legislation mandated (a) the development of centers targeted for research in the field of mental retardation, the mental retardation research centers; (b) training centers (university-affiliated facilities) to develop model interdisciplinary programs and to improve the training of new and better qualified personnel in the field; and (c) with the help of an accompanying legislation, the expansion of community-based services including those provided by community mental health centers. The Kennedy family, by acknowledging the existence of a mentally retarded daughter, also provided a psychological lift for and gave hope to families in similar situations.

Subsequent to the passage of PL 88-164 a stream of helpful legislation ensued, and categorical programs were established that benefited the mentally retarded (Birenbaum & Cohen, 1984). Subsequent modifications of the initial legislation added other disability categories to the legislation and, more recently, incorporated a functional definition for developmental disabilities (DD). The modified versions of what is now called the DD Act also added funds to develop new programs within states, to establish state councils to plan new services, and to determine the allocation of new federal funds under the DD Act; it created a bill of rights for the developmentally disabled and established protection and advocacy agencies in all states. Other important legislation of a categorical nature expanded Medicaid (Title XIX) to support improved care in state institutions by funding care in what were called intermediate care facilities for the mentally retarded (ICF-MRs). Subsequently, the ICF-MR rubric was applied to community-based facilities, expanding the states' ability to fund such facilities while concomitantly setting new and somewhat controversial standards for those facilities. Medicaid also became an important provider of hospital inpatient and outpatient care for the mentally retarded, particularly those who were being cared for by medically indigent families living in the community. In addition, another component of the Social Security Act, Supplemental Security Income payments, became an important source of funding to support mentally retarded persons living in the community.

Other key legislation and financial help for programs serving the mentally retarded came from federal education legislation, particularly PL 94-142, the Education for All Handicapped Children Act. This law established the right to a free public education in the least restrictive setting for all mentally retarded Children. By 1984 a federal expenditure of $1.2 billion was associated with the implementation of educational programs linked to this act.

Finally, vocational rehabilitation legislation evolved that in its more recent modified versions supported not only vocational training but independent living programs, as well as the right to access all federally supported programs and facilities. This was a much publicized component of Section 504 of the Rehabilitation Act of 1973 (PL 93-112).

All told, by 1983 an estimated $14.33 billion was being spent in the United States on mental retardation services, the major portion coming from state or local sources, with an estimated $6.93 billion emanating from federal entitlement or categorical programs.

UNMET NEEDS

Despite the enormous economic and psychological costs of a lifelong disability such as mental retardation, surprisingly little has been expended on preventive efforts. More vigorous primary prevention, and in particular expanded and improved prenatal care for high-risk groups and a reduction in the rate of prematurity, coupled with more vigorous early identification and intervention activities, could lead to a significant reduction in both the prevalence and cost of mental subnormality.

Another key issue is how to make services more effective in improving the lives and functional levels of the mentally retarded and in helping their families. Elements that are usually missing, even in communities with a relative plethora of services of the types described earlier, are case management efforts, coordination of services, and mechanisms for supporting families with a severely disabled child living at home. Families need help in negotiating the complex system of services that exists in most communities, a system that developed based on diverse funding streams involving components of different service networks (health, mental health, developmental disabilities, education, social service, etc.) (Birenbaum & Cohen, 1984). More often than not there is no designated fixed point of reference in most communities to assure overall case coordination, case management activities, continuity of care, counseling, and advocacy over the lifetime of many affected individuals.

For families who have kept their relatives at home, inadequate respite care, financial support, transportation, recreational activities, and day programs are the most frequently cited problems. If our society is to encourage the concept of maintenance of the mentally retarded within the community, preferably within a family unit, then provision must be made to relieve some of the extra burden placed on families. They cannot be parents, therapists, residential caretakers, and advocates without causing enormous stress on the respective members of the family. Currently, alternative residential placements are sought, primarily for psychosocial reasons, when parents or families feel they can no longer cope with the problem. Helping families to cope must become a more important priority in the future.

REFERENCES

Abramowicz, H. K., & Richardson, S. A. (1975). Epidemiology of severe mental retardation: Community studies. *American Journal of Mental Deficiency, 80,* 18–38.

Begab, M. J., & Richardson, S. A. (1975). *The mentally retarded and society: A social science perspective.* Baltimore: University Park Press.

Birch, H. G., Richardson, S. A., Baired, D., Horobin, G., & Illsley, R. (1970). *Mental subnormality in the community.* Baltimore: Williams and Wilkins.

Birenbaum, A., & Cohen, H. J. (1984). *Community services for the mentally retarded.* Totowa, NJ: Rowman and Allenheld.

Cohen, H. J. (1982a). Introduction: Mental retardation. *Pediatric Annals, 11* (5), 424–425.

Cohen, H. J. (1982b). Trends in service delivery and treatment of the mentally retarded. *Pediatric Annals, 11,* 458–469.

Cohen, H. J., & Kligler, D. (1980). *Urban community care for the mentally disabled.* Springfield, IL: Charles C. Thomas.

Crocker, A. C. (1982). Current strategies in the prevention of mental retardation. *Pediatric Annals, 11,* 450–457.

Doernberg, N. L. (1982). Issues in communications between pediatricians and parents of young mentally retarded children. *Pediatric Annals, 11,* 438–444.

Dupont, A. (1980). Medical results from registration of danish mentally retarded persons. In P. Mittler (Ed.), *Frontiers in knowledge of mental retardation.* Baltimore: University Park Press.

Grossman, H. J. (Ed.). (1983). *Classification in mental retardation.* Washington, DC: American Association on Mental Deficiency.

Gruenwald, K. (1979). Mentally retarded children and young people in Sweden. *Acta Pediatrica Scand., Suppl. 275,* 75–84.

Hagberg, B., Hagberg, G., Lewerth, A. & Lindberg, V. (1981). Mild mental retardation in swedish school children. *Acta. Pediatrica Scand.*, 441–444.

Kugel, R. & Shearer, A., (1976). *Changing patterns of residential care for the mentally retarded.* Presient's Committee on Mental Retardation (DHEW No. (OHD) 76-21015) Washington, DC: U.S. Government Printing Office.

Mercer, J. R. (1973). *Labeling the mentally retarded.* Berkeley, CA: University of California Press.

Mercer, J. R. (1979). In defense of racially and culturally non-discriminatory assessment. *School Psychology Digest, 8,* 89–115.

President's Committee on Mental Retardation (1980). *Report to the President: Prevention strategies that work* (DHHS Publ. No. (OHDS) 80-21029). Washington, DC: U.S. Government Printing Office.

Taft, L. T. & Cohen, H. J. (1977). Mental retardation. In H. Barnett (Ed.), *Pediatrics* (16th ed.). New York: Appleton-Century-Crofts.

Wolfensberger, W. (1972). *The principle of normalization in human services.* Toronto: National Institute of Mental Retardation.

Chapter 33

SPEECH AND COMMUNICATION DISORDERS

Mary D. Laney

The history of speech and language functions may be viewed from evolutionary, social, and psychological perspectives. From an evolutionary vantage, speech and language are intimately tied to the biological progressions culminating in a species requiring information-exchange capabilities. That is, in its most primitive form the human communication system provides specific and specialized capabilities for receiving, processing, and transmitting biologically essential information (Tinbergen, 1964). In accord with his line of thinking, communication capabilities facilitate and ensure the transfer of information that is essential to the preservation, growth, and adaptation of both the individual organism and society (Wilson, 1975). One need but recall the biblical account of the outcome of efforts to build the Tower of Babel to realize the pervasive and debilitating effects vain communication may have on societal homeostasis and growth.

The psychological view of the function of speech and language is based on human adaptation through the socialization of language and the psychological organization of the human experience. The construction of the individual's inner world, the internal representation of ideas and other people, as well as the development of ego and personal identity, occur through the use of both overt and internal symbolic language.

In view of the multiple functions of speech and communication, speech and communication disorders may be conceptualized broadly as impairments in receiving, processing, and transmitting information. In more pop-

SPEECH AND COMMUNICATION DISORDERS   361

ular terminology, a speech disorder may be defined as that which (a) interferes with communication, (b) draws attention to itself, and (3) causes the speaker discomfort (van Riper, 1978). Generically, disorders of communication include disturbances in the areas of speech, voice, spoken and written language, and language-based learning.

INCIDENCE, PREVALENCE, DEMOGRAPHICS

Exact figures regarding the prevalence and incidence of the number of people with communicative disorders are difficult to obtain because of imprecise classification of disorders, lack of agreed-on terminology, and problems of sampling and data retrieval. Historically, the most frequently cited prevalence study has been the 1952 White House Conference (Healey, Ackerman, Chappell, Perrin, & Stormer, 1981), which estimated that 5 percent of the population between the ages of five and twenty-one had defective speech. More recently, the 1984 Department of Education's Sixth Annual Report to Congress on the 1982–1983 Implementation of Public Law 94-142 revealed that during the period of the study 4,298,327 children in the United States were reported as being handicapped. Of the total school enrollment 2.86 percent were identified as speech-impaired. The frequency with which speech impairments were identified was second only to the frequency (4.4 percent) with which learning disabilities were reported.

Results of the Seventh Annual Head Start Report published in 1980 revealed that of the 11.9 percent of the Head Start enrollment of children diagnosed as handicapped, 53.2 percent or 21,988 children were speech/language impaired. Whereas some speech and language problems are more prevalent in young children, other communication problems occur with increasing frequency in older populations. Though precise figures are not available, extrapolations and demographic projections suggest that between 1980 and 2050 the numbers of persons with speech and hearing impairments will increase at faster rates (54 and 102 percent, respectively) than the total U.S. population (36 percent) as a direct result of aging of the U.S. population. By 1990, 2,879 per 249,731 are expected to have speech impairments (Fein, 1983).

ETIOLOGY, CONTRIBUTING FACTORS, PREVENTION

Aberrations in either the biological, social, or psychological foundations of speech and language may result in communication disorders affecting speech, voice, language, hearing, and fluency. Neonatal and congenital factors that have been shown to be associated with the development of subsequent communicative impairment include genetic disorders, neuromuscular and neurophysiological problems, and mental retardation. Among children aged zero to three years of age, impairments in central nervous system functions resulting in mental retardation account for 50 percent of speech or language delays. Cognitively based communicative disorders account for 3.3 percent, oromotor apraxia accounts for less than 5 percent, and cerebral palsy accounts for 5 percent of speech and language delays in young children (Coplan, 1983). Many of these disorders may be multiply determined: that is, a child may have speech and language problems as a result of both motoric difficulties and mental retardation.

Although some etiologies underlying speech and language problems may be amenable to preventive intervention, others are less preventable. Prevention with regard to communication disorders is defined as the elimination of factors that interfere with the normal acquisition and development of communication skills (Marge, 1984). Examples of factors that are preventable with regard to language delay or impairment include some types of mental retardation, familial factors, cultural factors, some genetic disorders, fetal alcohol syndrome, brain damage due to prematurity, and neonatal complications. Preventable factors related to disorders of voice and fluency include vocal abuse, drug and alcohol abuse, trauma and injury, faulty respiration, environmental and communicative stress, and cultural factors.

Primary preventive strategies include genetic counseling, immunization, family planning, prenatal care, and environmental quality control. Secondary prevention strategies are focused on the early detection and treatment of communicative disorders through mass screening. Typically, such screening occurs as a part of state and federal programs such as Early Periodic Screening, Detection, and Treatment programs (Moore, 1978), with physicians and nurse practitioners becoming increasingly responsible for carrying out communication screening in pediatric populations, especially among those populations that are at increased risk for developmental deviance (Laney et al., 1985). Tertiary prevention efforts are designed to reduce the effects of communication impairments through various interventions, which include, but are not limited to, early intervention programs, rehabilitative programs, speech-language therapy, and a range of case management strategies.

CLINICAL DESCRIPTIONS

Communicative disorders take many forms. Articulation problems, voice disorders, disorders of fluency, language disorders, and language-learning disabilities are considered major communicative disorders. Communication disorders associated with special populations include cleft palate, hearing problems, neurogenic disorders, cerebral palsy, and aphasia.

Articulation Disorders

In their most basic forms articulation disorders subsume those disorders caused by imprecise or inaccurate placement of the articulators (tongue, teeth, lips, hard and soft palates) in the production of speech sounds comprising spoken words. The production of "wabbit" instead of "rabbit" by a seven-year-old child is an example of an articulation error. Although articulation distortions, substitutions, additions, and ommissions occur as part of the normal language acquisition and maturational process, in cases where such phonetic misproductions perpetuate beyond the formative articulation-acquisition period, an articulation problem requiring treatment may be evident. Etiological factors underlying articulation errors may include physical abnormalities, environmental factors, or phonologic errors related to a specific feature of phonemic production such as voicing and learning (van Riper & Irwin, 1958; Winitz, 1975).

Children suspected of having articulation problems typically are referred to speech-language pathologists for evaluation. When an initial evaluation suggests the presence of an articulation problem, a second and more thorough evaluation is conducted to determine the scope of the problem and the individual's personality characteristics and social history. Essential to the assessment of articulation problems are the collection of speech samples and the administration of standardized articulation tests. Whereas speech samples allow the clinician to profile general aspects of the child's communicative competence as well as specific aspects of oral-verbal expression, articulation tests are designed to discern if an individual's phonetic productions are discrepant from the phonetic acquisition norms for his chronologic age. Although specific criteria for determining how many or what kinds of articulation errors warrant therapeutic intervention are not available, factors frequently affecting the decision to refer for speech therapy include (a) clinical judgments of overall speech intelligibility; (b) the frequency, type, and consistency of errors; and (c) the severity of the problem.

Voice Problems

Most of us have encountered an individual whose voice pitch, loudness, or quality call attention to the speaker's voice rather than the content of what he is saying. The woman who speaks in a high-pitched, whisper-like voice or, perhaps more unusual, the woman who speaks in a raucous or low-pitched voice are as discrepant to the voices we normally hear as is the voice of the young child who speaks as if he suffers from chronic laryngitis. Though incidence reports for such voice disorders are imprecise, it has been suggested that approximately 6 percent of the school-age population have voice problems (Moore, 1982).

Closely intertwined with respiration and the biological functions of the larynx and vocal folds in phonation, disorders of the voice typically refer to problems of vocal pitch, loudness, and quality. Psychogenic or functional problems of voice may result from underlying organic factors such as paralysis (restricting closure of the vocal folds), stiffness or fixation at the cricoarytenoid joint, laryngectomy, debilitating diseases and conditions, tumors, polyps, vocal nodules, papillomata and carcinoma, ulcers, and edema. Prob-

364 HANDICAPPED CHILDREN AND YOUTH

lems of resonance, hypernasality, and hyponasality also may result in voice quality that impedes understanding. The thorough evaluation of voice disorders usually involves observation of the vocal apparatus and careful listening to the various components of phonation and resonance. In view of the physiological etiologies that may be associated with voice problems, referral to an otolaryngologist is a critical component of a complete evaluation of voice and vocal functioning.

Disorders of Fluency

In addition to the aberrant use of pauses, hesitations, interjections, and prolongations, disorders of fluency include cluttering and stuttering. Cluttering, which usually is characterized by very rapid speech, is distinct from stuttering, which affects not only the fluent, smooth, and effortless flow of words but also the individual's concept of himself and views toward social interactions. Though diverse theories of the cause of stuttering have been available for quite some time (Johnson, 1933; Luper & Mulder, 1964; Orton & Travis, 1929; West, 1958), there is at present no definitive and universally accepted theory of the etiology of stuttering.

The diagnosis and evaluation of fluency usually involves careful listening to the child's or adolescent's speech under varied conditions (casual speaking, rote repetition, and emotionally laden or stressful situations). Stuttering is diagnosed on the basis of the integration of a thorough developmental history and the clinical analysis of the type of contacts made in word production, the frequency of fluent periods, the presence of secondary symptoms, and the level of emotionality or avoidance.

Language Delay and Language Disorders

Among various age segments of the population, language disorders comprise the largest group of communication problems. Disorders of language cut across chronologic age, educational background, cultural milieu, and level of linguistic proficiency to affect children, adults, and older people. Although some language disorders may go unnoticed, the more general and pervasive language disorders are usually evident to family, friends, and associates in the individual's immediate environment.

Many terms are used to refer to language disorder, language disability, and language delay. Since such terms are not necessarily synonymous, it is meaningful to differentiate among those terms most frequently used to refer to the language problems of children and adolescents. Language-delayed children or children with specific language impairment are characterized by a slower emergence and development of linguistic features (Leonard, 1982). Children who are mentally retarded are often similar to children with specific language impairment in that they too are often slow to acquire language rules and features. Like autistic children and children with acquired aphasia, these children may exhibit severe impairments in language.

A language disorder syndrome refers to a characteristic cluster of developmental or acquired language difficulties that encompass impairments of language comprehension and formulation, word finding, and language used in interpersonal communication (Wiig, 1982). A developmental language disorder associated with learning disabilities in school-age children is referred to as a language-learning disability.

It is estimated that children with language problems make up from 50 to 80 percent of the cases seen by speech-language pathologists serving preschool children. In response to the prevalence of language impairments, there are currently available numerous language assessments designed to measure comprehension and production as well as syntax and overall language competency.

Other Communication Disorders

The communication problems of individuals with cleft palate, neurogenic disorders, and cerebral palsy typically involve disorders of speech and voice. Language disorders also may be present in children with cerebral palsy and may be secondary to general delay, retardation, and some defect of functioning. A thorough oromotor examination (including the assessment of reflexes and coordination of the articulators) is used in conjunction with results of intellectual assessments and hearing testing to distinguish symptoms of immaturity from paralytic symptoms.

MANAGEMENT

The range and complexities of speech and communication warrant varied intervention strategies. Primary or preventive strategies have been addressed previously in this chapter. At the secondary level, efforts to facilitate the early identification of communicative disorders utilize screening programs and education strategies designed (a) to increase public awareness regarding communication disorders and (b) to educate physicians and other health care personnel regarding the etiologies, nature, course, and medical concomitants of various speech, language, and hearing impairments. Additional management strategies are designed to reduce the effects of the disorder and restore effective functioning through responsive interventions at the individual, family, and community levels.

Preschool Populations

As a result of Public Law 94-142 and funding for demonstration and outreach projects through the Handicapped Children's Early Education Program (1984) there are currently available many intervention programs and models designed to serve special populations (communicatively impaired, physically handicapped, emotionally disturbed, and preschool handicapped) residing in rural, urban, and community settings. Criteria for enrollment in federally funded programs usually are more flexible than criteria for enrollment in programs funded through state health and education agencies, with the latter programs usually requiring for program eligibility either (a) the presence of a condition that impairs or predicts impairment in normal attainment of developmental milestones, or (b) measurable delays of at least 25 percent below the child's chronological age (as verified by assessment) in two or more of the following areas: gross motor, fine motor, communication, sensory, cognitive, social-emotional, self-help, and feeding (Stromsland, 1984).

Most early intervention programs offer services that either have speech-language intervention as a major focus (Weistuch & Lewis, 1985) or include speech-language remediation and stimulation efforts among comprehensive intervention services. Transdisciplinary approaches to assessment and management of communication disorders in preschool populations use speech–language pathologists to train other professional members of the "team" in speech and language intervention strategies through "role release" (Woodruff, 1984). Many preschool programs provide parent training as either central or ancillary to programmatic efforts. Parent-mediated speech and language curricula (Laney, 1978) provide speech and language activities as well as strategies that parents may be trained to carry out daily to facilitate their child's speech and language development. Individual speech-language therapy may be available to children in need of such services through either free-standing or hospital affiliated speech and hearing clinics, university programs, or private-practicing speech-language pathologists.

School-Age Children

In response to the diversity of language and learning problems among school-age children, most school systems offer varied alternatives to regular classroom placement. Such alternatives include itinerant programs, resource room placement for a part of the academic day, self-contained classrooms, and the use of the speech-language pathologist as a consultant to the regular or special education classrooms. Specific factors influencing the decision to serve a particular student and the form of service provided include the severity of the speech, language, or hearing disorder; the effect of the disorder on the student's academic performance; the presence of additional handicapping conditions; and the chronicity of the problem.

Intermittent direct contact with the speech-language pathologists through itinerant programs are well suited to students with all types of disorders, varying in severity from mild to severe. The length and frequency of sessions selected are determined by *Guidelines for Caseload Size for Speech-Language Services in the Schools* (ASHA, 1984) and the student's individual needs. Individual and group therapy sessions typically range from 30 minutes to 1 hour per day from two to five times per week.

The resource room is used most frequently to serve children with articulation and language disorders that are severe enough to warrant the direct services of the speech-language pathologist and continued monitoring of the student's progress. Students in the resource room may receive direct individual therapy or group therapy with as many as five other children. The self-contained (or special education) classroom is composed of children who have severe or multiple communication disorders and whose needs are best met through a classroom for the communicatively handicapped. Finally, through consultation the speech-language pathologist seeks to facilitate the classroom teacher's functioning in ways that improve the speech and language of multiply handicapped children as well as children with various communication disorders (Frassinelli, Superior, & Meyers, 1983).

UNMET NEEDS

In view of this country's shifting demographics and increases in minority populations, future directions in services for communicatively handicapped individuals no doubt will involve sensitive and effective responses to service delivery in multicultural populations. According to results of the 1982 *Self-Study Survey of the American Speech-Language Hearing Association* (ASHA, 1985) 77 percent of the certified speech-language pathologists indicated a need for more knowledge and skills to serve bilingual-cultural populations. Inherent in the improved services to those populations will be the refinement of language screening and assessment procedures that insure the accurate identification of communication-impaired infants and children of all cultural and ethnic backgrounds. The suggestion that sociocultural background, like genetic history and prenatal or birth complications, may place a child at increased risk for communicative deviance emphasizes the need for careful screening of these children. Long overdue, the prevention and early identification of communicative disorders among minority language populations has behind it what Victor Hugo so germanely referred to as the power of an idea whose time has come.

REFERENCES

ASHA, Committee on Language, Speech, and Hearing Services in the Schools (1984). Guidelines for caseload size for speech-language services in the schools. *Asha, 26,* 53–58.

ASHA, Committee on the Status of Racial Minorities (1985). Clinical management of communicatively handicapped minority language populations. *Asha, 27,* 29–32.

Coplan, J. (1983). *The early language milestone scale.* Tulsa, OK: Modern Education Corporation.

Fein, D. (1983). Projections of speech and hearing impairments in 2050. *Asha,* *25,* 31.

Handicapped Children's Early Education Programs 1983–1984 Overview Directory (1984). Chapel Hill, NC: Technical Assistance Development System.

Healey, W., Ackerman, B., Chappell, C., Perrin, K., & Stormer, J. (1981). *The prevalence of communication disorders: A review of the literature. Final Report.* Rockville, MD: American Speech-Language Hearing Association.

Johnson, W. (1933). An interpretation of stuttering. *Quarterly Journal of Speech,* *19,* 70–76.

Laney, M. (1978) *Talk, talk, talk: Language curriculum for the preschooler* (Vols. I–IV). Johstown, PA: Mafex Corporation.

Laney, M., Byers-Brown, B., Downs, M., Northern, J., Kenworthy, O., Morgan, D., & Shonrock, C. (1985). *Communication screening and assessment in pediatric populations.* Miniseminar presented at the 1985 Convention of the American Speech-Language-Hearing Association, Washington, DC, November 22, 1985.

Leonard, L. (1982). Early language development and language disorders. In G. Shames & E. Wiig (Eds.), *Human communication disorders* (221–257). Columbus: Charles E. Merrill.

Luper, H., & Mulder, R. (1964). *Stuttering therapy for children.* Englewood Cliffs, NJ: Prentice-Hall.

Marge, M. (1984). The prevention of communication disorders. *Asha, 26,* 29–37.

Moore, B. (1978). Implementing the developmental assessment component of the EPSDT program. *American Journal of Orthopsychiatry, 48,* 22–32.

Moore, P. (1982). Voice disorders. In G. Shames & E. Wiig (Eds.), *Human communication disorders* (pp. 141–186). Columbus: Charles E. Merrill.

Orton, S., & Travis, L. E. (1929). Studies in stuttering IV: Studies of action currents in stutters. *Archives of Neurology and Psychiatry, 21,* 61–68.

van Riper, C. (1978). *Speech correction principles and methods* (6th Edition). Englewood Cliffs, NJ: Prentice-Hall.

van Riper, C., & Irwin, J. (1958). *Voice and articulation.* Englewood Cliffs, NJ: Prentice-Hall.

Status of Handicapped Children in Head Start Programs. (1980). The Seventh Annual Report of the U.S. Department of Health Education and Welfare to the Congress of the United States on Services Provided to Handicapped Children in Project Head Start. Washington, DC: Office of Human Development Services, Head Start Bureau.

Stromsland, F. (1984). *The guide to early intervention programs in New Jersey.* Trenton, NJ: New Jersey State Department of Education.

Tinbergen, N. (1964). The evolution of signaling devices. In W. Elkin (Ed.),

Social behavior and organization among vertebrates. Chicago: University of Chicago Press.

West, R. (1958). An agnostic's speculations about stuttering. In J. Eisenson (Ed.), *Stuttering: A symposium*. New York: Harper & Row.

Wiig, E. (1982). Language disabilities in the school-age child. In G. Shames & E. Wiig (Eds.), *Human communication disorders* (pp. 187–220). Columbus: Charles E. Merrill.

Wilson, E. (1975). *Sociobiology: The new synthesis*. Cambridge, MA: The Belknap Press of Harvard University.

Winitz, H. (1975). *From syllable to conversation*. Baltimore: University Park Press.

Woodruff, G. (1984). Project optimus (abstract), In *Handicapped Children's Early Education Programs 1983–1984 Overview Directory*. Chapel Hill, NC: Technical Assistance Development System.

INDEX

Huntington's Disease Foundation of
America, 73

Independent Living Act, 87
Individualized educational plans
(IEPs), 174, 217, 323–324
Institutional care, 27, 28, 239–232;
see also Residential facilities
IQ tests, 127, 348

Kennedy, John F., 46, 231
Kennedy family, 356

Language, 127, 187, 320–321, 326,
360–361, 364–365; *see also*
Communication disorders,
Speech-language pathology
Lead poisoning, 113
Leadership, 258–259
Learning disabilities, 135, 175,
317–325
clinical description of, 319–322
definitions of, 317–318
and education, 324
management of, 322–323
predisposing factors in, 319
Least restrictive environment, 60,
179, 192, 203
Llorens, Lela A., 170
Low birth weight, 135, 266, 350

Mainstreaming, 216
March of Dimes-Birth Defects
Foundation, 72, 74, 75, 78,
166, 307
Marriage, 225
Mass transit, accessibility of, 253,
254
Masturbation, 227
Maternal and Child Health Block
Grant, 51, 52, 65, 89, 266

Medecon, 185
Medicaid, 56, 92, 93, 101, 122, 197,
248
Meningomyelocele, 19, 298–307; *see
also* Neural tube defects
Mental retardation, 18, 22, 29, 30,
347–358
characteristics of, 351–352, 353
definition of, 347
early intervention in, 350
etiology of, 349–350, 351
funding for, 357
IQ tests in, 348
prognosis for, 353
programs for, 46, 231, 356–357
Mental Retardation Facilities and
Community Mental Health
Centers Construction Act,
356
Migrant workers, 67, 68
Moore, Marie, 84
Mosey, Anne Cronin, 170
Motor development, 127, 366
Muscular dystrophy, 309–316
diagnosis of, 311, 312, 313, 314
exercise for, 315
genetic counseling in, 315–316
management of, 315–316
statistics on, 319
types of, 309, 310–315
Muscular Dystrophy Association,
73, 75, 316

National Association for Retarded
Citizens, 46, 47, 73
National Center for Education in
Maternal and Child Health,
37
National Foundation for Infantile
Paralysis, 72, 74
National Foundation for
Poliomyelitis, 45–46
National Health Council, 72–73

DATE DUE

BRODART, CO.   Cat. No. 23-221-003